Social Networks,
Drug Injectors' Lives,
and HIV/AIDS

AIDS Prevention and Mental Health

Series Editors:

David G. Ostrow, M.D., Ph.D.
Howard Brown Health Center and University of Illinois / Chicago School of Public Health, Chicago, Illinois

Jeffrey A. Kelly, Ph.D.
Center for AIDS Intervention Research (CAIR), Milwaukee, Wisconsin

---

Evaluating HIV Prevention Interventions
Joanne E. Mantell, Ph.D., M.S.P.H., Anthony T. DiVittis, M.A.,
and Marilyn I. Auerbach, A.M.L.S., Dr. P.H.

Handbook of Economic Evaluation of HIV Prevention Programs
Edited by David R. Holtgrave, Ph.D.

Methodological Issues in AIDS Behavioral Research
Edited by David G. Ostrow, M.D., Ph.D., and Ronald C. Kessler, Ph.D.

Preventing AIDS: Theories and Methods of Behavioral Interventions
Edited by Ralph J. DiClemente, Ph.D., and John L. Peterson, Ph.D.

**Preventing HIV in Developing Countries:
Biomedical and Behavioral Approaches**
Edited by Laura Gibney, Ph.D., Ralph J. DiClemente, Ph.D.,
and Sten H. Vermund, Ph.D., M.D.

Psychosocial and Public Health Impacts of New HIV Therapies
Edited by David G. Ostrow, M.D., Ph.D., and Seth C. Kalichman, Ph.D.

Social Networks, Drug Injectors' Lives, and HIV/AIDS
Samuel R. Friedman, Ph.D., Richard Curtis, Ph.D., Alan Neaigus, Ph.D.,
Benny Jose, Ph.D., and Don C. Des Jarlais, Ph.D.

Women and AIDS: Coping and Care
Edited by Ann O'Leary, Ph.D., and
Lorretta Sweet Jemmott, R.N., Ph.D., F.A.A.N.

Women at Risk: Issues in the Primary Prevention of AIDS
Edited by Ann O'Leary, Ph.D., and Loretta Sweet Jemmott, R.N., Ph.D.

A Continuation Order Plan is available for this series. A continuation order will bring delivery of each new volume immediately upon publication. Volumes are billed only upon actual shipment. For further information please contact the publisher.

Social Networks, Drug Injectors' Lives, and HIV/AIDS

Samuel R. Friedman, Ph.D.
National Development and Research Institutes, Inc.
New York, New York

Richard Curtis, Ph.D.
John Jay College of Criminal Justice
New York, New York

Alan Neaigus, Ph.D. and
Benny Jose, Ph.D.
National Development and Research Institutes, Inc.
New York, New York

and

Don C. Des Jarlais, Ph.D.
National Development and Research Institutes, Inc.,
Beth Israel Medical Center, and
Albert Einstein College of Medicine
New York, New York

Kluwer Academic / Plenum Publishers
New York, Boston, Dordrecht, London, Moscow

ISBN 0-306-46079-3

© 1999 Kluwer Academic / Plenum Publishers
233 Spring Street, New York, N.Y. 10013

10 9 8 7 6 5 4 3 2 1

A C.I.P. record for this book is available from the Library of Congress.

Foreword

Friedman, Curtis, Neaigus, Jose, and Des Jarlais in their critically important, and timely publication on drug injectors' lives in the Bushwick section of Brooklyn, New York, combine epidemiological and ethnographic data and introduce social network concepts and methods to enumerate and explain co-occurring, inter-related, and epidemics of drug use and HIV/AIDS. The authors provide a historical perspective on the lives of drug injectors in New York City, the epicenter of HIV/ AIDS in the United States, and the city with the largest AIDS epidemic among IDUs anywhere in the world. The authors' crossdisciplinary theoretical perspectives, and the findings from this study create a methodological dialogue between epidemiological and ethnographic data about HIV/AIDS among drug users contributing greatly to our understanding of the spread and dynamics of HIV transmission in drug-using populations and the prevention of HIV and other blood borne infectious diseases, including hepatitis B.

To appreciate the considerable contributions of this book to help us understand drug abuse and HIV transmission as well as the prevention and control of the spread of HIV, I want to provide a brief contextual perspective on the evolving science related to HIV in drug-using populations. Earlier in the epidemic, researchers relied on traditional epidemiological methods to help better identify and enumerate risk behaviors of individuals, the relationship between risk behaviors (e.g., multiperson reuse of drug injection equipment) and the transmission of newly emerging infectious diseases, and develop prevention and control strategies for helping individuals change their behaviors. Friedman and his colleagues are among a small number of researchers who introduced and contributed to an expansion of the research paradigm that integrates social network concepts and methodology with traditional epidemiological methods. They focus on the following: the contextual factors—the context or where behaviors occur and the relationship between risk behaviors and the likelihood of acquiring and/or transmitting HIV infection, and structure and dynamics of drug-using risk networks and behavioral transaction that link IDUs in drug acquisition, preparation, and the injection process. They combine quantitative and qualitative data to describe the context of HIV risk among drug users and their sexual partners in Bushwick. Drug injectors in Bushwick were recruited through street outreach in areas with heavy drug use and through chain referral by other participants. They were interviewed from July 1991 to January 1993, and questions about their life histories, particularly about their drug-using behaviors, permit the researchers to report on changes in their patterns of drug use and risk behaviors over time. The authors' bibliography is extensive, crediting other researchers for their many contributions to our understanding of risk networks, drug abuse and HIV transmission, and they are careful to report the limitations of the methodologies used in their study.

How then have Friedman and his colleagues helped us to better understand the changing dynamics of the co-occurring and interrelated epidemics of drug abuse and HIV/AIDS and anticipate the challenges of emerging HIV-related issues in preventing the spread of HIV? Emerging from this very important study is the finding that the context of HIV risk, or the settings where risk behaviors occur, such as crack houses, shooting galleries, and other public high-risk environments, influence the probability of viral transmission. The compelling narratives of the everyday lives of drug injectors, describing the dynamics of buying and using drugs, and changes in the drug scene over the course of the HIV epidemic, help us to understand how more macro-level factors such as neighbor density, housing, and the economy affect the lives of injectors, influence the formation, mainte-nance, and/or dissolution of risk and social networks, and affect their risk behav-iors and, in turn, the probability of viral transmission. Specifically, context and the behavioral transaction linking IDUs in the multiperson use of drug injection paraphernalia (e.g., cookers, cotton, and water) and from injection practices related to transferring drug solution from one syringe to another, as well as multiperson reuse of syringes, helps account for the dynamics of HIV transmis-sion. Most importantly, Friedman and his colleagues discuss risk networks, the location of a person within the network, and the differential probabilities of engaging in high- and low-risk behaviors. It is their discussion of the concept of mixing and the findings related to behavioral transaction between HIV seronega-tive risk network members and HIV seropositive risk network members that helps the field understand how the merger of the social network paradigm with ethnogra-phy helps inform our epidemiological concepts of infectious disease transmission.

Friedman and his colleagues had hoped to provide the reader with informa-tion that can strengthen efforts to conduct useful research and develop or imple-ment effective prevention programs or policies. They were successful.

This foreword represents the expressed/written view of the author (Richard H. Needle, Ph.D., M.P.H.) and not of the National Institute on Drug Abuse (NIDA), National Institutes of Health.

Richard H. Needle, Ph.D., M.P.H.
National Institute on Drug Abuse

Preface

By early 1989, the senior author of this volume (Sam Friedman) had been working in the AIDS field for over 5 years. Most of his efforts had been spent in research based on individualistic models of epidemiology or prevention. Thus, he had worked on studies at the individual level of analysis of risk factors in HIV infection among drug injectors in drug abuse treatment (Friedman et al., 1987c; Marmor et al., 1987); on an experiment to determine whether providing social skills and AIDS knowledge and referrals to heroin sniffers would help them avoid becoming injectors (Casriel et al., 1990; Des Jarlais, Casriel, Friedman, & Rosenblum, 1992); and on an evaluation (with associated epidemiological research) of an AIDS outreach project that emphasized knowledge and HIV antibody testing and counseling (Friedman et al., 1989a–c; Neaigus et al., 1990). He had also been involved in helping to establish the World Health Organization Multi-Centre Study on Drug Injecting and Risk of HIV Infection, including having written the first draft of its individually oriented questionnaire (Stimson, Des Jarlais, & Ball, 1998). He also had been a major drafter of the individually oriented questionnaire for the multisite National AIDS Demonstration Research (NADR) project, which the National Institute on Drug Abuse sponsored and funded in more than 50 cities in the United States (Brown & Beschner, 1993). All the authors of this volume were involved in the Community AIDS Prevention Outreach Demonstration (CAPOD) project, which they organized as part of NADR. CAPOD, however, contained an effort to use supraindividual social forces as well as individually focused efforts to encourage risk reduction. Specifically, it aimed to use social pressures to "change the culture of risk," with a major thrust to help drug injectors establish their own organizations modeled after the Dutch *junkiebonden* and other drug users' unions (Friedman et al., 1987b, 1988, 1989b) that would attempt to mobilize social pressures and change norms from within the drug scene to support risk reduction. CAPOD in fact seems to have led to considerable risk reduction (Friedman, 1991; Friedman et al., 1991, 1992; Jose et al., 1996), although its attempts to organize drug users' groups were less than totally successful. Though part of the reason for this is that the subcontractor that carried out this phase of the project resisted its supraindividual focus and spent very little time trying to set up drug users' groups (Friedman et al., 1991), it is never easy to organize groups "from the outside." (Drug users' organizations have formed themselves in many parts of the world, including The Netherlands, Australia, and some cities in the United States. Several years after CAPOD ended, and in part due to our continuing efforts to encourage users to organize, and AIDS intervention projects to assist in, this effort, users' groups were established in New York City with the help of syringe exchange projects in the Bronx and Manhattan's Lower East Side).

As CAPOD was drawing to a close, our team spent considerable time soul-searching and trying to figure out how we could most usefully contribute to the battle against AIDS. It struck us that there were a number of key questions in the epidemiology of HIV and in the shaping of high-risk behavior and deliberate risk reduction that needed more study. Particularly salient in our minds were the following questions:

1. Why are African-American and Puerto Rican drug injectors consistently more likely to be infected than white drug injectors? These differences remained in most studies even after statistically controlling for different levels of risk behaviors (Friedman et al., 1997d, 1998b; Jose, 1996). It seemed to us that there would likely be two important contributors to blacks' and Puerto Ricans' greater probability of being infected: First, their social and injecting networks were likely to include primarily other African Americans and Puerto Ricans. This would mean if their infection rates were higher or began earlier, they would be likely to continue to have a higher HIV seroprevalence than whites for some years because the epidemics in the different racial ethnic groups would be socially separated, and thus would follow somewhat different trajectories (Des Jarlais & Friedman, 1989; Friedman, 1995). These network phenomena might explain why the epidemics remained semisegregated, but by themselves, however, would not explain why it was that African Americans and Puerto Ricans had higher seroprevalence than whites. To explain this, we looked at a second possible explanatory framework: As the victims of racial–ethnic oppression and subordination, African-American and Puerto Rican drug injectors would have access to fewer resources than white injection drug users, and the social organization of both their neighborhoods and their portion of the drug scene might be shaped by the stigma and police pressures of oppression in ways that would make it difficult for them to engage in sustained risk avoidance. This framework, of course, was rather vague. We hoped, in the course of the research, to be able to concretize and demonstrate it.

2. How did new injectors come to be infected? Our prior research had shown that new injectors in New York City were much less likely to be infected than longer-term injectors, even though they engaged in similar levels of high-risk behavior (Friedman et al., 1989a). In part, of course, this was simply a question of exposure time: the longer-term injectors

had engaged in high-risk behaviors for many more years, and thus had had many more opportunities to encounter HIV. Nonetheless, we were struck by the fact that if a group of uninfected persons began to inject drugs, continued to inject and have sex only with others who were new injectors, and whose circles injected only with others like them, HIV would never enter their networks and they would remain uninfected. This meant that new injectors would become infected only as the result of a *social process* in which their networks came to interact and intersect with those of infected persons. The SFHR project aimed, in part, to study this social process and show how it was related to the spread of HIV infection among new injectors.

3. How did the social shaping of drug injectors' risk behaviors take place? We and others had collected considerable evidence that peer influence was one determinant of risk behavior (Abdul-Quader, Tross, Friedman, Kouzi, & Des Jarlais, 1990; Friedman et al., 1987b; Huang, Watters, & Case, 1989; Huang, Watters, & Lorvick, 1989b; Magura et al., 1989, 1990). We felt it was important to develop a better understanding of how peer influence operated and how other social influences might shape risky behavior. In particular, we were impressed by a simple fact that seemed not to have been incorporated in most other researchers' theories or practice: The behaviors that put persons at risk for HIV were always *interactions* among two or more persons (Friedman et al., 1990). It is impossible (other than through physical violence or sneakiness) either to share syringes or to have unprotected sex with someone who refuses. Thus, high-risk behavior was a form of interpersonal interaction rather than a personal characteristic. (To clarify this: A personal behavior is something like picking and eating a strawberry, which is governed only by desire and by the availability of strawberries, whereas the interactive nature of some behaviors is exemplified by the absurdity of trying to understand the physical gesticulations of a prizefighter without taking into account the blows and dodging of her or his opponent.) To understand high-risk injecting and sexual behaviors better and to develop more effective intervention techniques we would have to study behaviors as characteristics of the relationships between those who were engaging in the behaviors and also the norms that guided action in their social circles.

These three issues (racial–ethnic difference in seroprevalence, the social pathways through which new injectors might come to be infected, and the social shaping of risk behavior) can, in part, be studied by looking at the social networks and risk networks of drug injectors. Here "social networks" can be understood as the pattern of social linkages among people, such as friendships, acquaintance-ships, kinship relations, and more formal relationships such as those with teachers or workplace supervisors. "Risk networks" are relationships that can spread HIV and typically involve sexual intercourse among two (or more) persons, or sharing syringes or other injection paraphernalia. Risk networks, however, can also include anonymous or even unknown linkages such as those that occur when people inject with the same syringe several hours apart in a shooting gallery, or that occur when a person is transfused with blood from an infectious donor whom they do not know. (This occurred frequently in the United States before 1985, and unfortunately still occurs in countries where economic incapacity or political unconcern have prevented adequate screening of blood supplies.)

Acknowledgments

Support was provided by the National Institute on Drug Abuse grant DA06723 "Social Factors and HIV Risk." The New York State Department of Health AIDS Institute assisted in drawing serum samples, HIV testing, and referrals. The views expressed herein do not necessarily reflect the positions of the granting agencies or of the institutions by which the authors are employed.

Other National Development and Research Institutes (NDRI) staff who participated in this research include Hector Guadalupe, William Henry, Mario Laboy, Lisa McCullough, Patrice Mota, Pablo Pabellon, Jany Quiles, Lourdes Rebollo, Bruce Stepherson, Nelson Tiburcio, and Thomas Ward. Theresa E. Perlis and Jo L. Sotheran assisted us with analytical and conceptual issues, and too many other NDRI staff to name provided useful advice, ideas, or other assistance. R. Terry Furst provided ethnographic assistance in the start-up phases of the project and, in particular, suggested that we measure role behaviors. Katherine A. Atwood, a student at Harvard University School of Public Health, has provided us with useful ideas in the course of writing a dissertation using data from this project. She also co-wrote Chapter 4, "The Very First Hit." Lisa Maher, now of the National Drug and Alcohol Research Centre, Sydney, Australia, provided field assistance and ethnographic insight while she was studying women crack users in Bushwick for her dissertation.

We would like to acknowledge assistance provided by hundreds of other scholars. Unfortunately, the list is far too long to include everyone who has provided ideas or assistance. Those who stand out in our memories include Stephen Q. Muth, John J. Potterat, and Donald E. Woodhouse, El Paso County Department of Health and Environment; David C. Bell, Affiliated Systems Corporation, Houston; Carl Latkin and David Vlahov, Johns Hopkins University; Martina Morris of Pennsylvania State University; Patricia Case, Harvard University and NDRI; Jean-Paul Grund, Lindesmith Center; Holly Hagan, Seattle Department of Health; King Holmes, University of Washington; Judith Levy, Lawrence J. Ouellet, and W. Wayne Wiebel, University of Illinois, Chicago; Sten Vermund and Ralph DiClimente, University of Alabama, Birmingham; Rodrick Wallace, The Institute for Health, Health Care Policy and Aging Research, Rutgers University and The New York State Psychiatric Institute; Mindy and Robert Fullilove, Columbia University; Richard Lovely, Battelle; Mildred Vera and Margarita Alegröa, Medical Services Campus, University of Puerto Rico; Gene McGrady, Morehouse School of Medicine; Alden Klovdahl, Australian National University; Nick Crofts, Macfarlane Burnet Centre for Medical Research, Melbourne, Australia; Alex Wodak, St. Vincent's Hospital, Sydney, Australia; Wouter de Jong, National Institute on Alcohol and Drugs, Utrecht, The Netherlands; Gerry Stimson and Tim Rhodes, Centre for Research on Drugs and Health Behaviour, London; Denise Paone, David Perlman, Nadim Salomon, and Alyse Bellomo of Beth Israel Medical Center; Eric van Ameijden of the Amsterdam Municipal Health Service; Jordi Casabona and Anna Rodes, CEESCAT, Hospital Universitari Germans Trias I Pujol, Barcelona; Rafael Nåjera Morrondo and Rafael de Andrês Medina, Centro Nacional de Biologia Fundamental, Majadahonda, Madrid; and Maria Victoria Zunzunegui of the Escuela Andalucia de Salud Publica. Brazilian scholars who provided useful ideas included Tarcisio Andrade, Francisco Bastos, Regina Bueno, Elson Lima, Fabio Mesquita, and Paulo Telles. A number of scholars employed by the United States government have provided assistance, including Barry Brown, Katherine Davenny, Peter Hartsock, Elizabeth Lambert, and Mario De La Rosa of the National Institute on Drug Abuse; Janet St. Lawrence, Centers for Disease Control and Prevention; and Judith Auerbach, Office of Science and Technology Policy, Executive Office of the President.

The staff of the New South Wales Users and AIDS Association, a large drug users' union in Australia, provided extremely useful feedback about network-based prevention approaches during a 2-day visit with them in 1996. Jude Byrne of the Australian I.V. League, David Burrows, also of Australia, and John Mordaunt of the United Kingdom, were other leaders of the international drug users movement who provided useful insight as we wrote this book.

Series Editors Jeff Kelly, University of Wisconsin, and David Ostrow, Howard Brown Health Center, University of Illinois, provided invaluable feedback. Mariclaire Cloutier of Plenum Press provided encouragement, good advice, and necessary leniency on deadlines. Other Plenum staff, including Tina Marie Greene and Nicole Turgeon, were models of helpfulness; and Susan Monahan provided excellent indexing.

Richard Needle, NIDA, and Richard Rothenberg, Emory University, deserve special recognition for their encouragement and intelligent ideas about networks and their analysis from the beginning of the project (and before) until now.

Finally, we would like to acknowledge the help provided to us by many hundreds of drug users who provided us with information in grueling interviews, and who underwent phlebotomy, in order to help us understand the HIV/AIDS epidemic better. Many of them also assisted us in our recruitment efforts, took part in additional ethnographic interviews, or assisted our ethnographic staff in their fieldwork. As is described later in this volume, some of those who helped us the most have since passed away. We mourn them deeply.

Contents

Chapter 4. The Very First Hit

with Katherine A. Atwood

Chapter 5. Network Concepts and Serosurvey Methods

Chapter 6. The Research Participants and Their Behaviors

Chapter 7. Personal Risk Networks and High-Risk Injecting Settings of Drug Injectors

Chapter 8. Syringe Sharing and the Social Characteristics of Drug-Injecting Dyads

Chapter 9. Sexual Networks, Condom Use, and the Prospects for HIV Spread to Non-Injection Drug Users

Chapter 12. Prevention and Research

Chapter 13. Appendix: Methods for Assigning Linkages in Studies of Drug Injector Networks

with Gilbert Ildefonso

Introduction

This volume presents findings from a study of drug injectors that was conducted in the Bushwick section of Brooklyn, New York, in the early 1990s. This study was the first one to use a "social network" approach to understanding which drug injectors engaged in behaviors that put them at particularly high risk of becoming infected with human immunodeficiency virus (HIV), the virus that causes acquired immunodeficiency syndrome (AIDS), and to look at "risk networks" to determine which of them actually did become infected. The Social Factors and HIV Risk (SFHR) study was the result of a number of years of prior research that had convinced us that existing research in the field was inadequate because it focused on the individual without looking at the individual's immediate social and risk relationships and, beyond that, without looking at the next level of relationships beyond that.

As will become clear in reading this volume, the network perspective is quite useful. It allows us to study relationships as well as individuals. It allows us to study individuals in the context of the people with whom they directly interact. It allows us to look at how the connections among individuals help shape the spread of HIV and other infections through a community at risk. And, perhaps most important, it allows us to think about prevention in new ways and suggests new forms of interventions to help drug injectors protect themselves and others against AIDS.

Before we can discuss this at any length, however, it is necessary to present some background about drug injectors and HIV.

HIV/AIDS AND DRUG INJECTORS IN THE WORLD, THE UNITED STATES, NEW YORK CITY, AND BUSHWICK

Drug injection has been a major route of transmission for HIV. Drug injection is itself a worldwide phenomenon. By 1996, there were at least 127 countries with injecting drug use, and HIV infection among drug injectors has been reported in 96 of them (Ball, Rana, & Dehne, 1998).

Although HIV/AIDS is often thought of as primarily a sexually transmitted disease, drug injection is the major route of transmission in a number of countries. For example, AIDS cases among drug injectors have been 68% of all cases in Italy,

68% in Spain, 44% in Portugal, 42% in Argentina, and more than half of the relatively few AIDS cases yet reported in Poland, the Ukraine, Yugoslavia, China, Malaysia, and Vietnam (UNAIDS/WHO, 1997). In other areas of the world, drug injectors have been a key route of initial entry of HIV into a country. For example, areas along the routes from the Golden Triangle where heroin is produced from local poppy crops have seen the HIV epidemic follow the drug transportation routes. Locales where this has taken place include Thailand, Myanmar, northeastern India, and southwest China (Stimson, 1994; Stimson, Adelekan, & Rhodes, 1996; Stimson, Des Jarlais, & Ball, 1998). Sexual transmission from drug injectors to others, plus perhaps autonomous sexually transmitted epidemics of other strains in Thailand, have then extended the epidemics in these areas. Similarly, although Brazil already had a large sexually transmitted HIV/AIDS epidemic among both "heterosexuals" and men who have had sex with men [United States terminology and ways of classification of sexuality have been shown to be inadequate to deal with Brazilian culture by (Parker, 1991)], this epidemic has been extended into new geographic areas along the cocaine-trafficking routes from Bolivia to Sao Paulo state and Rio de Janeiro (Bastos & Barcellos, 1995).

In the United States, as of June 30, 1997, there had been 604,000 cases of AIDS, of which 49% had been among noninjecting gay or bisexual men; 26% among heterosexual drug injectors; and 6% among men who both inject drugs and have had sex with men. In addition, 9% have been assigned to the heterosexual transmission category (although there is some doubt about the extent to which persons in this category have been misassigned either due to their not having been asked about their drug injection history or due to their having denied either such a history or having engaged in male–male sex). Among these heterosexual transmission cases, between 42 and 93% have had sex with drug injectors. Similarly, among the 7157 AIDS cases among children who were born to infected mothers, between 58 and 81% had either a mother or a father who injected drugs. [Since the Centers for Disease Control (CDC) report heterosexual and perinatal transmission risks in such a way that reports of "sex with HIV-infected person, risk not specified" and "Mother has HIV infection, risk not specified," there are unavoidable uncertainties in the extent to which we can determine the proportion of these AIDS cases that were related to drug injection.]

These statistics underplay the wide geographic variation in the ways in which HIV has been spread in the United States. The extent to which the HIV/AIDS epidemic involves sexual transmission versus drug injection transmission is highly variable by location. New York City has been the major epicenter from which HIV has spread to other drug injectors. As early as 1980, almost 40% of a sample of Manhattan drug injectors were infected (Des Jarlais et al., 1989b). The virus spread to Connecticut, New Jersey and then beyond from its base in New York (Caussy et al., 1990; D'Aquila, Peterson, William, & William, 1989). The extent to which drug injectors in different cities are infected (their "seroprevalence") is given in Table 1.

Table 1. HIV Sero Prevalence among Drug
Injectors in Selected Cities in the United States
and Other Countries

United States cities[a]	% HIV-seropositive
New York	58%
Paterson, NJ	52%
Newark, NJ	50%
San Juan	48%
Jersey City	46%
Miami	32%
Boston area	23%
Houston	8%
Long Beach, CA	6%
Honolulu	6%
Dallas	4%
Minneapolis/St. Paul	3%
San Diego	2%
Tucson	2%
San Antonio	2%
Columbus/Dayton, OH	1%
Laredo	1%
Portland, OR	1%
Cities outside of the United States[b]	
Santos (Brazil)	63%
Madrid	60%
Rio de Janeiro	34%
Bangkok	34%
Rome	20%
Berlin	16%
London	13%
Toronto	5%
Glasgow	2%
Sydney	2%
Athens	1%

[a]Data on street-recruited drug injectors as presented in R. A. Labrie,
W. E. McAuliffe, R. Nemeth-Cozlett, B. Wilberschield. (1993). The
prevalence of HIV infection in a national sample of injection drug
users. Brown, B. S., & Beschner, G. M. (Eds.). (1993). *Handbook on
Risk of AIDS: Injection Drug Users and Sexual Partners*. Wesport,
CT: Greenwood Press. p. 19. Data on cities with more than one
project site were averaged.
[b]Data on a mixture of street-recruited and treatment-entry drug
injectors as presented in M. Malliori, M. V. Zunzunegui, A.
Rodriguez-Arenas, D. Goldberg. (1998). Drug injecting and HIV-1
infection: Major findings from a multi-city study. In G. V. Stimson, D.
C. Des Jarlais, & A. Ball (Eds.), *Drug Injecting and HIV Infection:
Global Dimensions and Local Responses*. London: Taylor and
Francis. p. 74.

Clearly, the center of the epidemic among drug injectors remains the Northeast, with other key centers of infection being Puerto Rico, Miami, and Chicago, and a West Coast epicenter in the San Francisco Bay area. This geographic variability is reflected in AIDS case figures. In New York City, as of the end of 1997, 48% of total cases had been among drug injectors. Furthermore, between 66 and 95% of New York City cases among children born to infected mothers have had a drug injector as the source of the virus. In New Jersey, 53% of total cases had been among drug injectors. In Los Angeles, by contrast, only 13% of cases have been among drug injectors.

This volume deals with drug injectors and HIV in Bushwick, a section of Brooklyn, New York, that had a population of 102,000 in 1990. Thus, it is worthwhile to consider the history of the HIV epidemic among drug injectors in New York. The initial entry of HIV into drug-injecting populations in New York City probably was via a drug-injecting man who had sex with other men (Des Jarlais et al., 1989). Initially, black* drug injectors were more likely to be infected than whites or Latinos, but rates among Latinos soon caught up (Novick et al., 1989), although rates among whites still are lower (Des Jarlais et al., in press; Friedman et al., 1997b).

In the period from 1976 to the early 1980s, seroprevalence in New York rose from zero to about 50%. If there were 200,000 drug injectors in New York City, approximately 100,000 became infected in about 5 years (Des Jarlais et al., 1989a).

The epidemic then entered a period of dynamic stabilization. Prevalence levels for approximately 7 years were in the range of 50 to 55% for long-term injectors and 20 to 25% for injectors in their first 6 years of injection. During this period, incident infections tended to increase seroprevalence; but seroprevalence was held down by the arrival of new drug injectors on the scene, by the departure of older injectors (who were more likely to be infected) who either died or stopped injecting, by behavior change, and perhaps by network saturation (Des Jarlais et al., 1989a). Although mathematical models have suggested that network saturation may have been a very important part of the stabilization process (Blower, 1991), the sociometric analyses of drug injectors' networks conducted during the research for this volume suggest that the extent of network saturation may have been quite limited. [Nonetheless, network structures did affect which drug injectors became infected (Neaigus et al., 1996), with those in the cores of large connected components being at particularly high risk (Friedman et al., 1997a)].

Behavior change probably made a major contribution to the stabilization of seroprevalence. In spite of a popular image that would suggest that either "slavery to their addiction" or "hedonistic, selfish personalities that ignore risks and social

---

*We use the term "black" when referring to data in which this was the category used in the questionnaire or in the source article. Other terms, such as "African American," are usually used where appropriate and where the discussion is more general than a given data set.

responsibility," drug injectors in New York (and, indeed, throughout the world) have acted both to protect themselves and to protect others against the AIDS epidemic. Thus, by 1984, before there were any programs other than the mass media to inform them about AIDS or to help them to protect themselves, drug injectors in New York were engaged in widespread risk reduction. When we asked a small sample of drug injectors from treatment centers if they had done anything to protect themselves, 59% said yes and told us what they had done—mainly, reducing needle sharing or being more careful about needle cleaning (Friedman et al., 1987b). Furthermore, observations on the street confirmed this by showing that drug dealers were competing with others for business by offering free sterile syringes along with their drugs as AIDS-prevention techniques (Des Jarlais, Friedman, & Hopkins, 1985). In Bangkok, Thailand, in 1989, soon after HIV first entered the community, male drug injectors who knew they were infected were trying to protect their wives or lovers by avoiding sex altogether (Vanichseni et al., 1993). Later, we will present detailed data on both the widespread efforts of drug injectors to protect themselves and others and also on the limits of these efforts.

As shown by previous evidence (Des Jarlais et al., 1995a; Friedman, de Jong, Des Jarlais, Kaplan, & Goldsmith, 1987a; Neaigus et al., 1994), risk reduction was driven by small-group pressures toward mutual protection assisted by efforts by the infected not to infect others. By the late 1980s, such behavior change was both stimulated and reinforced by outreach interventions.

The following chart shows that the history of drug users' own behavior change and of public health prevention programming indicates that drug users were far quicker to respond than public health systems:

Date	Drug injectors	Health professionals
1976 or 1977		First retrospectively known HIV infection
1979	Drug injectors knew of new illness: "walking pneumonia"	
1981		Medical discovery of AIDS
1983	In-depth interviews: drug injectors increasingly demand new needles to protect themseleves	
1984	Drug injectors in methadone maintenance programs: 59% report risk reduction; about 30% each had reduced sharing and increased new/ clean needle use	
	Syringe markets expand; advertise clean syringes as anti-AIDS	

(continued)

Date	Drug injectors	Health professionals
1987		First publicly funded outreach
		Few treatment programs had AIDS prevention efforts before 1987
1992		First large publicly funded street syringe exchange

One of the great "what ifs" of the history of the HIV/AIDS epidemic is what would have happened if drug injectors were less stigmatized and less cut off from being active participants in public health discussion in the late 1970s in New York. It is possible that AIDS would have been discovered in 1979 rather than in 1981. It is impossible to estimate how many hundreds of thousands of HIV infections and deaths could have been prevented by knowing about the epidemic 2 years earlier than we did. Thus, in a world of rapid movements of people (and any infections they may have), localized repression and stigmatization can have global repercussions on human health.

Toward the end of the period of stabilized seroprevalence, the purity of available heroin and cocaine increased (in spite of law enforcement efforts at repressing the drug trade). This made possible a large-scale increase in the proportion of drug users who stopped injecting their drugs and also an increase in the number of long-term heroin users who did not inject (Friedman, 1996). This increased purity of drugs probably reduced the influx of new injectors into the scene and also removed old injectors from injecting. Although the effect on proportions of drug injectors who are infected is indeterminate, it clearly reduced seroprevalence among heroin and cocaine users.

A period of declining HIV prevalence began coincident with the introduction and expansion of syringe exchanges in New York (Des Jarlais et al., in press). Syringe exchanges were begun as illegal (but tolerated) volunteer efforts during the time that the study reported in this volume was conducted. It was later legalized, funded by the state of New York and by the American Foundation for AIDS Research, and massively expanded. It led to further reductions in such risk behaviors as receptive syringe sharing, distributive syringe sharing, indirect sharing, and syringe-mediated drug sharing (backloading, frontloading) (Paone, Des Jarlais, Gangloff, Milliken, & Friedman, 1995b). Continuing users of the syringe exchange had incidence rates of 1.5% per year, and nonusers of the syringe exchanges 5.3% per year (Des Jarlais et al., 1996). Trend data from 1990 (before the beginning of syringe exchange) to 1996 show large-scale increases in syringe exchange use, reductions in risk behavior, and reductions in HIV seroprevalence. Among new injectors, similar trends occurred. Thus, by 1996, seroprevalence overall had decreased to approximately 30% and among new injectors to approximately 10%.

This process has some tendency to be self-reinforcing, at least so long as risk-reduction efforts such as syringe exchanges remain large-scale, nonbureaucratic, and user-friendly. During the stabilization phase of the epidemic, a new uninfected injector entered a drug scene in which 20% or more of the other new injectors were infected and in which half or more of the older injectors were infected. Now, however, the proportions of infected partners (assuming random mixing) have shrunk to 10% for new injector partners and 30% for older injection partners. This will produce a corresponding decrease in the probability of becoming infected for each instance of a given high-risk behavior with a new injector or older injector partner.

Nevertheless, the possibility of a return of high infection rates remains. Even the 10% infection rate for new injectors provides a sufficient basis for rapid increase in infection if high rates of risk behavior, together with efficient mixing (for example, through injecting in shooting galleries), should increase. Furthermore, the absolute number of infected drug injectors could increase if there is a large influx to injection drug use by persons who use heroin or cocaine by other routes of administration.

Thus, for New York, great progress has been made, although progress deeply shadowed by the deaths of many thousands of drug injectors due to AIDS and other HIV-related illness and by the infection and illness of tens of thousands more. Continued prevention efforts are needed to maintain these lower prevalence rates and to decrease them even more. Furthermore, no one can be content with existing seroconversion rates (1.5% per year) among continuing syringe exchange users, much less the 5.3% per year among nonusers of the exchange.

INDIVIDUALISTIC PERSPECTIVES ON EPIDEMIOLOGY OF HIV AMONG INJECTION DRUG USERS

How did drug injectors come to be infected? Research has studied this question using the standard techniques of epidemiology to determine the risk factors that compare individuals to distinguish either (1) those who, in a cross-sectional study, have become infected from those who have not, or (2) those who, in successive observations and tests over a period of time, become newly infected from those who remain uninfected. These studies have isolated a number of specific behaviors that seem to be related to HIV infection. What they have shown is as follows:

1. Sharing of syringes is clearly a way in which HIV can be transmitted (Des Jarlais et al., 1994a; Friedman et al., 1995a; Metzger et al., 1993; Nicolosi, Leite, Musicco, Molinari, & Lazzarin, 1992). Drug injection

frequency is also often found to be related to HIV infection (Marmor et al., 1987; Patrick et al., 1997).

2. Cocaine injectors are more likely than heroin-only injectors to become infected or to be infected (in cities where both groups are fairly widespread). On the other hand, internationally, some of the areas of highest seroprevalence (like Myanmar) are areas where heroin is the only drug injected (Anthony et al., 1991; Chaisson et al., 1989b; Stimson, Des Jarlais, & Ball, 1998; van Ameijden, van den Hoek, van Haastrecht, & Coutinho, 1992).

3. People who inject in shooting galleries are particularly likely to be or to become infected (Friedman, Sterk, Sufian, & Des Jarlais, 1989d; Marmor et al., 1987; Vlahov et al., 1990). Shooting galleries are multiuser-injecting locations where people go to inject their drugs outside of the view of police or neighbors and where it is possible to use "house works" such as syringes and cookers as injection equipment. In shooting galleries, the sequential use of the same equipment by people who do not know one another can spread HIV from members of one friendship group to members of another (Friedman, Neaigus, & Jose, 1998a; Friedman et al., 1989d; Marmor et al., 1987).

4. Men who both inject drugs and have sex with men are more likely to be infected than other drug injectors. In some localities, they seem to have formed a bridge group through which HIV entered the drug-injecting population (Lima et al., 1994; Marmor et al., 1987).

5. Sexual transmission also occurs among drug injectors through unprotected sex, although different studies differ in whether they can detect this. This probably reflects a greater ease of transmission of HIV through shared syringes or other forms of contaminated injection than by heterosexual sex. To the extent that injection drug users (IDUs) have reduced their highest-risk injection behaviors more than their unprotected sexual behavior, then, heterosexual transmission becomes the source of a larger proportion of new infections, and thus becomes easier to detect (Schoenbaum et al., 1989).

There is also considerable evidence that other specific behaviors can transmit HIV. These include:

1. Syringe-mediated drug injecting (backloading, frontloading), in which the mixture in which the drugs are dissolved (and perhaps HIV) are squirted from one person's syringe to another's. This will be discussed at some length in Chapters 3 and 11 (Jose et al., 1993; Jose, Friedman, Neaigus, Curtis, & Des Jarlais, 1992; Stark, Müller, Bienzle, & Guggenmoos-Holzmann, 1996; Vlahov et al., 1995).

2. Sharing of cookers, rinse water, cottons, and other forms of indirect sharing in which infected blood from a syringe that one person has used may be transferred to some of the materials used in preparing a drug injection and then sucked up into another person's syringe (Centers for Disease Control and Prevention, Health Resources and Services Administration, National Institute on Drug Abuse, and Administration, 1997; Koester, 1989; Koester, Booth, & Zhang, 1996; Koester & Hoffer, 1994; Solomon et al., 1993).

3. Injecting in outdoors multiperson-injecting settings (Friedman, Jose, Deren, Des Jarlais, & Neaigus, 1995b). In these locations, because they are outdoors and thus in potential view of police, family, or employers, injectors try to spend as little time as possible during the injection process. This means, for example, that they are less likely to take the time to disinfect potentially contaminated syringes.

Several studies have shown that women IDUs who have sex with women are more likely to be infected with HIV (or to become infected) than other IDUs (Cheng, Ford, Weber, Cheng, & Kerndt, 1997; Friedman et al., 1995b; Jose et al., 1993; Ross, Wodak, Gold, & Miller, 1992). We suspect but cannot prove that this is to a large extent due to their injecting drugs (in ways that can transmit HIV) with male injectors who have sex with men or else due to the network properties of their drug-injecting relationships with each other (this is discussed more in Chapter 11).

INDIVIDUALISTIC VIEWS OF RISK BEHAVIORS

Parallel to these analyses of risk behaviors, there have been a number of studies of the characteristics of individuals who engage or do not engage in them. In these studies, the behavior is seen as a characteristic of the individual rather than as varying between social relationships. Thus, if a person engages in syringe sharing, this is seen as a consequence of his or her own characteristics. Explanations are then sought using theories such as the health belief model (Becker & Joseph, 1974, 1988), social learning theory (Bandura, 1977, 1993), the theory of reasoned action (Ajzen & Fishbein, 1980; Ajzen & Timko, 1986; Fishbein & Ajzen, 1975; Fishbein & Middlestadt, 1987), or the AIDS risk reduction model (Catania, Kegeles, & Coates, 1990). In these theories, then, lack of knowledge, skills, values, or internalized norms that prioritize other issues over safety are seen as leading people to engage in high-risk behaviors. For example, researchers studying syringe sharing in Madrid found that sharing was more common among injectors with lower education, who lacked legal income, who injected drugs more often, who inject cocaine, who began injecting at an earlier age, who had less knowledge about how

AIDS is transmitted, and who were gay men (Rodríguez Arenas, Zunzunegui, Friedman, Romero, Bellido, & Ward, 1996).

Similarly, condom use by drug injectors has been found to be associated with a number of individual characteristics. A number of studies have shown that drug injectors who know that they are HIV-positive are less likely to have unprotected sex than are those who are HIV-negative; they do this either by not having sex or by using condoms (Casadonte, Des Jarlais, Friedman, & Rotrosen, 1990; van den Hoek, van Haastrecht, & Coutinho, 1990; Vanichseni et al., 1993; Watkins, Metzger, Woody, & McLellan, 1993). Snyder, Myers, and Young (1989) found that cocaine injection is negatively related to condom use, and Malow et al. (1993) suggest that crack use may also be negatively associated with condom use. Malow et al. found that condom enjoyment, condom skills, self-efficacy, and sex communication skills are associated with condom use in a study of seronegative African-American cocaine users (primarily smokers rather than injectors).

The great bulk of AIDS prevention activity aimed at drug injectors has focused on them as individuals, with major emphases on providing them with knowledge about HIV and how to avoid it, on teaching them personal skills that will helps them resist pressures to share syringes or to have sex without condoms, and/or on helping them reduce or eliminate their drug dependency (Brown & Beschner, 1993).

SOCIAL AND RISK NETWORKS INFLUENCE HIV RISK BEHAVIORS AND INFECTION: OTHER RESEARCH

Many studies have found results that indicate that there is a need to increase our understanding of the social network and social influence aspects of (1) the determinants of risk and protective behaviors and (2) HIV transmission. Thus, in addition to the findings about individual characteristics related to syringe sharing cited above, many studies have reported that injecting with a used syringe is a function of social influence (Frey et al., 1995; Friedman et al., 1987b; Huang et al., 1989a,b; Magura et al., 1989; Tross et al., 1991).

Support from sex partners also affects condom use. Magura, Shapiro, Siddiqin, and Lipton (1990) found that in a sample of 211 drug injectors enrolled in a methadone maintenance program in New York City, greater sexual partner receptivity to condom use was independently associated with condom use. Higher levels of social support were associated with increased condom use among a cohort of 600 gay men who were followed-up between 1984 and 1987 (Catania, Coates, Stall, Bye, & Capell, 1989). Among a sample of women drug injectors in a methadone treatment program, El-Bassel, Gilbert, and Schilling (1991) found that higher social support was associated with feeling more comfortable in discussing safer sex with sexual partners and believing that one's sexual partner would not be upset at suggested changes in safer sexual practices.

Deliberate risk reduction, which has been found to be protective against seroconversion in Bangkok (Des Jarlais et al., 1994b) and to be associated with lower seroprevalence in Rio de Janeiro (Lima et al., 1994), is more common among those whose friends have reduced their risk (Abdul-Quader et al., 1992; Abdul-Quader, Tross, Friedman, Kouzi, & Des Jarlais, 1990; Friedman et al., 1987b; Tross, Abdul-Quader, Silvert, & Des Jarlais, 1992). Further, deliberate risk reduction is a product of social influence processes in New York, Rio de Janeiro, Bangkok, and Glasgow; in all these cities, talking about AIDS with drug-using friends was a predictor of deliberate risk reduction (Des Jarlais et al., 1995a).

Social network characteristics and processes also affect risk and protective behaviors. This has been shown experimentally by Latkin and co-workers (Latkin, 1995; Latkin, Mandell, Vlahov, Oziemkowska, & Celentano, 1996). They compared a "standard" education and HIV-testing intervention with a social network intervention that promoted mutual concern about risk reduction through peer-led group exercises and discussions among members of drug injectors' personal networks. They have provided evidence that research participants who were exposed to the social network intervention were more likely to have reduced their frequency of sharing needles, reduced injecting in shooting galleries, begun always carrying bleach, and begun always cleaning their needles before injecting than were members of a "standard" intervention control group. Zapka, Stoddard, and McCusker (1993) report that, in an intervention targeting clients in a short-term residential detoxification program, decrease in the level of drug-use-related HIV risk behavior was related to reducing the number of drug-injecting friends in subjects' social networks. In our SFHR data, both condom use and receptive syringe sharing in dyads are affected by the duration, type, and intimacy of the relationship (as well as by peer norms).

The spread of HIV is shaped by the networks of those engaging in risk behaviors (Friedman, 1995). Klovdahl (1985), for example, has argued that the "structure of a network has consequences for its individual members and for the network as a whole over and above effects of characteristics and behavior of the individuals involved" (p. 1204). Auerbach, Darrow, Jaffe, and Curran (1984), in a study of HIV infection among homosexual men during the early 1980s, found that a cluster of 40 patients with AIDS in 10 cities were linked directly or indirectly (via index patient O) through sexual contact. A study of networks in a combined data set of commercial sex workers, drug injectors, and their sex partners in Colorado Springs (Potterat et al., 1993; Rothenberg et al., 1995; Woodhouse et al., 1994), a city that has a low and stable seroprevalence of approximately 3% among drug injectors, found that those infected with HIV, most of whom were drug injectors, were located in small-risk networks rather than in a large connected component. Drug injectors were not centrally located within these networks. They suggest that the potential for HIV spread in a city may be influenced by the structure of the risk network. Klovdahl et al. (1994) also reported from the Colorado Springs data that, in a core composed of 106 persons, the average distance between those infected with HIV and those who were susceptible was 3.1 steps, and that everyone in the core was within 6 steps of infection with HIV.

Frey et al. (1995) found that drug injectors' social networks affect the extent to which they share syringes, and Trotter, Bowen, and Potter (1995b) found that network characteristics were related to drug injection frequency. Price, Cottler, Mager, and Murray (1995) showed that drug injectors' social networks affect such sexual risk behaviors as condom use, number of sex partners, soliciting sex from commercial sex workers, and whether or not they worked as a commercial sex worker. Neaigus et al. (1994) found that the relative proportion of interaction with drug injectors and with noninjectors in drug injectors' egocentric networks was related to syringe sharing, shooting gallery use, renting syringes, borrowing syringes, and sharing cookers. They also found that peer norms affected the probability of syringe sharing.

SUMMARY

Although the HIV epidemic has been quite severe among drug injectors, both drug injectors and researchers have taken a number of positive steps to fight the spread of HIV. Drug injectors themselves have engaged in considerable risk reduction both to protect themselves and to protect others. Researchers have made considerable headway in understanding the behaviors that drug injectors engage in that can transmit HIV and some of the individual characteristics that make drug injectors more or less likely to engage in such high-risk behaviors.

On the other hand, many issues in both the epidemiology of HIV and in the determinants of high-risk behavior remain unexplained. Furthermore, our appreciation of the extent of risk reduction by drug injectors needs to be tempered by recognition that far fewer drug injectors have achieved sustained long-term avoidance of all high-risk injecting practices than have achieved risk reduction in such practices; and that even less sexual risk reduction has occurred among them than injection-related risk reduction.

Thus, this volume focuses on understanding two things: the lives and social situations of drug injectors, which form a context for understanding their networks; the social networks and risk networks of drug injectors, which can help us understand why some engage in high-risk behaviors that others avoid; and why some are infected and others are not. Our deeper goal in this volume is to provide the reader with information that can strengthen efforts either to (1) conduct useful research in this area or (2) develop or implement effective prevention programs or policies.

"Learning from Lives"

The more than 800 drug injectors who were interviewed for this study came from an extremely wide variety of social, cultural, and economic backgrounds. As such, there was no "typical" injector and many assumptions that the field staff initially made about "users" were constantly being overturned by the reality encountered in the field. Of course, the researchers did not get to know all 800-plus injectors equally well. Those injectors who came to the neighborhood only briefly to buy drugs and then quickly disappeared remained somewhat mysterious to us, but the many brief conversations that we had with them suggested that heroin and/or cocaine was perhaps not the centerpiece of their lives that it appeared to be with some of the other injectors we got to know over the research period. Many of these occasional visitors to Bushwick seemed to be embedded in complex social lives consisting of family, neighborhood, and jobs, and in that respect they could not be sufficiently understood without immersion into those contexts. But following these occasional visitors into their myriad nondrug domains was too daunting a task for the resources we had, so we concentrated on injectors who occupied the crossroads of the heroin–cocaine scene in Bushwick. These injectors, too, came from a wide variety of backgrounds, as the following descriptions reveal, but they also shared several characteristics.

First, drug injectors are people and not the demons whose image is popularized by antidrug ideologues. Some were people we liked; others were not. Some were mild-mannered, but others were obnoxious or even dangerous. Some did horrible things to themselves and some did them to other people. Some were smart and others were not too bright. In other words, we found that most drug injectors were in many ways like anyone else, and our positions in life could very easily have been reversed.

The six people described below (whose names have been changed) began as research subjects in 1990, and with one exception, they remain of interest to our research today (4/97). But with the realization that they are people whose lives have meaning to others and ourselves, they have become more than research subjects; and as the accounts will suggest, our involvement with them extends beyond the boundaries of research. Anything less and we would become the very demons that they were initially suspected of being. Before presenting these six people, however, we will briefly describe the ethnographic techniques used in this study.

ETHNOGRAPHIC METHODS USED IN THE SFHR STUDY

Ethnographic fieldwork was conducted in Bushwick, Brooklyn, from 1990 to 1993. During the course of conducting fieldwork, hundreds of drug users (including many noninjectors) were contacted and observed by the ethnographic staff. The ethnography included extended observations in shooting galleries, crack houses, shanties and shacks, street corner hangouts, abandoned buildings, vacant lots, rooftops, cars, trucks, public parks, fast food restaurants, and apartments. Many hours were spent observing injection events and discussing the procedures and protocols surrounding those events with individuals and groups. Observations were also made of the interactions between drug injectors and drug distributors, family members, neighborhood residents, and various types of law enforcement personnel, including beat officers, members of the Tactical Narcotics Team (TNT), and the warrant squad. After 3 years of ethnographic fieldwork, several hundred pages of observational notes had been written and more than 210 open-ended interviews with 68 drug users in the neighborhood were conducted. Ethnographic interviews were designed to elicit information on a wide range of topics including demographics, childhood and family background, education and work history, drug use history, current drug use, social networks, knowledge of distribution and sales, income generation and expenditures, participation in criminal activity, impact of law enforcement, injecting practices, knowledge of HIV and other blood-borne viruses, and experiences of treatment and/or quitting.

Ethnographic fieldwork conducted in other Brooklyn neighborhoods, including Williamsburg, from 1989 to 1990, and Flatbush, from 1989 to 1991 (Friedman, Sufian, Curtis, Neaigus, & Des Jarlais, 1991; Sviridoff, Sadd, Curtis, & Grinc, 1992), also has informed the analyses and interpretations in this volume.

One enduring feature of ethnographic research is an attempt to situate the observed behavior of research subjects in the context of a wider community. As such, neighborhoods as a whole are examined, and the direct observation and analysis of behaviors and practices at both the individual and group level are thus able to be placed in the context of a community that gives them meaning. Research participants are observed in public and private domains, allowing for descriptions of the intimate, mundane, or extraordinary details of their everyday lives, the social contexts that frame them, and manner by which they comport themselves and construct identities.

One strength of ethnography is that it allows for the combination of different data sources and permits information to be cross-validated and targeted for follow up and/or clarification. The research team spent many hours discussing and reviewing field observations, information gathered through ethnographic interviews and data from the structured questionnaires, which form the basis for the analyses in Chapter 4 and after. Findings that seemed unusual or appeared to contradict prevailing wisdom became the topic of further ethnographic inquiry. For example, when the structured questionnaire revealed that backloading was associated with higher rates of HIV infection, ethnographers began to spend more time observing such events and asked respondents more pointed questions about the topic. Similarly, when it appeared that there were racial–ethnic differences in HIV statuses among respondents, the ethnographic team reinterviewed many respondents about the problem of ethnic–racial bias in various neighborhood settings, including shooting galleries and crack houses.

SIX LIVES

Pat

Pat was a 31-year-old African-American woman who had been injecting for 5 years when we met her in January 1991. Her father was a chemistry professor who she did not meet until she was 12. Pat's mother was abusive and she was raised by her maternal grandmother in the South until she was 8. She subsequently moved in with her mother in the eastern end of Bedford Stuyvesant, not far from Bushwick. The fifth of eight children, Pat felt that she had been largely ignored as a child, and she gave a heart-wrenching account of suffering a miserable childhood at the hands of an abusive and mentally ill mother. It was often difficult to know whether the childhood recollections that we recorded on tape were truthful or fictionalized rationalizations of a drug injector's present situation; but Pat was horribly scarred on her back and forearms, so that whatever the truth, she had endured great pain earlier in her life. The first few interviews we did with Pat, interviews that normally consisted of a brief life history, were quite difficult to complete. The emotional release that the interviews triggered in her required a whole box of Kleenex, and she and the interviewer found themselves dipping into the box at regular intervals. Although Pat was uncertain about why her mother singled her out for the most severe punishment, she felt that it might be because she was the "blackest" of the children and her paternity was unclear. Pat told us about her mother's constant verbal abuse—usually centered around her blackness—and about spending days locked in a dark closet:

> I was taken from my mother by BCW (Bureau of Child Welfare). My teacher was trying to show me a math problem; she touched my back and I started screaming. All my skin was off my back; my mother had beat me. She beat me everyday but I never told anybody. And she would put me in the closet too. That's where I used to sleep. She used to beat me with extension cords. They'd be dirty yellow ones; she used to bring 'em together and make me get naked. My sisters and brothers used to sneak me food and throw it in the closet and close the door so I can eat.

On at least one occasion, her mother poured boiling water on her arms and back, resulting in the permanent scarring that Pat took great care to hide from even her closest friends. So self-conscious about the way that she looked, Pat wore long-sleeved shirts in the middle of summer to hide her arms. Many injectors reasoned that she wore the shirt to hide track marks and abscesses, but they had never seen her arms and did not know that she could never "hit" herself there.

Shortly after being scalded with boiling water, Pat was placed in foster care in a group home in Williamsburg, Brooklyn. She was the only black girl at junior high school, and few students befriended her. But while school was unpleasant, the hardest part was listening to the other kids in the group home talk about going home to visit their families for the holidays, knowing that she would be stuck in the group home alone. It was during this period that Pat began to attract the attention of young boys from school. Even though she felt self-conscious about her blackness, she had a pretty, round face, a beautiful smile, and budding protrusions in all the right places. One boy who had taken a liking to her convinced his mother to allow Pat to visit them for a long Easter weekend. Mrs. W lived in the projects on Marcy Avenue, behind Woodhull Hospital. She was a meticulously clean woman whose apartment was jammed full of neatly placed knick-knacks, photos and mementos, and plastic-covered furniture. By Pat's account, she got along quite well with Mrs. W, who quickly became a second mother to her. Soon thereafter, Pat became pregnant with her first daughter and Pat moved in with Mrs. W and her son. The relationship with Mrs. W's son eventually soured when they were still both teenagers, but they had had two daughters who lived with Mrs. W (their grand-mother) until moving out in their late teenage years.

Pat was a quick-witted, personable young woman. Despite an awful start in life, she lived a fairly conventional existence through her early 20s:

> I finished school and 9 months at New York Community College in downtown Brooklyn on Tillary Street. My major was accounting. I wanted to change to nursing and I found a private nursing home where they train you. I went there and finished. That's really what I wanted anyway. I was a licensed practical nurse, so I was required to give out medication. First I was a nurse's aide for like 6 months, until I got my license and paid my malpractice insurance and stuff like that. I was a floater, meaning that I worked all over. My main base was Hillside Manor Nursing Home. I dealt basically with nursing homes.

Not long thereafter, Pat married an African-American housing police officer who lived in Bedford Stuyvesant (Bed-Stuy), not far from Mrs. W's housing complex. Pat never talked much about her two marriages, except to say that she loved both men and that they both died about a year after she was married. Her first husband was struck by a car and killed while he was jogging in Bed-Stuy. The driver was never identified. Though grief-stricken, Pat continued to plod along through her daily routines without many visible signs that his death had exacted a toll on her too.

Her second husband was a firefighter, and he too lived in Bed Stuy. Pat said that he was shot in the head during a robbery of a bodega where he had gone to buy groceries. His death was too much for Pat to bear. Unable to work, she quit her job and for several months took the drugs prescribed by a doctor to ease her pain. She traces the beginning to her subsequent history of drug use to this period of her life when she simply "no longer cared." But she had the presence of mind to realize that she was losing control over her life and she made sure that both husband's death benefits went almost entirely to her two daughters who remained with their paternal grandmother in Bed-Stuy. When her share of the life insurance money came, Pat's drug use skyrocketed.

> I never sniffed dope, I started out shooting. I was in love or infatuated with this dude. He was a drug addict. He knew I had money; I spent up $70,000 from my husband who was a fireman. And I got bank books and checks to prove it—it's all in black and white—in less than 6 months.

When the money was gone, she found herself homeless and separated from family and friends. In 1987, she entered her first of many detox facilities.

> My first detox was 21 days at Queens General Hospital. I stayed clean for 2½ years after comin' out of there. I got a job, and I was doing good. Just this March right here I started back shooting drugs every day. I was weighing like 158 pounds. I started coming around here when I was working construction. I was the only girl so I was carrying debris out the building. But even though I was working, I was still homeless.

When we first met Pat, she and her boyfriend, Tommy, were living in a rusty bread truck that had been abandoned in a garbage-strewn field located about a mile from the main Bushwick drug market where she spent the majority of her days and nights. The field was near the top of a hill, stuck between several old factories and overlooking a filthy, foul-smelling shipping canal that juts into Queens and ends near the edge of Bushwick. When the wind blew in the wrong direction, the rancid smell sometimes seemed enough to peel the remaining paint off the side of the truck. In the summer, the smell was especially bad and the truck, which had baked in the sun all day and had become saunalike, seemed to funnel in the smell and the mosquitoes, making sleep virtually impossible. In the winter, the wind often pierced the inside of the truck so that no matter how many blankets Pat and Tommy used, they could not manage to get warm. But we did not know about the truck for nearly a year. Tommy never took anyone to his secret lair. He feared that other drug users might try and muscle him out of his rent-free palace if they saw how cozy and secure it could be made. Pat, on the other hand, never took anyone there because she was embarrassed to be living in such primitive conditions and she was scared to death of Tommy.

In 1990, while working in Bushwick, Pat had met Tommy in the neighborhood. Tommy, a muscular crack smoker of Jamaican parentage, had a variety of hustles in the neighborhood. But while Tommy was adept at earning money, Pat quickly discovered that he was also extremely abusive. She lost her construction job and found herself working the local stroll (engaging in commercial sex work) under Tommy's watchful eye. While she resented the way he treated her, she found herself unable to escape his powerful hold.

> He would hit me for nothing sometimes. It brought back memories of my childhood, and I would ask him, "why are you hitting me?" And then he'd say the same thing my mother said, "Just shut up." And I couldn't take it. (Sobbing)
>
> One time we were in the street going home and he goes, "Oh, you said something bitch, you wanna be smart?" He grabbed me and slammed me up against the wall and banged my head. I had a seizure. He took and kicked me. I said, "Please don't let me swallow my tongue, just help me, don't let me die." He said, "Bitch I can't care if you die tonight." He kicked me in my side. Even this morning, he said, "You see bitch, I don't give a fuck about you, I'll let you lay there, I don't give a fuck if you swallow your tongue or not. What the fuck do I care."
>
> Every time that I would go out, Tommy was like clockin' me. And my luck was so fucked up that I could not get a fuckin' car date. Tommy was watching me to the point that I had to already have the money I was gonna give him separated. If I had money in my hand, he'd actually say, "Let me see what that is." The nerve of him. I thought everything was down the middle. Well, wasn't nothin' down the middle when I was working.

By the end of summer 1990, Pat was not only firmly entwined with Tommy and the wide range of crack smokers with whom he associated, but she was also a member of the core network of injectors in the neighborhood and she became a familiar face at many injection locales. Because her forearms were scarred from childhood burns, she had difficulty finding a vein and often solicited the assistance of other injection drug users (IDUs) in the neighborhood. Pat had a large number of injection partners during this period and strongly suspected that she might have contracted HIV. In 1991, she confirmed what she had suspected.

> About a week after I got tested, the results came back. Nothing happened to me when I found out 'cause I had an idea anyway. Even though I have been tested a number of times, I never went back to pick up the tests because I knew inside what the results were going to be. After they told me the results, they gave me a list of services, but they only do but so much. They don't have any major concern about what really happens to you. They give you a piece of paper, and they tell you about all these people's places that you can get involved with if you want to. And that's it. That's it. I wasn't too upset when they told me. I think I psyched myself out to believe that I already knew. The counseling they gave me was bullshit I had heard already, and I told them that.

At the time, the news that she was HIV positive did not compel Pat to seek treatment. She continued with her daily routine of working the stroll, helping Tommy with his various hustles and visiting shooting galleries as if nothing had changed. She did, however, begin to inform her injection partners of her status and began to develop resentments toward others who were more careless or dishonest.

> Susan is in the same boat as me (HIV positive), but I don't plan on sharin' works with a sick one. She asked if she could use my works and I said no. I still don't feel comfortable

sharin' works. And she's goin' around making a national announcement. I'm not. I told the people I wanted to know. She's going around tellin' everybody that she's got the virus. And she's still usin' everybody's sets and all.

Near the end of 1992, Pat had been so worn down physically and emotionally that she found it difficult to make money. Perceiving herself as no longer competitive on the stroll, she and Tommy fought over diminishing returns from each evening of work. She tried to compensate by putting together a variety of hustles— selling dope, "looking out," copping (buying) for others, selling scrap metal, selling works—but they yielded far less income. As the pressure from Tommy grew, she planned ways to break away.

So I was slowin' down from giving money to Tommy and his friend B. I was gonna start goin' back to the street makin' my own money, then I wouldn't have to ask him for anything. I didn't want to hustle with them no more 'cause I see what they do. They turned on me. They started that whispering shit. And they took everything that we got and split it between themselves. I didn't get a penny out of it.

Tommy was crazy. I told him, "I'm fuckin' leaving you." He says, "After you make the last of my money, okay. I want all the money I gave you when I was workin'. After you make it, bitch, then you go, okay. And I don't never want to see you again. If I see you, I'm gonna fuck you up every time I see you. I don't care who you with." On my way out he smacked me. He snuck me too, 'cause I really wasn't expecting it. And he told me, "Bitch, I don't know where you're going, but when you come back, you better have some drugs. If you don't have drugs, I'll beat you so bad you gonna wish you fuckin' never seen me." I was standing on the little hill by our truck and he smacked me so hard I almost fell. And you know if I fall on that cement, I'm fuckin' dead.

After this frightening experience, Pat called her eldest sister who lived in Staten Island and with who she had not talked in many months. Her sister, an occasional drug injector herself, invited Pat to her apartment.

I just made up my mind to go, but my intentions was to come back. But when I got to my sister's, she says, "I know you know you're not going anywhere tonight," because it was raining. I was tired—dead tired. I said, "Well, I'll stay." But my intentions was to get up the next morning and leave you know. She says, "I can give you $25 in the morning." She already had the money. She showed it to me and shit. She said, "But I will not give it to you tonight. If you leave tonight, I'll give you carfare and that's it. You can eat as much as you want and whatever you want before you go." I said, "Okay, at least I'll be able to get straight in the morning." But I got dope sick out there. I had brought my shit out there, okay, but since I thought I was goin' home, and she was givin' me $25 I did it.

One bag of dope cost $25 out there. And it's a dime bag, but it's not even a whole dime. It's like a half. And three of us was down on that. My sister had works because she used to be a drug addict. I told you she dips and dabs. Her man dips and dabs too, but he does his shit outside the house because she doesn't allow drugs in her house every day of the week. She doesn't use every day. She tells him that if he wants to use drugs every day, all well and good, but don't bring it in the house every day. Only on Sundays when she gets high. And not every Sunday, okay. At any time during the week he's not allowed to bring any drugs inside her house. If he does it without her permission, he got three strikes and he's out. And he already used one, so he got two more.

After more than 3 months at her sister's apartment, during which she sought medical treatment and opened a welfare case, Pat returned to the Bushwick, driven by mounting pressures in the household and because she "was bored and missed the neighborhood."

When Pat returned to Bushwick in early 1993, she took up residence in an apartment shooting gallery, assisting the owner in return for "tastes" and supplementing her income by helping outsiders make purchases in an increasingly closed market. Pat had a large number of injection partners while living there. When eviction proceedings finally managed to permanently close the gallery in the fall, Pat moved in with a downstairs tenant with two teenage children who she had befriended. Two months later, with her ability to sustain a daily habit limited, she tried unsuccessfully for several weeks to enter a methadone program. But Pat's Medicaid card had expired 6 months earlier and with the increasingly stringent eligibility requirements effectively weeding out the most needy and desperate, she was unable to secure coverage. A friend offered to pay cash in lieu of Medicaid for a spot in a methadone program, but the program refused the check, saying that Pat would have to show her own pay stub to qualify for "sliding scale" payment.

Psychologically beaten by steely-eyed social workers, deeply depressed, and perpetually nauseous from withdrawal, Pat heard about a detox facility in Queens that would accept clients without Medicaid coverage. Uncertain of whether they would admit her, Pat took a trip of desperation to Little Neck Community Hospital in Queens where she was admitted to their 21-day detox unit. While there, Pat met Odie, a 36-year-old African American from Harlem who lived in Washington Heights. Shortly after she was discharged from the hospital, Pat moved in with Odie. They both enrolled in a methadone program on 125th Street in Harlem, and she began a period of relative stability in her life. Attending her program regularly, she continued to occasionally inject heroin and cocaine, but had settled into a routine and had virtually severed all her previous ties with Bushwick and the IDUs she knew there. While her health and T-cell count continued to decline, with Odie's support she managed to see health care professionals more frequently than when she was living in Bushwick.

In November 1997, Pat was admitted to Columbia Presbyterian Hospital where she was treated for pneumonia and several other serious health problems, including abscesses on her lower legs that needed to be drained. Told by doctors that she also had heart disease, Pat was advised that, short of a transplant, there was very little that they could do. Her condition improved incrementally while there, but after a week, she was unceremoniously discharged when one of the doctors accused her of using drugs in the hospital after reviewing the results of her most recent blood work. Pat insisted that she had not used drugs while there (other than the methadone they were giving her, which would register "positive" on a nonspecific opiate test). Nonetheless, unable to walk, she was sent home without the six different medications that had been prescribed. Without money or Medicaid, she could see no way to get the medicine that she so desperately needed. Odie was outraged that she had been discharged in such a fragile condition and he vowed to complain to Patient Relations at the hospital. But Pat's week in the hospital also caused problems at her methadone program. After being absent for several days, the program would not automatically medicate her, and they insisted that she be reinstated, a process that caused a delay in receiving her usual dose. So, after hobbling to the program weak and out of breath, Pat discovered that they refused to give her methadone and she remained "dope sick" for the rest of the day.

Within a week after her discharge, Pat's condition began to deteriorate. Unable to walk, Pat spent her days calling friends and relatives on the phone, confiding in them that she was afraid that her health was not going to improve. At midnight, November 28, Odie called the ethnographer at home screaming into the phone, "she's dead, she's dead," and the crackling of police and EMT radios in the background said that, this time, there was no hope that she could be saved. Unable to breathe, Pat had died of cardiac arrest in Odie's arms. At the wake held in Bedford Stuyvesant a week later, family members who had not seen her in many years grumbled when the ethnographer brought IDUs from Bushwick to pay their respects, but no words were exchanged. Pat was buried at a cemetery in New Jersey on a sunny winter day. The wind kept blowing over the flower arrangement, interrupting the few speakers who came to pay their final respects, and Odie commented that Pat was getting in her last two cents before being left in peace.

Honey

When we first met her in 1990, Honey was a 40-year-old Italian-Irish sex worker who had been working the stroll in Bushwick regularly since 1988. The second of three daughters, she was raised in an ethnically mixed section of Williamsburg's southside. Her father worked in several manual labor jobs in Williamsburg. Her mother worked in a local ice cream factory "putting the sticks into popsicles."

Even though Honey had a large extended family in the neighborhood, it was less tight knit than other Italian families in the area. When asked about her parents, she was quick to point out that she never knew her father too well. During several interviews, she retold the story of how her father raped her in the shower when she was 8 years old. Even though she said that she "got over it," that incident clearly had a profound impact upon her life.

> (My father) tried to (rape me) once, but my sister told my grandfather. My grandfather beat the shit out of him. He, he moved. We got out of the house. I was afraid to say anything because he told me, you know, that if I did he would kill me just like he'd kill a dog. Because he killed my dog too. He took my dog away and poisoned it.
> Then my mom ... she started going out and stayed out nights and, uh, leave us alone and this and that. And I was having little nightmares: I went to the bathroom or

something and my father would be in there, you know? So we got out of that apartment.
But I got over it, you know.

Honey was unsure why her mother started going out at night and leaving her
and her sisters alone. She speculated that her mother never really had a childhood
since she had the three of them when she was still a teenager. After her father
moved out, she felt that her mother saw an opportunity to live the teenage years
which she missed and grabbed the opportunity. Shortly after that, neighbors called
the Bureau of Child Welfare and Honey and her sisters were placed in a series of
group homes before age 10. Honey and her sisters were never returned to their
natural mother and they remained in foster care until they were 18.

Honey, who bore the brunt of the family's tragedy, and her older sister began
experiencing serious problems even before being removed from their mother's
home by the state. Honey recalled being beaten by her mother for neglecting minor
household chores. When asked why her older sister was not given chores to
perform and was not beaten, she replied that she was always running away and that
her mother could never control her. Her sister drifted into the streets and drugs long
before she turned 18. Honey eventually lost touch with her, but later learned that
her body was found buried on the estate of a religious cult in upstate New York in
the 1970s.

Honey's younger sister was more fortunate. She was too young to experience
all the trauma that the others experienced when the family broke up. Even though
she too went through the foster care system, according to Honey, she "grew up
OK" and eventually married and settled in Long Island. Honey had not seen her
younger sister for more than 10 years.

Honey started using various types of drugs at the age of 12. She recalled
"trippin', smoking, snortin' dope," and so on. To make money, she would skip
school and work as a prostitute on the stroll on Manhattan's Lower East Side.
When asked who had introduced her to that—who had "turned her out"—Honey
replied that she had begun prostituting on her own. "After all," she replied, "my
father raped me when I was 8, so, what the hell."

When she was discharged from the group home at 18, she moved in with a
Puerto Rican man who lived in her old neighborhood, the Southside, and they had a
son together. Honey noted that, "He was always doing it [heroin]. There was never
time for me. There was no sex, there was no nothing." Nevertheless, he introduced
Honey to injecting heroin. Soon after this, Honey and her boyfriend separated.
With no place to stay and no support network, her son was eventually taken by the
Bureau of Child Welfare. Honey was bitter because she had gone to visit her
mother when she became homeless, but her mother, who was living with another
man at the time, refused to take them in. Honey noted that they "were flesh and
blood, but he was just a piece of shit." Honey did not see her son again until 1991,
more than 15 years later.

At 23, Honey married a Polish man in the neighborhood. He beat her and she left him several times. On one such occasion, she started selling drugs. She was also working as a barmaid in Queens and prostituting on the side. When she and her husband reunited, they sold drugs together, but as the two of them drifted farther into drug dependency, they drifted farther apart, and eventually she left him for another man.

Honey's heroin habit developed to the point where she could no longer hold a legitimate job, and she began to work various strolls full time. She recalled that at first the business was not too bad:

> Many moons ago, when I started out (in Bushwick) there was three girls out there: Flo, Irene, and myself. Right there by the train station, the LL train station. There was three of us out there. Blow jobs had been 5 dollars and 10 dollars for many moons. Everything goes up but the meat rack business. It's still the same. That was about, maybe, 12, 13, 14, 15 years ago when it was more discreet.
>
> There's so much difference, you know? And it was more fun back then too. Those [other girls] were friends. Yeah, now these girls out here are just for the drug and themselves. There's no friendship. Everybody's out to cut everybody else.

Honey had a heroin habit for many years. It was the only drug she did until the early 1980s, when cocaine and crack became enormously popular. She also had periods of several years when she stopped injecting or sniffing just heroin.

> I was shooting heroin for 16 years and never even thought to say, "what's a speedball," and do it with speed. I never started the speed—doing coke—till about 6 or 7 years ago.
> I have three abscesses going at one time—here, here, and here—you see them? You see, my legs full of abscesses. I never had—look at my breasts. I never had fuckin' abscesses in my life. All the years doing dope, and here I go starting shooting [coke].

The introduction of cocaine into her repertoire of drugs was extremely damaging to Honey's health and paralleled the development of the crack epidemic in New York City. It was probably no coincidence that around the same time that she started using cocaine regularly (both injecting and smoking it), many of her drug use and personal habits changed, and she developed her first case of syphilis, which went undetected for 6 months. Honey also developed a heart condition (mitral valve prolapse), and her asthma worsened to the extent that she occasionally required hospitalization. All the while, she worked the stroll in Bushwick, working longer hours for less money.

Many of Honey's "dates" were steady customers with whom she had had relationships for months or even years. Her relationships with these men were cordial but businesslike.

> If I'm going out with a client for a couple of months and he comes to me and he says, "I'm a little short this week, can I pay you next time" or, "I'll give you a few dollars now," I'll go for it. It's like having a grocery store and you give credit. If they don't pay you, they don't get no credit no more.

But changes in the conditions on the stroll undermined many of those relationships.

> I let a lot of my steadies pass me up. They say, "I'm not going out today." Meanwhile, 20 minutes later, you see them passing by with another bitch in the car. So you just don't look right today. Now you're starting to think, "What's going on here?" A lot of johns are afraid today because of the diseases going around.

Even though Honey accepted it as part of the business that a "steady" might opt for another woman on any particular night, she nevertheless perceived such behavior to be a breach of their relationship. In retaliation, she might not give him credit on their next "date" or she might decide to demand more money than their usual price. If truly angered, she might decide to take all of his money when he was in a vulnerable position. For example, on one occasion when she was "dope sick," a local man offered her $5 for oral sex. Honey said that she was insulted, and ordinarily would have turned him down, but she was so sick that she had little choice but to take the offer. In the middle of being aroused, the man decided that he wanted to have "straight sex" rather than just oral sex and he proceeded to take his pants off. At that point, still seething from his stingy offer, Honey noticed that he had a considerable amount of money in his pocket. She snatched his pants and ran off with them, leaving him standing in an empty lot in his underwear. Honey laughed wondering how the man was going to explain this to his wife. Later she explained:

> I don't want to rip anybody off. I don't make it a habit. But that guy got me so pissed off. Sunday morning, I was hungry, I was stressing like a son of a bitch. And here comes this sucker offering me 5 bucks, and he got a pocketful of money. Shit! That's a guy that's insulting you and, you know, I don't like that. Yeah, I mean, you going to get off on me? I'm going to get off on you!

During the winter of 1990, Honey was raped again by a Polish man on the Southside. She also got another case of syphilis.

> I was working the street [in Bushwick], and this guy called me and he was all nice and I quoted to him my price. And then he decided to go where he wanted to go after I told him not to go there. [He] took me to the waterfront outside and beat the shit out of me. He took me down on the Southside to the waterfront where there's a view of the sea, so pretty. Oh, the man was a horrible sight though. He just beat the hell out of me. My father raped me when I was 8 years old and I was looking at his face and I saw my father at the same time. You know, it sounds queer, but we were by the waterfront. Okay, water again. I got raped, I was in my shower, taking a shower and he, my father, raped me, you know?

Honey had stopped injecting drugs for several years and felt that she had gotten a handle on her habit. She began injecting again after the rape.

> Why? Because I, I found out I was pregnant. And I found out about 4 months ago, 3 or 4 months ago. We go down to the [just a pause, then continuing awkwardly] with a client of mine and, uh, we went to the hospital and they wanted to do X rays, but they said they had to take tests to make sure I wasn't pregnant before they X rayed. And I said it was impossible, because I use Trojans for everybody. But a blow job, you can't get pregnant

from a blow job. And that thing came back positive and I near about died. And then I
remembered the rape.

Honey was shocked to discover that she was pregnant. After much agonizing,
she decided to keep the baby, despite all the obstacles she knew lay ahead. At 41
years old and looking every day of it, it had already become more difficult for
Honey to make money on the stroll; being pregnant compounded those problems.

When you're pregnant, these guys don't like it. You know, I mean, I'll dress sometimes,
you wouldn't even know I was pregnant. And then I'll walk with my hands in my jacket
and I'll hold it out so you can't really tell. And then, when I get in the car, once I get the
money, man, I don't give a shit what they know, if I'm pregnant or not.

The baby was born remarkably healthy, but had a positive toxicology for
drugs and tested positive for HIV. A beautiful-looking boy, he was placed with a
foster care agency in Queens who found a stable, white family in Long Island to
take him. Honey had named the boy Richard, after the ethnographer on our project,
and expressed a desire that he would grow up to do the kind of work that we did.
Though flattering to us, Honey's choice of a name for her child reflected her
profound sense of isolation from family, friends, and the "straight" world. The
foster care agency could never get hold of Honey to make the parent–child visits
that they were required to arrange. They occasionally called the SFHR storefront to
inquire about her, and once they sent a few pictures of baby Richard, but Honey
could not bring herself to make the meetings. She blamed her addiction for not
seeing her child, but she was keenly aware that she would never be in a position to
get him back, and seeing him would only compound her pain. When the pictures of
Richard came to the storefront, Honey was eager to see them, but tears quickly
welled up in her eyes and she could not bring herself to look at them for very long.

Honey returned to working the street but said that it was many months before
she was able to stop thinking about her son. In 1993, as the streets of Bushwick
became less lucrative for sex workers, Honey began to work other strolls including
the Southside of Williamsburg and in Queens. Even though she did not receive
regular medical attention and her health continued to deteriorate, she survived
when many other HIV-positive street-level sex workers were succumbing to the
virus. When we last saw Honey, in April 1998, she had returned to Bushwick to
work the stroll. She had developed cervical cancer, which had rapidly spread and
was literally eating holes in her flesh. No longer able to get "high" from heroin,
she used as many bags as she could buy simply to dull the pain. During the
February freeze, Honey, who suspected that she would soon be dead from the
cancer, went to a local hospital emergency room for help. During her week-long
stay in the hospital, she was put in touch with a Manhattan-based agency that
provided housing for people with AIDS. Within a few weeks, she had her own
apartment in a new facility that had recently been built in East New York,
Brooklyn. But even with the opportunity to slow down a bit, Honey found it

difficult to divorce herself from the street and she spent little time in her new home, going there only long enough to sign in and change her clothes. Unable to explain why she could not manage to separate herself from the street lifestyle, Honey continued to spend the majority of her time hanging out in Bushwick, smoking crack and shooting dope.

Celia

Before the SFHR project began, senior staff members surveyed north Brooklyn to search for the best place to set up a research storefront. Our previous project, Community AIDS Prevention Outreach Demonstration (CAPOD), had been located in Williamsburg, but beginning in late 1988, the neighborhood began to change in response to gentrification and a massive police presence that displaced drug distributors and users to several other areas. We kept hearing about Bushwick, which is farther into the interior of Brooklyn and less accessible to highways and public transportation than Williamsburg. In early December 1990, we located a major street-level drug market centered at the corner of Knickerbocker Avenue and Troutman Street. Hundreds of injectors openly participated in this busy street-level drug market and it did not take long for us to decide that this was the spot for our project to set up shop.

Two blocks from the epicenter of the drug market, there was a short street—Melrose—that specialized in crack sales. When we first came to the neighborhood, we were reluctant to stop our car in the middle of the busy heroin-selling block. We did not want the dealers to think that we were the police, nor did we want to get stopped ourselves by the police who might think that we were there to buy drugs. When we turned onto Melrose Street that first afternoon, we saw a crowd of eight to ten drug users milling about. We decided to park the car and try and talk with a few of them. As we (one white and two black men) got out of the car, several of the users began to walk quickly in the opposite direction, fearful that we were plainclothes police. To allay their fears, we quickly began to give out condoms to those who would stop. Three women from the stroll immediately recognized the currency of outreach workers and returned to the car to see if we had any unlubricated condoms. The women were seldom paid for "straight" sex; oral sex was more than 95% of their business and dry condoms were the best type to use in those situations. Several street-level sex workers from the Kent and Wythe Avenue stroll in Williamsburg had told us that most of the working women had recently been displaced to the Flushing Avenue stroll in Bushwick, so we began asking the three women who crowded around the car if they had seen any of several women we know from CAPOD. Of course, the three Bushwick women knew them, since they were well-established and somewhat-respected street workers-so our credibility and trustworthiness were redeemed.

Most of the people we met that day were injectors and crack smokers in their mid-20s to early 30s. Among them was a 19-year-old Latina, Celia, and her 20-year-old brother, Luis. Celia was a newcomer to the stroll, and at that time, crack and cigarettes were her only vices. Luis was a shy, somewhat moody, young Puerto Rican who was working a daytime shift for a Dominican-owned white-top crack organization whose main outlet was near the corner of Melrose and Knickerbocker. Luis smoked crack too. He was also limping rather badly. He had run off with a couple of the organization's "bundles" of crack (24 $5 vials per bundle) a week earlier. When the managers had finally caught up with him, they shot him in the thigh with a small caliber gun. The bullet was still in his leg, bulging out just above the knee. When asked why he had not gone to the hospital, he simply shrugged his shoulders. Luis was never very communicative about himself or what he was doing; he was not a good candidate for the ethnographic interviews we were interested in conducting. Even if we could not always decipher Luis' motivations or predict his movements, however, it was clear that he was very close to Celia. As the only remaining members of a family that had disintegrated several years ago (both parents had died), Luis and Celia had a visible bond that somehow seemed terribly fragile in the context of the street scene.

Celia rarely talked about her childhood, but the bits and pieces that came out were disturbing:

> I live at Broadway and Myrtle with my mother's brother. My mother died. She had an asthma attack. Yeah, there was a asthma pump in her hand, but we could tell by her eyes she was hard as a rock. And that day I was crackin' up.

Before the SFHR project ended, in early 1993, Luis had been sentenced to prison for drug distribution. Celia had begun distributing and injecting drugs, had contracted HIV, and subsequently died of sepsis in Woodhull Hospital.

There was something strangely likeable about Celia. She was a young lady who seemed to have stopped maturing at about the age of 12. Dropping out in junior high school, she never learned to read. She seemed to be similarly unsuccessful on the streets and was not very adept at hustling or living by her wits on the street. But her waiflike manner made her seem innocent in a way that the other street people were not. More than the others, it seemed clear that the awful situation that she was caught in was not of her making, but was the product of the poor choices that significant adults in her life had made. Though Celia sometimes proved to be just as sneaky as many of the other injectors and crack users, somehow it seemed easier to overlook her transgressions. Celia claimed to live with her uncle in the projects about half a mile from Bushwick's drug markets, but she rarely slept there. She did not start hanging out in Bushwick and smoking crack until after her mother died in 1988.

> I used to steal cars too. That's why I really came here [to Bushwick]. I was 16. My brother teached me how to steal cars when I was 14. We used to go to Coney Island every

winter. We used to break all the games, all those stores, all those new stores in Coney Island, we used to break them up. The rides, the go-carts, we used to steal them. We used to steal a lot of shit, then we started stealing Buicks, real cars. We used to take hangers and pull them through the window and open the doors, take the screwdriver and pop the lock from the ignition key, put two wires together, turn on the car, and take off with the cars. We'd bring the cars to Bushwick and the junkyard man would give us $100, sometimes $125.

Most of her time was spent on Melrose Street, where she smoked crack, occasionally selling it, and prepared herself for working on the nearby stroll. She was often seen sleeping on the sidewalk or in some other outdoor location. Some IDUs, like Patricia, prided themselves on being able to talk people into giving them money or drugs or on being able to talk their way out of potentially dangerous situations. Celia, on the other hand, was not good at expressing herself and frequently asked for the meaning of relatively simple words. Unlike the other IDUs described in this chapter who were able to effectively describe events in their lives, Celia had difficulty conveying her thoughts and feelings. But even though the many formal and informal interviews with her failed to generate the type of rich descriptive accounts that are important to ethnographic research, daily observations of Celia and extensive discussion with those around her provide a compelling story.

On that first day, Celia's story already seemed tragic but easily explained: She was another young woman who had been seduced by a "blast" of crack. While that was partly true, her story turned out to be far from simple and involved a web of other people. What went unnoticed by us on that first day we parked on Melrose Street was a drab, two-story house—the only house on the block—set back about 20 yards from the curb. We later learned that Celia's two children were cared for by their paternal grandmother, Maria, in that house. Their father, Roger, lived there too, but seemed largely uninvolved in his children's upbringing and was verbally abusive toward Celia. Selling crack and herself right outside the gate to Maria's house, Celia was both connected to and disconnected from the family living there.

> Today I start selling blue tops [crack]. Since six o'clock in the morning all the way to about three o'clock. I sold three packages and made about $300. With the money I bought dope, I bought my son more pampers, and I bought him extra things, you know, in case he runs out. If he runs out, his father comes and tell me to buy some things for him. But I can't read minds. They have to tell me when they need things. I just try to show him I love him. A lot of times I help him, but when I am hungry and I ask for food he won't give me any. One time I bought a gallon of milk, eggs and juice. I figured that two eggs were mines and my brother's. And when I took a little bit of milk she told me to get out of the house. I said, "Come on, I just finished buying a whole gallon of milk." So anyway, I just put the milk and the eggs down and left. I said, "What kind of shit is that?" I mean, she acted like she bought it.

In talking about how she contributed food to the household, Celia portrayed herself as a concerned mother who tried to support her children even though she was not their primary caretaker. But her chances to make significant (or even insignificant) contributions to the household were rare. More often than not, Celia was tired, hungry, and broke.

Celia's relationship with Maria and the rest of the family was complicated and never as straightforward as it seemed on the surface. On the one hand, as the mother of two children who lived in Maria's house, she was part of the family, and Maria tried to make sure that Celia remained so, however marginally. On the other hand, Celia sold and used drugs, sometimes with members of the family, and because of that, Maria held her at arm's length, often preventing her from coming in the house and thereby giving the appearance of condoning her behavior. Also, Maria feared drawing the police into her house in their aggressive pursuit of crack dealers on that block. Below, Celia talks about her position on Melrose Street, describing the constant Ping-Pong between the streets and jail.

> I was selling white tops every 2 days. I'd usually sell a whole pack [240 $5 vials] in a day and would make like $100. I'm still staying on Melrose too, across from 384 Melrose [where Maria lived]. I sleep in a little hut, a little wooden house I built up. But the cops have been hassling me a lot; they go in there and break up the house and tear it up. I'm not sure where my brother is; I haven't seen him for 2 days. I was in jail; they put me in jail on prostitution charges. I wasn't even working at the time. I was getting ready to walk to the yard to take a hit of crack. I saw the cops in a van, but I kept on walking. That cop DeLaskis jumped out and grabbed me. He said, "I told you if we catch you, we are going to lock you up." I started to struggle with them and they put the handcuffs on me. They didn't take me to the 83rd. They took me to some other precinct and then to central booking. Finally, I saw the judge. He gave me some kind of community service.

Despite Celia's lifestyle and Maria's inability to intervene in her life in a significant manner, she continued to hold onto the hope that someday she would straighten out and want to reestablish a meaningful relationship with her children. When Celia was arrested in the summer of 1991 for selling crack, Maria and the project ethnographer tried to visit her in Rikers Island, bringing Celia clean clothes, soap, shampoo, and deodorant.

> Maria and I went to Rikers Island, but we never did get in to see Celia. I picked her up in my car at 6 AM on Sunday morning. We drove to the gate and parked on the street, waiting for the bus to bring us the rest of the way. When we finally got to the control building, we waited on line for an hour before we were told that Thursdays were her visiting days and not Sunday like she told us. So both of us were pretty annoyed when we left there, and it was a terribly taxing experience: the expense, the noise, the crowds, the bullshit you have to go through to get in. And not to get in was pretty infuriating. Maria wasn't nearly as bothered about making the trip as I was. Since Celia isn't her biological daughter, I was surprised that she wanted to make the trip in the first place. [field-notes-6/30/91]

Celia was not the only family member involved with drugs that Maria worried about. In addition to her son who smoked crack, her eldest daughter, Carmen, was a multiple substance user who had one foot in the house and the other in the street. In

the summer of 1991, Maria began to worry about how much heroin Carmen was
using and she pushed her to try and stabilize her life by enrolling in a methadone
program. But in some ways, the methadone seemed worse.

> Maria expressed concern about Carmen being on methadone. Her concern is that
> Carmen's been coming home, lying in bed and nodding out with a cigarette in her hand.
> The day before yesterday she burned a big hole in the mattress the size of a grapefruit.
> Maria wanted us to find out what was going on with the methadone. Carmen had come
> by the storefront yesterday and told us that she had been reduced from 50 mg to 40. She
> told her mother that she had been reduced from 60 to 50. Obviously there are two stories
> here, and we don't know really what the truth is.
>   I spoke with Carmen and told her that her mother was worried that she had become
> involved with selling heroin on Troutman Street. Carmen was quick to reply that she
> wasn't selling heroin, she was selling crack for the blue tops, as if to say that selling
> heroin was bad and selling crack wasn't so bad. She came in yesterday all decked out
> with about a half a dozen gold chains and gold rings on every finger, a new outfit she was
> wearing, and a new outfit in a bag. She told us that the previous night she had worked
> from about one o'clock to about five o'clock in the morning. She had made $155. She
> told us the previous week she had made nearly $1000. So she's making pretty good
> money out there. She's only been arrested once, and she says that she's been very
> cautious lately so as not to get arrested again. But today we saw her working for the first
> time during the day, and it was pretty unusual because we had never seen her selling blue
> tops before.
>   Maria and I also talked about going to see Celia who had recently been transferred
> to Forbell Women's Prison on Conduit Avenue. Apparently Celia's bail is about $500,
> which nobody's going to pay. So she's going to end up having to stay on Forbell until
> she's served her sentence. So she goes to court for sentencing, and we're going to see
> what happens at that time. [fieldnotes 7/8/91]

Maria's fears about Carmen were well founded:

> Carmen got arrested last week selling blue tops. The day after we saw her wearing that
> bathing suit she got arrested that night after telling us that she wasn't going to get caught.
> She was in Rikers Island for a couple of days before they let her go. I don't think she had
> to post bail. She went to court yesterday, the 17th, and they're going to send her to a
> rehab facility upstate for 18 months. If she doesn't go to the rehab facility, she's going to
> get 3 years in jail. She's not happy about going, but she's going to have to. Maria's not
> happy about Carmen going for only 18 months. She was hoping that she'd get 2 years
> and give Maria a chance to get her act together and move out of the neighborhood in the
> meantime. [fieldnotes 7/18/91]

Carmen felt that she was fortunate when the court did not remand her to a
residential treatment facility upstate. Instead, she was allowed to attend an outpatient program in the city, maintaining her enrollment in the methadone program.
But even with Carmen being closely monitored, Maria's ordeal was far from over.
Just as Carmen was being forced into supervised treatment, Celia was released
from jail and within a few days she was back selling crack on Melrose Street.

> I'll take my chances, even though they told me if they catch me selling again or doing
> anything wrong, they'll give me 5 years. I am out here on parole. Whatever you call it,

parole? On probation, you know what I mean. I have to go see my parole officer. I'll probably go see him tomorrow.

The experience of being in prison for the first time seemed to have little impact on Celia. It was no longer a place that frightened her and she never visited her parole officer. Completely detoxed when she came out, she immediately picked up where she had left off. Indeed, her heroin use grew and she began mainlining for the first time.

I had been skin popping before I went to Rikers. I still am. I'm not sure when I began. It was around when the summer started ending. I started to learn how to shoot up and do it my own self. You know I couldn't do it on my own. Now I am beginning to be hooked on it. I clearly got hooked on it. Lately I've been mainlining it. By mainlining you feel it more, more faster and it gets to your head real quick. By skin popping it, it takes you a long while to feel the highness, that's why I started to mainline. My brother was the first to hit me that way. He showed me how to do it. He's been doing it for a long time, since he was 16.

In early August 1991, Maria's house burned down. She later reported that Carmen had nodded asleep in bed with a cigarette in her hand and blamed the methadone (see Chapter 3 for an account of what happened to the house after the fire). But while the house was severely damaged by the fire, the garage in front went unscathed. Within days after the fire, Celia began to explore the garage as a spot where she could live, work (selling crack for the white tops organization on the corner), and make money or drugs by charging people to use the premises. Because of her relationship to Maria, no one contested her claim to the garage when it became obvious that this was evolving into a spot where people could go and use drugs.

I took over the place; now people pay me anytime they go in there. To use the place they either give me half a bottle of crack or give me half of their dope, or they give it to the others, you know, like that, whatever works. If they're going to shoot up, they bring their own works, but I've got the cookers there. A lot of people are coming there.

By December, Celia's garage had become a "hot" location because it was one of the only sheltered locations in the neighborhood. At first, because the block had a reputation for crack sales and use, crack users dominated the garage. Even though Celia was mainlining by this time, she kept scant injection equipment on the premises. Crack was still her drug of choice and she made no attempt to influence injection routines in the garage. Because it was primarily a crack-smoking and -selling site, needle exchange volunteers nervously avoided the area and AIDS outreach workers left fewer bleach kits there than at other injection sites in the neighborhood. Because drug taking here was dominated by rapid-fire crack smokers, IDUs who also used the spot were invariably rushed in their preparations and many of them neglected to take adequate precautions before injecting. For example, Susan, a white sex worker who had recently arrived in the neighborhood, talked about using drugs in Celia's garage.

Yesterday I didn't buy anything all by myself. I would buy like a dope and somebody else would put the coke. I got high with Celia, the one that runs the garage on Melrose. That's a tough place to get high 'cause after you do the one and one, the crack's right outside. So you can't really get away from it. I spent a lot of money over here yesterday. I had a dope and a coke, and I asked her if she wanted to down so she gave me the money for it. She gave me the money for the coke. But it wasn't just the two of us, there were a bunch of other people in there too. Some people were smoking, some people were getting off. I had my own works all day because I bought a couple of sets. Celia had her own set too, but we used my cooker. Everybody came to my cooker. I hung out here a while, I went and bought nails and put nails on my hand, fake nails. And then I took them all off because they didn't look right. After that, I bought some hits and I smoked, and I don't know, hours just seem to go by. I kept coming up by there, but I never seemed to get off this block.

Despite the preponderance of unsafe injection practices that occurred there, within a month of opening, injectors began to flock there in large numbers. And the police were never far behind. Between the police and vindictive crack managers looking for wayward workers, the front and back doors to the garage were quickly demolished, the building mysteriously caught fire a few times, and the usable space steadily shrunk until the building was virtually reduced to rubble. Celia found herself back on the street by the time cold weather arrived.

In late 1992, Celia met Jose, a Puerto Rican IDU a few years older than herself, and moved to the Bronx with him for several months. Jose had injected for many years and Celia, who up to that point had been an occasional injector and skin popper, immediately found herself following his lead. When the two of them returned to Bushwick in early February 1993, Celia looked like she had been injecting for several years. Her arms and hands were covered with track marks and sores where she had been poked with needles. With no place of their own, they spent their entire time in the several makeshift shooting galleries that dotted the neighborhood during this period. Never having been taught proper injecting technique and shooting up under the most unsanitary of conditions, Celia quickly developed abscesses that she tried to ignore by injecting more drugs to dull the pain. She came into the storefront on one occasion to get injection supplies (cookers, cottons, etc.) and several staff members advised her to go to the emergency room to get her abscesses lanced by a doctor, advice she ignored until 2 days later when her limbs began to swell. Knowing that something was wrong, Jose finally called an ambulance to pick her up from one of the shacks near Flushing Avenue and Celia was taken to Woodhull Hospital. Two days later, her body swollen like a balloon, she died of sepsis. Maria, her mother-in-law, took on the grim task of making final arrangements for Celia. Her body was laid out at a local funeral home, but the only visitors were Maria and a few of her children and the ethnographer. Celia's younger son was brought to the funeral home, but he did not recognize the puffy body as his mother. Maria made the long ride with the body to a New Jersey cemetery.

Bruce

Bruce was a brooding Othello, a dark, pensive, intelligent man who always appeared to be thinking. Though hard on the surface, he was capable of great tenderness and he was close with several of the women who worked the sex stroll. He did not appear particularly friendly at first, but he had a dry wit and was widely respected for his no-nonsense approach to his relationships with other injectors in the neighborhood. Born in 1959, the eldest of three children, Bruce was raised in a stable household by his mother in the Flatbush section of Brooklyn. His father maintained contact with the family but lived in Philadelphia. A smart child, Bruce dropped out of Erasmus Hall in the 9th grade, but went on to earn a GED degree.

Like many young men in Flatbush in the early 1980s, Bruce was attracted by the fast money and glamour associated with cocaine. Working in a local bar, he sold $20 aluminum foil packets of powdered cocaine to patrons to supplement his income. By this time, he was married and had a daughter. The routines associated with being a successful drug dealer strained his marriage, so he and his wife separated. By then, he had been sniffing heroin for a couple years after being introduced to it in 1985 by older family members. The breakup of his family pushed him to plunge headlong into uncontrolled use via injection.

> Separation from my family was a real traumatic thing. It fucked me up. At one time I wanted to die and [injecting heroin] was a cowardly way of doing it. And things would get worse. I wanted to make her feel guilty. It was a stupid thing to do.
> I was socializing a lot. Trying to move with the crowd. I sniffed dope for 3 years before I mainlined it. Oh, that was one self-destruction thing. Me and my wife had broken up, so I went into that. It was a cowardly way of self-destruction. That's exactly why I did it. I'd had the opportunity to shoot drugs years and years and years ago [but never did]. [When I finally did it] it was a stupid thing. I was at my stepfather's place. His roommate was pushing drugs. I sorta forced him to do it, you know. He refused the first time. A couple days later I came and gave him an ultimatum: If he doesn't do it, I go up on the street and find someone to do it. It made it feel like sniffing was a waste all those years. I loved it. After that, I did it all the time, In the streets. Roof tops. At my stepfather's house. But I, you know, I'd hide it from him.

Bruce moved to the Bronx where he took up residence in a shooting gallery and discovered that he was able to make money by helping sex workers on the local stroll.

> I actually got into pimping without the heart of pimping. Women are just drawn to me, I don't know why. I'm not dressed like a pimp, and I'm not sexually involved with any of them. Nah, can't be. The minute you sleep with them, that's when you get nothing from them. I mean, that's the way I've always interpreted things. I find that to be true. These womens are looking for someone to take care of them.

By the late 1980s, as drug markets began to reconfigure throughout the city and the situation in the Bronx deteriorated for Bruce, he eventually found his way to Bushwick. At first, he came there just to buy dope, and he injected primarily in a shooting gallery run by Bootsie, a former sex worker from the Southside of Williamsburg who was visibly dying of AIDS.

> Bootsie was the proprietor of that place when I first came out here in 1989. It was filthy. Half-naked people begging. It was atrocious, man. I used to come from Manhattan where I was robbing people, come over here and cop, and then get back on the train and go back to Manhattan. I used to like commute six times a day over here. And as I got to know Bootsie I started getting to know other people by being here. I got to know who the snakes were, who the lowlifes were, you know.

As he became familiar with the scene in Bushwick, Bruce found opportunities to make money there, especially working with sex workers, so he quickly gave up pulling robberies in Manhattan to be closer to the heroin markets. He first made his mark by defending women who were regularly robbed of their money and drugs by local, Puerto Rican stickup boys. Bruce quickly gained a reputation on the street as someone who would defend women and other vulnerable drug users. Many tried to take advantage of him, but he was no pushover.

> I help the girls out. When they're sick, they come to me. When their deals don't go through, they come to me and say, "Bruce, I'm sick." And I gotta give them $15 outta my pocket. And they don't even appreciate that sometimes. No sex and violence from me. I don't wanna fuck them, just pay me my money back. And some of them abuse that. Sometimes to the point where I have to snatch my money from them. I don't have it easy. It's hard to be straight up about it, but I continue to keep my standards. Believe me, it's hard to be straight up in this game. The one thing I've got is my morals, the way I was raised. It's hard where I am.

Though Bruce was close to many sex workers, he was by no means a pimp and could not rely on them to sustain his habit. To make money he began selling syringes, buying drugs for outsiders, and by 1991, as he got known by local drug managers, selling drugs. But while selling drugs provided him with a steady source of income, he was in a precarious position, pinched between his employers and the police. Many local drug businesses preferred to employ Latinos in positions that required them to handle product and/or money, but in 1991, as police focused on Bushwick's blatant drug markets, race–ethnicity and/or nationality became far less important as a condition for lower-echelon employment in the local drug businesses.

> The owners would prefer to hire Dominican guys or Puerto Rican guys or something like that. In my case I think it's different because like I said I'm a part of the neighborhood now. I'm accepted. The street workers, the guys that actually pitch the stuff, those could be all kinds of different guys. But it's highly unlikely that a guy like myself could become a manager. They have something against anyone who uses drugs even though they sell it. It's very illogical; but that's the way they are.
>
> The owners of these crack and dope businesses were Dominicans. Basically I didn't like them. They didn't like me either. Their attitude. Their general attitude. They think they are better than the other minority groups around here, and they look down on people who use drugs and sell drugs. They don't see anything wrong with supplying it. They despise drug users even though that's what was putting bread on their table. It was very hypocritical. Not only did they despise them, they openly criticized them. They'd

say stuff like, "You crackhead, get away from me," like you got some kind of disease that they're going to catch by being in the same vicinity.

They have people that work blue bag [cocaine] that they don't even know where the hell they come from. They don't really care whose hand they put their product in as long as they can stand over them and watch them. A lot of times, guys who work for them are getting cheated. The managers charge them 5% off a bundle. Guys are workin' out there for like $10 off every $100 when they're supposed to get $20. It's dog eat dog. If it was up to some of the managers, they wouldn't hire anybody because of their greed. Until he sees two or three cops and then he says, "Hey Bruce, come here. You want to work?"

Knowing that drug businesses were taking advantage of them in an environment where most street-level operatives lasted for a brief period before being arrested, many workers like Bruce began to run off with their supplies to enjoy a moment of pleasure before the police or vindictive managers caught up with them. As the police waged a relentless war of attrition with drug organizations, the resulting tensions between workers and managers led to many nasty confrontations and violence.

They demand all their workers to stay in one spot on that corner. But I refuse to do that. I let them know that I've been in this game too long and that you might as well just turn yourself into the 83rd Precinct if you're gonna stand in one spot. They asked me to work because I know a lot of people, but also, at that time, nobody wanted to sell it cause they was too scared.

I got myself a broken left arm after I took it upon myself to slip off with their material, two bundles [of powered cocaine]. 100 bucks, really, it was no real money. I could have worked that off in 45 minutes. If they were to take everybody off and just let me sell for about a hour, I could have made that 100 bucks back. But I think they wanted to set a example. He [the manager] hit me with a baseball bat. This bat was like sitting there for days with my name on it. I knew they were after me, and I wasn't really worried. My drug habit kept me in the area like an asshole. I knew a beatin' was comin'. It was just a matter of time. I'm not gonna pay none of that shit back. You know this is payment enough—this broken arm. You know, for me to pay them a couple of hundred dollars, that means it's a broken arm for nothing. But I won't say that because it wouldn't be in my best interest.

In the summer of 1992, the local police presence was so heavy that many sellers, faced with almost certain arrest, refused to work, especially during daylight hours. Bruce had been working for several organizations desperate for workers when he ran off with one manager's bundles of cocaine. This immediately affected his relationship with other employers.

In the process of getting my arm broke, I was selling dope for these guys on Knickerbocker. Now this is strictly coincidence. When the blue bag managers caught me, I had two bundles of this guy's dope money. But in the process of gettin' my arm broken, I had to immediately disappear. So now I have these dope dealers down here thinking that I cut out with their dope. I'm walking around with a broken arm, and now I got these guys to deal with. They caught up to me about last week and they gave me a beatin' too. They all figure that I owe them money. I don't have to run anymore, but if they see me and I got money, they'll take it. They scared the shit out of me. They had took me around to this basement on Jefferson and pulled a .45 on me. They beat me, kicked me, and stomped me. I'm a hard nut to crack, ain't I? I guess the guy, he got pissed off because all the kicking and stomping and punching … I don't bleed 'cause I used to box. So after they didn't see me cry, he fuckin' must have got frustrated. So this guy gave him a ring. He put the ring on his finger. And he got one good shot and he cut me. After that, I guess he was satisfied.

When he wasn't selling drugs, Bruce continued to make money from a variety of other hustles. For example, when the underground syringe exchange program began operating on Jefferson Street, Bruce became a regular participant. At that time, the exchange marked the barrel of each syringe with red nail polish (an extremely time-consuming chore) and monitored which clients exchanged the same syringes given to them during previous visits. Bruce rarely returned the same needles. He sold most of his sterile syringes either on Troutman Street or, during the summer of 1992, in a makeshift shelter that he and Manuel, another IDU, erected as a shooting gallery. It was in an empty lot near the subway station to catch the heavy foot traffic in and out of the neighborhood. The police demolished this shooting gallery several times before finally burning the pile of debris from which it was repeatedly put together and fixing the fence that surrounded the lot. Prior to that, Bruce had primarily supported his habit on "tastes" from gallery customers; drug selling was still a sideline occupation. Once the gallery was gone, he had to rely more on drug selling to support his habit. The recipient of far fewer "tastes," he now chose to inject in private rather than public spots. Bruce began sneaking up to the roof of a local factory building across from the empty lot to inject. The building watchman allowed him to use the building and even provided him with a broom to clean up after himself. Bruce noted that "it's a nice warm building, but I won't take a lot of people around there. I keep it discreet."

In the fall of 1992, Bruce's luck finally ran out and he was arrested by under-cover police for selling drugs. Physically and psychologically worn down from 5 years on the street, Bruce was almost grateful for his "vacation paid for by the state" and "cold turkey" (abrupt, complete cessation of an addictive drug) withdrawal period while at Rikers Island. Though he drew a sentence of 3–6 years in prison, Bruce opted to participate in a "shock" program that lasted a mere 6 months. When he arrived at Summit Shock in upstate New York, Bruce was by far the oldest inmate there. In many letters, Bruce wrote that the boot camp regimen and hard manual labor was especially hard for older inmates who were not as resilient and were more set in their ways than their younger counterparts. But the rigors of the shock program did not appear to compromise his health, even though he was HIV positive and received minimal health care there. Allowed the oppor-tunity to reflect on his situation, Bruce wrote that he wanted to move back to his mother's house upon release and asked our assistance in finding a job. And though he did move back to his mother's house in the fall of 1993, he was there only a week before he was back in Bushwick permanently.

In 1993, Bruce returned to a much-changed urban terrain. The busiest heroin markets in the city had were now located in East Harlem, the South Bronx, and the

Lower East Side. There were still many heroin and cocaine sellers in Bushwick, but the markets were much more discreet, selling only to known customers. Since outside buyers were now a small percentage of the overall number of customers, there were far fewer opportunities for IDUs like Bruce to earn money or sustain a habit. Because transactions had moved indoors, on the few occasions when IDUs like Bruce were afforded the opportunity to sell drugs, they were much more exposed and vulnerable. A more reliable source of income for Bruce and others was copping drugs for users who could not buy for themselves because dealers would not sell to them or they were too afraid of being arrested.

With the only indoor shooting gallery in the neighborhood on hotly contested ground, Bruce took up residence in "the dumpsters," two blocks from the major heroin copping spots. About a dozen steel, covered bins (dumpsters) were parked in a dirt lot behind a newly opened tortilla factory. The dumpsters appeared to be used primarily for paper refuse, so they remained relatively clean. And because they had a roof and a door, they were well-suited to serve a variety of needs for drug users. A convenient place to smoke crack or inject drugs, they became a popular meeting spot for users looking to share drugs—"do an angle"—with others. The dumpsters were also ideal for drug buyers who drove into the neighborhood to meet up with someone who could procure for them. Located in a no-man's land between police precincts, buyers in cars could park at the curb and call out from the window of their car to users inside the dumpsters. Several IDUs, including Bruce, had moved into the dumpsters to take advantage of the many buyers who were eager to pay for their services.

Scarcely 6 months after moving into the dumpsters, Bruce was arrested while making a run for a customer. This time he spent a year in Rikers Island, withdrawing from drugs cold turkey when he got there. While serving his sentence, Bruce learned that an uncle in Philadelphia had died and left him a modest inheritance. Like his previous stay at Summit Shock, Bruce vowed to stay straight and get a job upon release, and this time he had a nest egg to support his efforts to do so. But suspecting that he would be unable to honor his commitment and would instead spend the entire amount on drugs, he put the bulk of the money under his mother's control (so as to protect his daughter's interests), limiting his own ability to spend the money foolishly. Not surprisingly, upon release from Rikers Island in early 1995, Bruce quickly found himself shooting drugs in Bushwick and he enjoyed several months before the smaller share of the money that he had set aside for himself was gone and he had to begin "hustling" again.

Throughout the rest of 1995 and early 1996, Bruce used several outdoor locations to inject, including the dumpsters. Though his resolve to "go straight" dissipated quickly, he seemed eager to avoid selling drugs again.

I did my time for selling. I am not going to jail again. No, not me, I know that. They probably would hire me again and I probably wouldn't even have to ask to work.

> They're kind of in need of warm bodies. Sellers don't last too long out there. I'd give
> them about 2 weeks before they're arrested.

Bruce's primary hustle remained procuring drugs for others and he built a fairly stable clientele of 12–15 injectors. In February 1996, Bruce opened a shooting gallery in an abandoned brick building on the edge of a local park, outside the window of the police antidrug trailer that served as their mobile command post in the neighborhood. Despite its location, the gallery became a magnet for injectors, especially outsiders who needed help in getting drugs. Bruce's habit ballooned to more than 15 bags of heroin a day. The police made repeated visits to the gallery and arrested many people, but they were unable to close it for very long. But as police attention began to decrease the number of customers coming into the neighborhood, Bruce began selling heroin inside the gallery to compensate for the loss of business as a market intermediary. In February 1997, the building burned and took two adjacent ones with it. Bruce was back on the street.

Jerry

Jerry was a magnificent liar and everyone knew it. The problem was that mixed in with the lies was an amazing rags-to-riches-to-rags story. As a white injector who spent most of his time hanging out in Bushwick, he was at a great disadvantage. Even dressed in tattered clothing, he stood out from the crowd of shabbily dressed injectors. His high visibility made him largely ineligible for even the most demeaning work in the drug trade. Dealers sometimes refused to sell him drugs since he was so easily spotted by the police. But despite all these disadvantages, Jerry persisted, and his unwillingness to back down earned him considerable respect among his peers.

Because of his widely known reputation as a prevaricator, it is difficult to be confident about Jerry's account of his past, but interviews and conversations with him between 1991 and 1997 included many cross-checks of internal consistency and he held up remarkably well. And just when some stories seemed too fantastic to be believed, other IDUs occasionally and unwittingly verified his accounts during their own interviews. But still, it was hard to know when Jerry was telling the truth or taking us for a ride. For example, when he was first interviewed in 1992, Jerry told us that he was 37 years old. In a 1996 interview, he said that he was 44. We were unable to check the accuracy of the story he told of growing up in Queens and his early adulthood, but even if it was not the entire truth, it nevertheless spoke volumes to his current mindset on the streets of Bushwick.

> I was born and raised in Queens, New York. I lived there until I got married in my early
> 30s. I grew up in a middle-class to upper-class mostly white neighborhood. Counting
> me, there were three kids in our family. I was the youngest. I did good in school and
> graduated a year early. For elementary school, I went to Holy Family. I was always
> picked on [by the nuns] for no reason. Once, the nun asked my father to scold me and

gave him an example of how she would do it. She grabbed me by the sideburns, pulled my sideburns, and slapped me in the face in front of my father. I looked at my father's eyes, and he made a gesture. From that day I didn't really hate my father, but I hated that he stood there. I wanted him to hit me instead. I was 7 years old and in the second grade. In third grade I was always getting 100 on the math. I was very good in math. The teacher thought I was copying, so she put me in the first seat, the fourth or fifth row. I got 100 on that test, and I was the only one in the class to get 100.

I went to NYU in premed. Before that, I took a year of computer technology at Queensboro. I graduated with a degree in radiology. Then, I went to Cornell on 73rd and York. Eventually, I went to work at Bellevue and later I worked at New York Hospital. In the beginning, I enjoyed working there. I had a lot of business sense, and I wanted to run my own business. I thought of ways of incorporating, but it was truly risky to have a partner that was a radiologist. You got to have contracts with health-related facilities and nursing homes. You have to have portable machines.

When I left that job and went into my own business I failed twice. The first time I made it, I made it really big real fast. It skyrocketed. I published a manual. I didn't publish it, McGraw-Hill did, a manual, *The Art of Mail Order*. I made it real good. It took off like a skyrocket. I remember going there my first day. It was a Wednesday. I went home to get my little post office box. I had the cheapest one because I couldn't afford anything else. There was a little note inside, "please see clerk." There were three or four boxes with mail, the ones with the handles on the sides. There were two rows of envelopes. Each box had two long rows.

My first success was with people ordering merchandise that I put for sale in the *TV Guide*. I picked *TV Guide* because I figured people would hold onto it for a whole week. They're always going through it. Every time there is a commercial on TV, they might pick it up. The farther back in the *TV Guide* you are, the better off you are. I advertised full-page ads. I couldn't afford their national issue which is 108 issues. That's how many they have. So I picked the cheapest one which was Greensboro, North Carolina. A subscription of 300 people. It cost me $300 to advertise in all of them for one week for black and white four pages. New York is $7,500 just for New York. So anyway that's why I took off like that. I was selling those cheap, inexpensive digital watches called Chicklets. It had a real leather band. I got them for 75 cents in Hong Kong and sold them for $1.99 plus 50 cents shipping and handling. I made money on the shipping and handling. The thing is, I put shipping and handling. You've got to make sure you put that word handling in there. If you didn't, you were guilty of mail fraud and you could go to jail. Thirty-seven cents it cost me to ship. So I made 13 cents on the postage, legally, because I put handling in.

According to Jerry, his meteoric success in the mail order business made him a millionaire almost overnight. He and his wife started several other businesses and bought a large house in Long Island. (Several IDUs in Bushwick later told us that they had once visited his Long Island home, where his wife still lived, when they went there to retrieve some electronic items—TVs and VCRs—that he resold in Bushwick so they could buy more drugs.) Before becoming successful, Jerry claimed that he never used drugs.

I didn't smoke any pot at high school. I only smoked in high school parties and stuff. I was married and we had just bought a house in Long Island. I started with freebasing [cocaine smoking]. I ran into an old friend one day and they had some. I did base for about 6 months before I tried heroin. At first, I was doing drugs in the garage. My wife didn't know; I did it by myself. The base got me too wired up. I wanted something to bring me down a bit. The first time I used heroin, I smoked it. I first injected about 3½ or 4 years ago [around 1990] at a friend's house in Huntington, Long Island. It was their dope, but my works. I had lots of them. One of the requirements of being a radiologist is identifying all the gauges and kinds of syringes. In the beginning, hitting myself was a little bit uncomfortable, but I quickly got the hang of it. In the beginning it was like twice a day. Then it went to four to six times. Eventually, I was doing four bags, five bags at one time. Now, I only do one at a time; financial reasons. I inject about 8 bags a day now, but I use almost exclusively speedball. I never shoot dope by itself unless I don't have money and I'm dope sick.

I originally came to Bushwick through people that I met out in Long Island where I grew up. They knew about this place, and we came together one time. Little by little I found myself here more and more. I foresaw the disaster coming. Everything of wealth I sold. There were a few things that I refused to sell like my jewelry, which a lot of it was hand-me-downs from people that I love. I had such bad luck; instead of selling it, I went to a pawn shop and pawned it for 6 months, eventually losing it all.

When we first met Jerry he had already exhausted all the available resources from his previous life and he was trying to develop a niche in the Bushwick scene. As a white injector without street-hustling experience he was fortunate that the *Daily News* went on strike and replacement workers were hired to sell the newspapers on the street and in the subways. Jerry claimed that during this brief period he was able to make about $150 a day selling the newspaper near the subway entrance. When the strike ended, he continued selling the *Daily News* for a few weeks, eventually selling them on the L train rather than at the entrance. Even though supplies of the *Daily News* eventually dried up, Jerry discovered his niche: a fairly lucrative and reliable source of cash selling newspapers on the subway, usually local papers that were free on the news stand.

To support myself, I sell newspapers on the subway. It all started when I ran into the owner of a newspaper, a publication in the city. I get these newspapers that are marked $1 each. I incorporated a little speech, and I sell them. People hit me off with anywhere from a $1 and some people $5, you know, for the homeless. I usually make about $150 for 4 hours of work. I'm a nonprofit organization for the homeless. No problem, I spend it all. When I'm done, I've got no money.

Selling newspapers on the subway was convenient for Jerry since the trains were no person's exclusive territory and his whiteness did not work against him as it did in Bushwick where his obviousness made him a poor candidate to be a drug seller, lookout, or even a market intermediary for outsiders who could not make their own purchases. But even once he found a way to make money and survive, Jerry often had a more difficult time on the streets than other injectors. His situation was further undermined by his bizarre reaction every time he injected a speedball. He would immediately freeze up like he was having a grand mal seizure, twitching and unable to speak for about 10 minutes. This behavior made him an object of ridicule among other IDUs. Louie called him "space base." On one occasion, after

Pat "hit" Jerry in the neck with a speedball while in the back seat of a car, she became annoyed with his convulsing and started yelling at him to "stop faking it." When he persisted, she opened the car door, yanked him into the street where he lay jerking back and forth in a fetal position, and instructed the driver to speed away.

Jerry's situation in the neighborhood grew worse when the police began stepping up their war on drugs during the summer of 1992. Determined to regain control of the streets, they began to hassle many drug users, especially the more obvious ones like Jerry.

> The policing of the area has gotten a lot more thorough. It's like they're using this area as some kind of testing ground, I don't know; but they're determined to clean it up; and they're not leaving one stone unturned—if you're white especially. If you're white, you're automatically a candidate to be pulled over and shook down because in their view you have no business being in the area; and if you can't show any local address, they make you clean out your pockets and everything. The cops think I don't belong in the neighborhood and they sometimes make me leave. And I've gotten beat up a few times by police in the street.

Because Jerry was, in some ways, in a more precarious position than other drug users in the neighborhood, he often made an extra effort to curry favor with other IDUs, hoping they would take care of him on those occasion when he was "sick." Though he denied consciously attempting to build up "markers" that could be called in at a later date, his behavior suggested otherwise.

> I got blisters on my feet from walking in the rain, so I can't walk too good. So I'm very slow. I can hand my money over to Gus, he'll run up and go cop for me and bring it back. There's not many people that you can trust with money. He's not one who looks out for other people. But what I've done was, I showed him something. I look out for him like in the morning right after I do my newspapers. He's still sleeping when I come back. I give him some cookies and a drink. I call it the Gandhi syndrome. I overload him with a little bit of friendship, doing things for him and not asking anything in return. And all of a sudden, I started getting these things in return like, out of the blue, he bought me a drink. And out of the blue bought me something to eat. He gave me a set of works or something. Totally against his nature, because he's a businessman on the street. People say he's cheap, but he's just a little cunning, that's all. I look at it this way: if I turn somebody on or I give somebody a gift, it's not because I want it returned, it's because I'm doing it for them. So if I get something in return fine and dandy, but I'm not asking for anything.

Curiously, even though Jerry was in many ways more dependent on other IDUs—and one might guess that this made him more vulnerable to sharing drugs as the second partner in a dyad—he never admitted to sharing drugs in a risky fashion nor was he ever observed doing so. Despite a shabby appearance that made it seem like he did not care about his health or well-being, Jerry told a very different story.

> I don't share nothing with anybody. I'll let them share from me, but I won't share with them. I will not take anything from anybody's works or anybody's cooker. I will not borrow anybody's water, I will not borrow anybody's cooker. I won't do any of that shit.

I went to school for radiology, so I know a little bit about … you don't even have to go to school for radiology. You don't even have to go to school period. All you have to do is have common sense and intelligence to realize. I don't want to get AIDS, that's why! I rarely get to use bleach. I've got two cookers, three cookers. I got one for myself in case I have to do something, and I always carry a backup, because if somebody needs one and they don't have it, they'll fight with me because I won't give them mine.

Jerry was something of a hypochondriac, always complaining of some ailment or another. In early 1992, he told people that he had terminal colon cancer. Three years later, still alive and apparently well, the story changed to another disease. He never complained about HIV, but even though he denied sharing drugs in a risky fashion, few were willing to believe that he did not have the virus. Still, more than any other IDU in the area, Jerry was a loyal patron of the syringe exchange, often trading in more than 50 sets at once.

I try to go to the exchange on Putnam [Avenue] to get my works, or I buy them from people, diabetics that sell them. There are a lot of diabetics in the neighborhood. They need that money. So they'll sell them, and you've got the exchange twice a week. So if you bothered to work at it and go to the exchange, you're going to get them for nothing. But a lot of people don't think that far in advance. Sometimes I'll exchange several dozen.

Of course, Jerry did not use all the clean needles himself, and many of them were sold on the street or in local galleries. It was hard to know how many of the sterile syringes Jerry actually used himself. And he was always rather cagey about his HIV status. In an environment where most IDUs were upfront about having the virus, Jerry neither confirmed or denied. He usually claimed not to really know, but offered that he had tested negative several times. For someone who claimed to be afflicted with other terminal ailments (like colon cancer) it seemed odd that he would not admit to one that so many of his "associates" did.

Unlike many of the other IDUs who the project followed over the last 6 years, Jerry was remarkably consistent in many ways. He did not follow the familiar pattern of moving between jail, detox, and the streets that characterized so many other Bushwick IDUs. Except for short stays in the precinct lockup or central booking, Jerry was a constant presence on the streets. Always in trouble with someone, he often fought with other IDUs and took beatings from local dealers. On one occasion in 1996, Jerry was whacked on the arm by Dominican heroin dealers who he had shortchanged in a business deal. After telling us that his arm was broken, he refused a ride to the hospital because he would inevitably get "dope sick" and he feared that more than the throb in his forearm, a pain he thought might disappear if he could use enough dope.

Unlike many other IDUs, Jerry rarely talked about detoxing, seemingly willing to push his habit up at every opportunity. Where other IDUs sometimes used detox as a respite from the streets and/or a way to whittle down large habits, Jerry seldom opted for treatment.

The first time I went in [to detox at Beth Israel Hospital] was because of medical reasons. I got stabbed by these two black twins. They were prostitutes. Then I detoxed again at Beth Israel, and that's when I realized there is only one way to really, really lick it and that is to detox and not come back into the street. Go into your second half of the detox, detoxing the mind! Detoxing the body is just one thing. Physical is nothing compared to the mental.

Jerry was not ready to detox, physically or mentally. He liked shooting speedballs too much to stop. Dope sick half of the time, he was in for the long haul. When seen in March 1997, he was selling free newspapers on the L subway line. He revealed that recently he had been released from Beth Israel where he was diagnosed with endocarditis. He worried about the long-term antibiotic therapy needed to combat the condition, but happily, in one hand, he gripped a slip of paper which said that he had tested negative for HIV.

After his last stay in the hospital, Jerry's health never improved. Lethargic much of the time, Jerry often could be seen sleeping on a bench in the subway station or slumped in a chair in one of the local shooting galleries. Unable to hustle as he once had, Jerry found himself suffering from withdrawal pains much of the time. By the second week of December 1997, Jerry had developed several serious health problems. One day he was semi-comatose inside Bruce's gallery and the other injectors called the ambulance to come and get him. Jerry never fully regained consciousness in Wyckoff Heights Medical Center where he was placed in intensive care. In addition to his heart problems, Jerry experienced complete kidney failure. When the ethnographer visited him, Jerry's eyes rolled around as if he was aware someone was with him, but, bristling with tubes and hooked up to several machines, Jerry never woke up. When the ethnographer pulled the sheet back to look at his legs, both of Jerry's feet were coal black: gangrene had set in. The fact that the doctors had not amputated his feet immediately told the ethnographer that they did not expect Jerry to leave the hospital. On December 18th, he died in the hospital. No one came to claim the body. Aside from the questions asked the ethnographers by a few IDUs who were curious about what had happened, it seemed almost as if he had never existed.

Louie

Louie was a muscular Puerto Rican IDU who grew up in Bushwick. He had a variety of hustles, but his primary occupation was running shooting galleries. He had several of them over the duration of the project. Hardworking, he was one of the most widely known IDUs in the neighborhood despite a glaring lack of interpersonal skills. By all accounts, Louie had an unremarkable childhood in a stable family with both parents present.

By the time we met Louie, at age 31, he had been injecting for 11 years. He was almost completely estranged from his four brothers and four sisters. Both parents had died and only a sister who lived in East New York maintained any contact with him. Louie's path away from the security of family and friends began as a teenager. Two older brothers had "shot dope" when he was quite young, but he said that they had very little to do with his later involvement with the drug. But Louie disliked school.

> I went to P. S. 25, Junior High School 57, and Boys High. But I never liked school, so I was always out. All we used to do is go to homeroom or official class and just cut out and go to Highland Park and play wink, 7 minutes in heaven, and other games. We'd also be drinkin' beer, smokin' reefer, you know. We weren't using any hard dope then. I made it to the 11th grade before I called it quits. After that, I lived at my Mom's house for a couple of years. My parents didn't really pressure me to get a job. They kind of accepted that I didn't like school.

Louie wanted to be a "family man" and lived at home while he tried to make it in the world of work. But never having learned to read, Louie was at a distinct disadvantage in a depressed job market; and after dropping out of school, he took a series of menial jobs.

> Soon after that, I got married—common law. She was a virgin and 16. I was 18. She was livin' with me in my mother's house. I started workin' at Super Notion on 34th Street as a messenger, but I only worked there for a few months. I had a daughter with my wife. She's now 12 years old. The last time I saw her, she was 3 months old.

Frustrated by his inability to make money or find a better job, and missing the freedom and attention he received as a teenager with multiple girlfriends, Louie began spending more time hanging out in Bushwick where the lure of the drug business enabled him to earn money and chase the ladies. But his involvement with drugs had begun several years before he started hanging out everyday.

> Back when I was cutting school, I used to trip on acid mostly every day. We used to buy it on Putnam from a Spanish female. It was blotter acid: Snoopy and Mickey Mouse on paper. Back then I liked it.
> I first tried dope in 1980. I was in a friend's house, and he told me, "You want to try this?" and I said, "Yeah." So, he hit me with dope and I liked it. That friend is dead now. He died of AIDS. I never really sniffed dope. I hate that taste. But after about 10 or 12 years I just learned how to hit myself last year. I used to get homies to hit me. In return, I'd give them a taste.

After his initiation into injecting heroin, Louie quickly developed a taste for speedball and stopped using other drugs. He dabbled in selling drugs, but because of his habit he found it difficult to make money or advance in the business. As a stickup man he was not much better, and by the early 1980s was doing time in Sing Sing for armed robbery. While in Sing Sing, Louie continued to use heroin but complained that a "jailhouse bag" was not only twice as expensive but half the size of what he was buying on the street. Sing Sing also introduced Louie to body building, and by the time he was released, he described himself as being "big as a house." Released from prison in the late 1980s, Louie returned to Bushwick where he quickly regained his speedball habit and became a well-known figure among

IDUs, dealers, and police. To finance his substantial habit Louie had several hustles.

> To make money I either sell works or help the dealers, look out for them when they're selling dope, look out for the cops. Plus I've got a lot of friends, a lot of white guys. They come lookin' for me when they want to cop. And they give me a bag, or they give me a nice taste or a couple of dollars. I've sold coke, but not dope. I can't take that chance 'cause I'm gonna leave with it. I might get tempted. I might step off with it.

Though Louie had a variety of hustles, his reputation was made as the operator of shooting galleries. Once police began cracking down on outdoor drug consumption in 1991, Louie's galleries were among the busiest places in the neighborhood.

> With all these cops around, it's a lot harder to get off in the streets now. Now, they're going to [my gallery in] the tire shop. Yesterday, for example, there were about 25 or 30 guys in there at once. Last year, we were getting high right there on Troutman. Now it's hard to do that. We used to get high right there in the public in front of anybody. But now we're going down to the tire shop. Now, you got a lot of people that never been there 'cause you can't do it on Troutman no more. When you go into that garage, people are doggin' you for a taste.

The pressure to share drugs in these places was considerable. Sharing drugs in these contexts could mean any (or all) of several things, including physically splitting the powder before cooking, sharing syringes, cotton, cookers and syringe-mediated drug sharing, which is often called "backloading" [see Jose et al. (1993) and Grund et al. (1996), for a complete description of this process]. Louie describes his preferred method of sharing drugs:

> To give someone a taste, I'd first put a 40 in a one and one. It's gonna grow because of the coke. We're gonna heat it up. It's gonna go up to about a 50. I probably give them a 20 and I take a 30, you know. I'd squirt the 20 into his works.

When the tire shop opened in early 1991, located three blocks from the major buying areas, it was the only public "taste" gallery in the area. By public taste gallery, we mean it was a place where virtually anyone could gain entry by giving a "taste" of drugs to an "owner." It was operated by Louie and Gus, another Puerto Rican IDU in his mid-30s. They disliked each other, but the business was lucrative and allowed each of them to inject more than 30 times a day. So many people came to the tire shop that many injectors preferred to stay out of this gallery for fear of being robbed (and several reported that they had been) or because they didn't want to share their drugs with other injectors who hung out there. As a result, the spacious yard behind the tire shop also became a popular injection spot and there were many shacks hastily erected that served IDUs who wanted to avoid going into the gallery.

The tire shop was notorious both for the number of IDUs who used it and also for being a place where uncontrolled injection behaviors took place. Until summer 1991, when AIDS outreach workers began to visit the tire shop to educate IDUs and deliver bleach kits and condoms, with the exception of refusing to share drugs with others, virtually no harm reduction techniques were observed being used by injectors there. Pope (another local IDU discussed several times in this volume) describes how careless injection behaviors were inside the tire shop:

> I take care of business as far as cleaning my works and all that stuff, but a lot of the people that were coming in there were disgusting. I tell you, the cookers are so filthy and people don't bother to wash them out before they use them. They'll just leave all that cut in it, and add more stuff to it. And many of them share works too. There's a lot of people that has AIDS or the virus and lend works and do not say anything. That is very fucked up.

Louie and Gus were among the worst offenders in this regard. They were often observed practicing hazardous injection routines: sharing cookers, water, backloading, and occasionally using syringes whose sterility was highly suspect. Louie bragged on several occasions that he would inject more than 25 times per day inside the gallery and on several occasions professed not to care about his or anyone else's HIV status.

> I was in the tire shop most of the day yesterday, from like 10 [AM] to 10 [PM] or 10 to 11. When I first went in, there was like 15 guys in there. Later, 30 or 35 showed up, in one room, in another room, in another room. I be getting off like crazy man with all kinds of guys, black, white, Spanish. Any of them. I know them all. I have a hell of a habit. Shit, I shot a storm man. I was gettin' busy yesterday. I'm telling you. I shot up 20 or 30 times or something and every time was in the garage. Not one of those times was by myself, I was always getting tastes. Everybody goes to the garage. There's no other place in the neighborhood to go that I can think of. The garage is like Grand Central Station. It's like that. Everybody goes in there to get high.

Ultimately, the tire shop became a victim of its own "success." Reviled by many IDUs for the "wild west" reputation that it undoubtedly deserved, on some days business was too slow to sustain the habits of those IDUs who had come to rely on the "tastes" they got there.

> I was sick this morning, so Gus gave me a taste. He gave me like a 20, which he left in his cooker. It didn't really get me straight, but it took the edge off. Then I met this other guy, a black guy named Manuel. He gave me a taste 'cause I hit him in the neck. He gave me a 20, too. I always got to hit him first. I had hit Gus in the neck too. After that, I was chillin' for a while. A couple of people came, but they kept comin' with coke, coke. I stayed there the whole day. People were lookin' out for me: "Here's some coke, yo. You got a cooker? You got the works? You got a piece of cotton?" In all, I was given coke about eight or ten times over the day.

As the biggest magnet for injectors in the neighborhood, the tire shop became a familiar stopover for police, emergency medical technicians, and AIDS outreach workers. It lasted for about a year before it was finally closed down with great difficulty by the police and the landlord, who threatened to shoot any trespassers found on his property. For a few weeks after the tire shop closed, many IDUs continued to crowd into its back yard to inject, but it proved to be a temporary and largely unsatisfactory solution.

Within a week of being displaced from the tire shop, in mid-October 1991, Louie and Gus found a storage lot next to a factory building where piles of wooden pallets provided them with ample building materials. Thrown together with wood, nails, rope, and plastic sheeting, their new gallery was clearly not as sturdy as the brick and mortar of the tire shop, but as shacks went, it looked fairly sturdy. Once it was built along the east wall of the factory, the new gallery was not as spacious as their previous digs (5–6 people was its capacity) and it lacked the kind of protections afforded by the first and caught on fire twice before it was closed. The shack forced IDUs who went there into such close proximity that it was virtually impossible to avoid sharing drugs with others, and without a regular supply of bleach kits and other harm reduction materials, high-risk injection practices were commonplace. Even though it was somewhat closer to the major drug selling blocks than the tire shop and therefore was more accessible to IDUs, the shack was not nearly as "successful" as its predecessor.

Within a month of constructing the gallery, several IDUs broke through a brick wall to the factory, which they discovered was actually a storage facility for a lamp wholesaler. For the next several days, before the hole in the wall was discovered by employees, hundred of lamps were sold on the streets of Bushwick. The police came immediately upon notification, and after two IDUs were arrested, the gallery was demolished, the yard was cleaned of debris, and a sturdy fence with a locked gate and topped with razor ribbon was quickly erected. For the next few weeks there were no large public galleries in the neighborhood and despite a heavy police presence many IDUs used the streets to inject. John, another local IDU, lamented the gallery closing and talked about how difficult the scene had become for many IDUs.

> Since the tire shop closed, some of the customers have been injecting outside the building in the back there by the corner. Then some people go by the gasoline station on Flushing where all the pallets are stacked up. But that got burned out two times already. There's no new places, so people are goin' back to the street like to Jefferson [Street] by the factory. The cops have been around hassling people but not me. I happen to be unfortunate not to have no money to be bothered. Since the galleries have closed I haven't been able to make money. Nothing.

In finding the lamp factory location, Louie and Gus were more fortunate than Pope, who after being evicted from the tire shop spent the next few months injecting primarily in the streets. The clientele of careful injectors (which Pope had cultivated in his minigallery; see Chapter 3) were reluctant to go into Louie and Gus's shack, and they too spent the winter injecting in public venues. Over the duration of the winter there were several public locations where core network members could go when they wanted to inject, including the subway station and the park bathroom (mostly for women). Less accessible to many IDUs were two crack houses (Chantel's and Pop's) where injectors were tolerated as long as long as they did their business somewhat discreetly and the owner of the apartment was paid in crack. Missy and Earl, both African Americans, had apartments in the area where IDUs who were close friends, who were capable of respecting the place as a living space, and who were willing to share their drugs could find a place to inject. But these places and several others like them never drew much of a crowd. During this winter, secure and warm indoor spots remained at a premium and many core network members, like Bruce, who used the tops of stairwells in nearby factory buildings, kept good spots to themselves.

As was discussed above in Celia's story, in early August 1991, a house burned down on a major crack selling street in Bushwick. The house remained virtually inaccessible to anyone until the spring thaw. In March, the partially burned house at the back of the lot, a place that had looked entirely inhospitable during the winter when it was frozen over with visible ice, began to attract the attention of Louie and his new girlfriend, Carmen, who were eager to get another large gallery going. After being displaced from their gallery on the side of the lamp factory just when the weather was getting cold, Louie and Gus's fragile partnership quickly dissolved, and they both spent the winter making money from a wide variety of hustles and injecting in most of the places scattered around the neighborhood, including Celia's garage. When the cold weather began to moderate, Louie was one of the first IDUs to venture into the burned out old house with the intention of finding a space that might be transformed into a new gallery. He and Carmen spent several days cleaning out a bedroom on the second floor of the house, throwing all the waterlogged and/or burned refuse either out the windows or into adjacent rooms. At first, conditions were very crude in their gallery as Louie notes:

> We don't have many supplies in the house 'cause it's really all messed up. You see we haven't cleaned it. But we got a couple of [bleach] kits stashed around, you know. Mostly everybody comes with their own water, their own shit, you know.

Despite these drawbacks and the lack of many amenities desired by IDUs, by spring 1992, Louie and Carmen's gallery was the busiest spot in the neighborhood, but it was not until they had been in operation for several months that the gallery began to be visited by AIDS outreach workers and injection events began to develop a noticeable routine. By summer 1992, at least 50 bleach kits a week were being dropped off by outreach workers and syringe exchange took place there each Wednesday evening. But supplies of injection equipment could not keep pace with demand, and to make the bleach kits last until the next delivery they were kept in a plastic milk crate and stuck under the bed, out of public view. Even though safe injection practices were not strongly advocated by Louie, Carmen, or many of the core network members who injected there, many visitors asked for bleach kits and used them to clean their injection equipment.

The summer of 1992 was the peak of the supermarket period in Bushwick and injectors from throughout the New York metropolitan area came to the neighborhood in unprecedented numbers. Louie and Carmen's shooting gallery quickly became the busiest place in the neighborhood, especially early in the morning when IDUs with jobs would crowd into the gallery for their "wake up" before going to work and after 5 PM on their way home from work. The gallery also attracted the attention of the police. Louie talks about one encounter with patrol officers from an adjacent precinct.

> Yesterday, a fuckin' cop went in the gallery. I don't know this guy. He's from the 90th Precinct. I was ready for him. He hit me with his stick, but I didn't really feel it. When he went in he asked me, "What you doin' in there?" I said, "I just finished getting high." I've got works on me and cooker and water and everything. He just said, "Stay out of here." He grabbed me and hit me with the stick. I was waiting for it. After he left, I went back in.

In early August 1992, after repeated visits from the police who were frustrated by their unsuccessful attempts to close it down and officials from the Departments of Sanitation and of Housing Preservation and Development who "evaluated" the property for demolition, Louie and Carmen's gallery was burned down under somewhat mysterious conditions. Louie claimed that the police, who had become tired of visiting the house, burned it down early one morning. When he went to the local police precinct to complain, he was arrested for violating the conditions of his parole and spent the next 9 months in Rikers Island. Carmen, who was 7 months pregnant, had a premature baby weighing 3 pounds and 10 ounces. The baby was taken by child welfare workers, but was placed with Carmen's brother and his family. Carmen was referred to a drug detox program through the SFHR project and subsequently to a residential drug treatment facility where she lived for the next 18 months. IDUs who had come to rely on the house were now left to search for another location, and for many of them, the winter of 1992 left them with frightfully few options.

With police cracking down on drugs in the neighborhood, the visitors' waiting room at Rikers Island resembled a Bushwick block party. Like many young Latinos in jail during this year, Louie joined the Latin Kings. As someone with experience in prison, he quickly rose to leadership—"crown"—positions in the various buildings he lived in while on the Island. Membership in the Latin Kings was not about joining a gang to better pursue criminal enterprise, it was about personal transformation and improving the welfare of the Latino community. To many, including Louie, this was a laudable goal. But for Louie, the Latin Kings' renunciation of drugs—especially injecting—proved to be too much for him to comply with, especially once he was released from jail the next summer. Once out of Rikers Island, he briefly moved in with a Latin Queen he had met through jail contacts, but within one week he was shooting speedballs in Bushwick and found himself robbing her apartment for redeemable electronic equipment.

When Louie returned to the neighborhood, he attempted to wedge his way into an apartment shooting gallery that was run by several IDUs. When he could not force his way into a controlling position within the apartment, he erected a small shack in a yard enclosed by cinder block walls and began attracting IDUs who had grown tired of all the fighting at the apartment and/or were tired of being pressured to share their drugs with so many other IDUs. But as bad as the apartment had become, the yard was worse in many ways. No one person consistently controlled this spot; whoever happened to be there at the moment often assumed the role of "proprietor" and demanded tastes from visitors. Because it was outside and exposed to the elements, IDUs were not encouraged to inject at a leisurely pace and they often rushed to complete their business. Once AIDS outreach workers realized that a gallery was forming at that location, they began to deliver bleach kits, but given the instability that characterized the yard, materials often disappeared within an hour, leaving no harm reduction materials there for days at a time.

Forced out of the apartment gallery and unable to sufficiently control the yard, Louie took up residence in what was to become the hottest injection spot in the neighborhood for the next 3 years: the dumpsters. The dumpsters were located in a large lot behind a tortilla factory. The symbolism of shooting galleries located in garbage bins was lost on no one and it was hardly surprising that the dumpsters and harm reduction did not mesh well. In some ways, because they were more susceptible to being taken over by particular people or groups, they represented an incremental improvement over the almost total chaos found in the yard, but there were several sources of pressure that mitigated against safe injection practices being regularly employed by IDUs in the dumpsters. Even though the dumpsters were visited regularly by AIDS outreach workers and needle exchange volunteers, the turnover of IDUs in them was such that there was no regularity in people or behavior. And because there were several dumpsters from which IDUs could pick and choose, constant fragmentation occurred among the IDUs who went there. Police actions also fragmented groups in the dumpsters.

Louie controlled one of the dumpsters for himself and his many customers found it convenient to simply drive up to the curb and yell his name. Louie would come out, take their money, and go to a nearby purchasing spot and buy what they had requested. For this, he was usually paid a combination of cash and drugs. Within a few months, Louie was again arrested for making buys for other drug users and sent to Rikers Island.

Over the next 2 years, Louie shuffled between the dumpsters and Rikers Island, never staying in one place long enough to get comfortable. In 1996, during his last visit to Rikers Island, he was finally accepted by the Division of AIDS Services (DAS) as a client. Upon release from Rikers Island, Louie was given an apartment in the South Bronx where he lives with another DAS client. He continues to visit Bushwick, but no longer spends much time in the neighborhood.

CONCLUSION

Those who inhabited the center of the drug injector universe in Bushwick came from extremely diverse backgrounds. They differed by gender, race, ethnicity, education, and socioeconomic background, and had very different person-alities and outlooks on life. Yet, despite their many differences, they also recognized that they shared a sameness. Largely cut off from their own families, they formed compensatory communities from which they usually eked out a bare minimum of human intimacy and compassion, but where they also sometimes found deep empathy and lifesaving help. For most, heaped upon their profoundly felt tragedy of descending into unchecked drug use, the specter of AIDS and death left them deeply pessimistic. While we are increasingly told that people are learning to "live with AIDS," these victims had no such illusions. They were told that they were not like the rest of us, they were the "other." Scorned by the medical professions, disenfranchised by social workers, and hunted by the police, the message they received was that they were expected to die and when it happened it was entirely their own fault. But, of course, they are not the "other" after all.

The Drug Scene and Risk Behaviors in Bushwick

OVERVIEW

To some extent, the lives of these drug injectors have taken place and have been shaped by the drug scenes they were part of. In this chapter, we look at the Bushwick drug scene, starting from the context of what Bushwick is like as a community and then looking at the history of the drug scene within Bushwick (and how it has been shaped by wider events). Then, we turn to the variety of specific settings in which drugs are injected. One type of setting is the "shooting gallery." We describe the history of shooting galleries in Bushwick during the course of this research. Then we turn to one specific shooting gallery and describe its history, physical layout as an injecting setting, and some of the activities that occur during the day, along with some of the activities that its managers and clientele engage in when they are not there. These descriptions exemplify some of the behaviors and network or relationship properties discussed throughout this volume

THE DRUG SCENE IN BUSHWICK: THE MAKING OF A STREET-LEVEL DRUG SUPERMARKET

Bushwick is located on the eastern edge of Brooklyn. It has long been one of the poorer neighborhoods in the borough. (Like other New York "neighborhoods," Bushwick has a population of over 100,000). Bushwick's northern edge is dotted with small manufacturers and was once a major employer of neighborhood residents. The first Europeans to settle in Bushwick were Dutch. In the 19th century it became largely a German community noted for its beer breweries. The early 20th century saw waves of Italian immigrants expand the neighborhood. By the early 1960s, African Americans and Puerto Ricans had established a significant presence. Blockbusting, a technique used by real estate speculators to capitalize on racial and ethnic bigotry and fear, was the primary tool of large-scale neighborhood reorganization. Blockbusting triggered the flight of whites from Bushwick and simultaneously signaled the beginning of a long period in which arson-related fires demolished entire blocks and led to the abandonment of thousands of buildings. By 1992, when we were conducting this study, one fifth of the lots in Bushwick lay vacant. Unlike central Brooklyn, whose prewar buildings were generally solid brick structures, most houses and apartment buildings in Bushwick were hastily constructed structures with wooden frames. As whites fled the neighborhood in the 1960s, many torched their unsellable houses to collect insurance moneys, and ended up burning down entire blocks as rows of connected wooden frame houses went up like match books.

By the late 1970s, the process of ghettoization was nearly complete. The New York City blackout of 1977, during which Bushwick was the most severely ravaged neighborhood in the city, nearly ended the long period of devastation. In the following year, a local newspaper (*Daily News*, 12/24/78) noted that:

> Despite a significant drop in fires and the arrest of hundreds of arsonists and building strippers by fire marshals and police from the Mayor's Arson Task Force, abandonment goes on at an estimated rate of 30 to 40 buildings a month in this relatively small neighborhood of about 10,000 homes and apartment buildings. Later this winter, when the city takes over its latest batch of tax delinquent properties, 1,500 in Bushwick are expected to fall out of private hands, an estimated quarter of them occupied apartment buildings.

As the neighborhood was physically transformed, the population changed dramatically; non-Latino whites decreased from 38% in 1970 to 5% in 1990, and Latinos increased from 27% in 1970 to 65% in 1990 (New York City Division of Planning, 1993). By the time that this research began, the northern end of the neighborhood was dominated by Latinos, while the southern end had more African Americans. The northern end contained mostly four-story walk-up rental apartment buildings (many of which were owned by Italian landlords who had once lived in the neighborhood), while the southern end was predominantly owner–occupied attached and detached wooden frame houses. There was one public housing project in the center of Bushwick, but it had fewer of the problems that are typically associated with public housing projects, as much of it was low-rise housing spread over several blocks.

The northern end of the neighborhood had many small factories that manufactured a variety of items, from sheet metal to scented cleansers. Several garment "sweat shops" employed women doing piece work. The western edge of Bushwick, along Broadway, had once been a thriving retail market and had many large stores and several movie theaters. The construction of the elevated subway track along the length of Broadway diminished its attractiveness as a commercial area, and looting during the 1977 blackout wiped out many of the remaining businesses. By the early 1990s, small businesses had begun to reappear on Broadway, but many buildings remained in shambles or boarded up. The most viable commercial area in the neighborhood was along Knickerbocker Avenue, a one-way avenue that ran north through the center of the neighborhood. This area had a wide variety of retail shops and was always crowded with pedestrian traffic and double- and triple-parked cars blocking the flow of traffic.

While the 1977 blackout represented a low point for Bushwick, it also marked the beginning of a new wave of immigration into the neighborhood by Dominicans, Central Americans, and especially Mexicans. Between 1980 and 1990, the population of Bushwick rose from 92,500 to nearly 103,000 (New York City Division of Planning, 1993). The 10,000 new residents had to squeeze into a shrinking housing stock, since the number of available housing units decreased by another 760 during the 1980s (New York City Division of Planning, 1993). Even though the neighborhood was no longer burning down like it had during the late 1960s and early 1970s, the large number of new inhabitants faced a severe housing shortage.

The median household income increased from $11,657 in 1980 to $16,285 in 1990, but remained barely half that of the New York City median household income of $29,823. Likewise, although the proportion of families in Bushwick who were officially listed as "below the poverty level" shrank from 45% in 1980 to 39% in 1990, it remained well over double the New York City average of 16%. Indeed, in 1990, 72% of all occupied housing units in Bushwick had a telephone as compared with nearly 93% citywide.

Bushwick has a long history as a neighborhood where drugs are bought and/or consumed. In the 1950s and early 1960s, African Americans dominated retail trade from the western edge of the neighborhood where it joined Bedford Stuyvesant. Since the mid-1960s, however, Latinos have controlled street-level drug trafficking in Bushwick: first, Puerto Ricans, and since the mid-1980s, Dominicans. By the time this research began, street-level drug markets extended throughout a wide area: from Flushing Avenue (the northern end of the neighborhood) to DeSales Street (near the southern edge), from Broadway (the western border) to Wyckoff Avenue (the borderline with Queens).

From 1989 to 1992, several sites in Bushwick saw a steady increase in the amount of street-level drug trafficking to become major "hot spots" for drug distribution and consumption. The marketplace described in this chapter was the biggest and most notorious and was the location of our research storefront. It spread over a four-block area, with the most lucrative selling spots located near the corners of blocks. The market was completely dominated by corporatelike organizations. Freelancers were strictly forbidden from working in the area.

The market was enormous, but it was difficult to estimate its volume of business because many different organizations had workers on the street around the clock. To gain some measure of the size of the market, between 1991 and 1992, the ethnographic team conducted systematic observations of the number of street-level drug distributors and users in these four blocks. It normally took two ethnographers about 30 to 45 minutes to complete the daily route that we followed. We counted only those drug distributors and users we knew, those who were visibly working or those who were seen buying, holding, or using drugs. We did not count people who could not be visibly associated with drug distribution or consumption on the street, like people who were simply sitting on the stoops of their buildings. We were conservative in our methods to ensure that the size of the market would not be overestimated. One way we decided to limit our estimates was by conducting our observations every day at noon. Early afternoon was characterized by a lull in the market, but by late afternoon business picked up considerably and the number of distributors and users were often doubled and tripled. There was also a higher ratio of consumers to distributors during late afternoon hours as people getting off work swarmed through the neighborhood buying drugs.

In 1991, the average number of distributors in the area at noon was 35. The average number of drug users during this lull period was 25. By 1992, with street-level drug markets dramatically withering away in many other neighborhoods (like Flatbush and Crown Heights), this section of Bushwick witnessed a substantial increase in the size of the market. Over the same observation period in 1992, the ethnographic survey counted an average of 65 distributors and 53 users, so the visible increase in street-level distributors in the neighborhood coincided with an increase in street-level drug users. Many came from other neighborhoods to take advantage of Bushwick's greater quality and availability of drugs (Curtis et al., 1995). Thus, this chapter describes a period when this section of Bushwick became a drug supermarket. It also describes how law enforcement interventions affected the drug scene and the distributors and consumers who comprised it.

The Bushwick drug market had been more typical during the 1960s and 1970s. Like nearly every neighborhood in northern Brooklyn then, it had a variety of spots where local residents could purchase heroin, cocaine, marijuana, and other drugs. Many of these were indoor locations—bars, bodegas, pool halls, apartments, and so forth—where a personal connection to the dealer was necessary to obtain access. Jose, a long time heroin user, describes what it was like:

> At that time [1970s], they wouldn't sell drugs in the street too much. You would have to go like to a house. At that time there were black and Spanish guys selling it. Years ago they used to sell drugs in a bar on Halsey Street. You could go there, right, and they would sell to you. And then they had a house connection across the street from the bar. If they didn't know you they wouldn't sell. It's lot different today. They'll sell to anybody today. Even if you are a cop, they'll still sell to you.
>
> Drugs first started coming to Troutman and Jefferson Street about 12 or 13 years ago. Over here was just pot buildings. These guys were selling inside of apartments so you can't see who they are. They served you through the hole. You might know one of the workers, but you wouldn't know the owner.

Outdoor drug-selling during this period was nearly always confined to public parks. There was virtually no trafficking on residential streets. Freddy and Pope discuss how police actions spread drug trafficking onto residential blocks.

> FREDDY: I used to buy dope in Putnam Park for $2 a bag in 1970. Puerto Ricans and Blacks were selling it then. They were from the neighborhood. I didn't have no idea about the owners. I wasn't even interested in who the owners were. I would buy the dope and go home and do it. I wouldn't do it in the streets.

POPE: I was living on Troutman about '85. There was no drugs on the block. All the drugs came from the park. When the police took everybody from the park out, then the people started goin' into the side blocks. At that time, it was Puerto Ricans selling the drugs. Dominicans are just getting here in the last 2 years. In '85, it was Puerto Ricans selling in the park; people that used to sell joints 10 years ago. You know, from reefer to pills, from pills to coke, from coke it came to dope. They had police in the park practically ... not practically, but you could say from the morning all the way into the night. And they would have a police in every entrance. So they drove everybody out of the park into the factories. As they came out of the park, they started in the corners like where Blimpie's is at, Star Street corner, they started there. They drove them out from the park to the corner of Star Street. Then they started pushing and they didn't want them hangin' out on that corner. So they came over to this corner, to Troutman.

In the late 1980s, street drug markets dramatically expanded and attracted distributors and consumers from surrounding neighborhoods. This development should be viewed in light of citywide changes in street-level drug markets during this period, where the process of market shrinkage (particularly crack markets) in some neighborhoods led to their growth and intensification in others. Crack markets in central and northern Brooklyn began to shrink beginning in 1988, but this led to the emergence of an ethnically heterogeneous street-level drug super-market in Bushwick.

Unlike Williamsburg, which was a "closed" marketplace, Bushwick was a neighborhood where new organizations could open a business alongside established organizations. For example, Bruce talks about a group of black men from Bedford Stuyvesant who began a street-level drug business in Bushwick during summer 1992.

They have black people dealing on the street over here. Yeah, two stamps called the Chosen One and Nine Lives. And it's pretty good. If you got a group of guys who's willing to protect their interests, they could bring their stamp here. It is an open market, but not basically on Troutman, but they work on the corner—they really don't go on the block 'cause that would cause trouble. You can't sell where somebody else has got their stamp. A certain stamp has a certain area.

BUYING AND USING DRUGS IN BUSHWICK DURING THE RESEARCH PERIOD (1990–1993)

Many types of drugs were available in Bushwick. Storefronts selling marijuana were widely spread throughout the neighborhood, and despite the raging popularity of crack in the mid-1980s and the supermarket bazaar atmosphere of the early 1990s, these discreet storefronts continued to operate without major interruption. They serviced a steady and relatively stable population of smokers. Powdered cocaine for sniffers and crack for smokers also could be readily bought in various neighborhood settings. Nonetheless, drug injectors and the markets that catered to their needs dominated the local drug scene. Our research storefront was located in the heart of these thriving markets.

Buying drugs in Bushwick was easier in some respects than using them. During the research period (1990–1993), there was never a problem finding someone to buy drugs from, although the large number of street-level dealers posed a problem of deciding which one was likely to have the best drugs (later, we discuss the implications of this problem with respect to injectors). But once buyers had purchased their drugs, unless they were willing to wait until they got home or to some other safe location to use them, it was sometimes not so easy to find a place to use them.

Of course, people who were simply smoking a joint or sniffing a bag of cocaine or heroin had many relatively discreet options. The boisterousness of the marketplace and the audacity of injectors' behaviors provided ample cover for drug users who were content to sit somewhere quietly and smoke a joint or casually pull out a bag and sniff it in a doorway.

Injectors, on the other hand, because of the process they go through to use their drugs, could not so casually sit on a park bench and "cook up" a "speedball" or stand in a doorway jabbing at a throbbing vein in someone's neck.* We observed drug injectors doing these things and more, but they were far from casual, laid-back events; they were done in great haste and were overlaid with tension, fear, paranoia, and uncertainty. When possible, injectors avoided public situations in favor of places where they were not so rushed, where they could take time to do it right and where they could seek help if and when it was needed. In Bushwick, several types of settings provided more convenient places to inject drugs than on busy residential or shopping streets. Several of these settings are described.

Many people who are unfamiliar with drug injectors and with how drug markets and injection routines have changed since the early 1980s believe that the injectors typically frequent shooting galleries where they use drugs in macabre rituals of a subculture hell-bent on self-destruction. To be sure, there were shooting galleries in Bushwick and they were often quite crowded, but it would be a mistake

---

*An often heard comment from many quarters (neighborhood residents, social service professionals, and many colleagues) was that "dope fiends" did not care about concealing injection behavior except, of course, from the police. While it was certainly true that many of their activities were carried on in plain view, most injectors expressed great shame about what they were doing, especially with regard to children seeing them. They generally took care to hide their drug-taking behaviors. Not coincidentally, we found out about their nearly universally held shame because we were interested in observing how drug injectors used drugs. When we would try to see exactly what they were doing, most injectors tried to turn away from our prying eyes. In every case, the explanation that was immediately offered was that they were "ashamed" of what they were doing, and because they "respected" us (by that time, we had usually become quite friendly with someone who was observed that closely) they felt that they should "hide" their drug taking, especially injections. Because they knew that our research was about AIDS, it is quite likely that their sense of shame was even more pronounced. But we met no injectors over the duration of the research who were in any way proud of their drug use or whose use of drugs in public was intended to model such behavior (as perhaps may be true for the mid-1990s generation of heroin users).

to characterize them as the center of a drug-injecting subculture or even as the most frequently used injection locale in the neighborhood. There was a wide variety of settings where injectors used drugs in Bushwick and the injection routines we observed were remarkably devoid of ritual or subcultural bonding. The most frequently mentioned injection spot and the place that afforded the most comfort, convenience, and safety was "home." But for those injectors who could not use drugs at home, sites other than shooting galleries also attracted users. For example, many side streets in the neighborhood were lined with factory buildings, and thus were relatively isolated. Injectors with cars would frequently park on these blocks and shoot up at a leisurely pace, without too much concern for pedestrians or patrol cars. Injectors who came to the neighborhood on foot could also easily walk to these blocks and find shelter (behind a dumpster or loading dock, in a doorway, etc.) to prepare their drugs without being rushed.

Injectors who feared the police or other drug users, or who simply became too paranoid after using drugs to want to be around other people when they were "high," sought secluded locations. Particularly popular, especially during the summer, were the sides of the railroad tracks that sliced through the factory section of the neighborhood and the banks of the foul-smelling canal at the edge of Bushwick. In these places, it was not uncommon to see huts hidden in the bushes that had been thrown together with bits and pieces of industrial refuse. They were often furnished with car seats or mattresses dragged down from the neighborhood. Because these sites were some distance from local drug markets, only the most paranoid or privacy-seeking injectors would bother to make the trek to inject there. This area was also popular with sex workers, who would sometimes have "dates" who wanted more than quick oral sex.

The far end of a subway platform was a popular spot both for drug injectors who came to the neighborhood via subway and for many neighborhood "regulars." At some platform ends, sturdy wooden boxes (which contained sand for the stairs in winter) were used as tables on which to prepare drugs. Using the subway platform had several advantages, including: (1) shelter from the elements, (2) lack of control by anyone (no fees or "tastes" had to be paid), (3) ample warning of anyone who might approach, since people had to walk the entire length of the platform to get to these spots, and (4) a fair amount of injection equipment lying about, including syringes, cookers, water, and sometimes even bleach kits and condoms. A major disadvantage, however, was increased vulnerability to being robbed (or worse) or arrested.*

Several outdoor spots within a block or two of the major drug buying streets were also used. One was behind a large dumpster pushed up against the side of a wall in the middle of a factory-lined street, one block from the major buying spot in

---

*In mid-1992, stepped-up police enforcement, especially in the subway stations, dramatically reduced drug injectors' use of public spaces in the neighborhood.

the neighborhood. Because traffic on the street was one-way and there were very few pedestrians, a couple of drug injectors could easily hide behind the dumpster; and since it was in the middle of the block, there was usually ample time to react to approaching police or others. Because it was so busy in 1991, this site was chosen by the underground needle exchange when they expanded services to Bushwick.

The most blatant outdoor injection spot was just across the street from the busiest drug market in the neighborhood. There, many injectors (generally, those who were deriving income by performing some role in market transactions) sat propped up against a factory wall or, even more visibly, across the street on a loading platform and injected quite near a busy intersection whose traffic light allowed motorists to wait long enough to more than just glance at this activity. Though the corner was especially busy during summer months, injectors often injected drugs there even during the coldest days of winter. One reason Bushwick gained a reputation as a neighborhood whose drug markets catered to injectors was because of the audacity of users who shot up on the sidewalk, especially on this corner. Groups of injectors were often seen sitting on the sidewalk with half-filled needles protruding from their arms and legs, "nodding out" from a particularly good bag of heroin, injecting one another, cleaning out their crack "stems" (pipes) or injection equipment, or seeking another injector to "throw down on an angle" (split the cost of an injection). During the summer, injectors would spend days at a time at these locations without moving. Between 5 and 6 AM, police officers would often walk through the block and kick awake the half dozen injectors who had fallen asleep on the sidewalk. Told to move along, they would grumble, rub their eyes, pull together their few possessions, and walk around the block, only to return a few minutes after the police disappeared to reclaim their spot.

SHOOTING GALLERIES OVER THE RESEARCH PERIOD

As busy as some outdoor spots were, the highest concentration of injection events clearly occurred in local shooting galleries. This section examines the major shooting galleries that existed in Bushwick.

Throughout the 1970s and 1980s, many abandoned buildings in Bushwick were taken over by drug injectors who converted them into living spaces and shooting galleries. By the mid-1980s, however, with the influx of many Central Americans and a steady rebuilding of the neighborhood, the availability of empty buildings decreased dramatically and so did the number of shooting galleries. Jose, a Puerto Rican injector who predominantly injected in the street, described this:

> There used to be a lot of shootin' galleries on Jefferson Street. One of my brothers had a gallery in the abandoned buildings that they fixed. That gallery—that was the number one gallery on Jefferson. He ran the gallery because the apartment was his first of all. Man, the way it is now they shoot up anywhere. There's this garage on Flushing,

the old tire shop. Sometimes I go in there because I don't want to do it in the open. See, a lot of these guys—which include myself—I shouldn't be doing this because I should know better. Sometimes I go in the street.

By the early 1990s, there was such a shortage of stable indoor locations where injectors could inject without trouble from police, neighborhood residents, or other injectors that when they found such a spot, they would often keep it to themselves. Bruce would sneak up to the roof of a local factory building to inject. The building watchman not only allowed him to use the building, but even provided him with a broom to clean up after himself. Bruce noted that "it's a nice warm building, but I won't take a lot of people around there. I keep it discreet."

During the period covered by this research there were several shooting galleries in the neighborhood, all run by a relatively small group of drug injectors from the core network. But in the summer of 1991, there was only one "taste" gallery in the area. By taste gallery, we mean it was a place where virtually anyone could gain entry by giving a sample, or a taste, of drugs to the "owner." This taste gallery was in an abandoned tire shop three blocks from the major buying areas. Louie and Gus, two Puerto Rican drug injectors, ran it. For injectors who were new to the area or lacked connections, this was the only indoor location available to them. Yvette, a 20-year-old Puerto Rican injector from Hoboken, New Jersey, was not new to the neighborhood and knew many other local drug injectors, but she still found herself drawn to the tire shop:

> I went to the garage over there.... That place is crazy these days. There weren't a lot of people there when I went in. I don't know how many 'cause I just stood towards the front. I didn't dare go inside. I went there with a friend. I had the stuff and I gave him some because I just didn't want to go there by myself. I was scared. I told him I'll give you something, you know. I gave him a 15 shot [15 cc] from a two and one [2 bags of heroin, 1 bag of cocaine].

In Yvette's case, the fear of going into the gallery alone prompted her to take another person with her and to share drugs with him. They were not regular drug-sharing partners or even good friends, as her payment for his company suggests. Like many injectors, Yvette's drug-sharing behavior was not driven by psychological weakness or governed by the rules and norms of a deviant subculture, but rather by a lack of choice and by fear.

Like Yvette, Melody, a 29-year-old Puerto Rican injector from Williamsburg, Brooklyn, sometimes went into local shooting galleries, but found them too dangerous and crowded with people with whom she did not want to share drugs:

> I don't have places at all to go to get off. I try and find a good spot where I can do it 'cause sometimes you got to pay $5 in some places. Or I got to pay my friend a bottle [of crack] so I can do it in her house, and they rob you. It's hard. They locked up all these buildings. You don't find no buildings at all anymore. They have one spot that I know of, two. Two spots that I know of, but I don't go there. Too many crowds, too many people. You meet up with people you don't want to.

But despite the fears that many injectors harbored about going into local galleries, many continued to do so, especially when the weather was cold or the neighborhood was hot with police.

The Tire Shop

Louie and Gus had often injected together, but they had never been "ripping and running" (i.e., drug users who hustle money and use drugs together) partners. The tire shop was their first business venture. They ran a fairly efficient shop, but were not friends, and even expressed a considerable amount of dislike for each other. Though the business allowed them each to inject more than 30 times a day, they were always angling for more. Neither would hesitate to steal a customer away from the other, even if it would lead to heated arguments and potentially violent confrontations.

Louie, the dominant partner, was 35 years old when the tire shop first opened. Puerto Rican by descent, he grew up in East New York and Bushwick but had spent half of his adult life doing prison time, mostly for stickups and burglaries. Though he was not tall, Louie had developed quite a physique in Sing Sing and other correctional settings, even while maintaining a heroin habit behind bars. His imposhing presence allowed him to control the gallery, but this same appearance of virility and strength also led him to pay little attention to the effects of HIV. This same attitude—that he was a model of health—later led him to stop taking tuberculosis prevention medication initially prescribed for him in Rikers Island. Louie was an HIV prevention worker's nightmare.

Gus was 37 years old when he and Louie became partners, but he had already been injecting heroin (primarily speedball) for 24 years, the first time in the bathroom of a local park. Much of his family lived in the neighborhood, but except for occasional visits to his sister's apartment where he "caught up" with family members, there were few signs that he had any ties but those forged in the gallery. As the junior partner in the gallery business, Gus was always second in line to receive any tastes from customers, except from those who were his personal clients. Gus's main function was to keep the place running when Louie was not around and thereby prevent other drug injectors from laying a claim to the tire shop.

The tire shop started when Louie smashed through the cinder blocks in a wall sheltered from street-view. He set up shop in the largest room of the building. (Later, Pope started a minigallery in a storage closet in the next room.) Louie covered the hole in the wall with a piece of corrugated tin roofing, but it hardly concealed the well-worn path that a steady stream of injectors had beaten to the door. The gallery quickly became known to injectors and police alike.

Peeling back the tin and peering into the darkness of the tire shop, it initially seemed that only the most hearty or dope-sick injectors would venture into such a place, but once one's eyes became accustomed to the dim light, the room bustled with activity and it seemed far less ominous. Still, many injectors stayed out of this gallery for fear of being robbed (and several reported that they had been) or because they did not want to share their drugs with other injectors who hung out there. As a result, the spacious yard behind the tire shop also became a popular injection spot. Many shacks had been hastily erected that served injectors who wanted to avoid going into the gallery. Nevertheless, there were sometimes as many as 20–25 people inside a single room of the gallery, and while injecting drugs was clearly the main activity occurring there, the gallery was also a center point for hustling. For example, one drug injector who regularly stole sneakers, shoes, and boots from a local factory to finance his habit spread out his wares in one corner of the room and sold them to other injectors. If people did not see the size or style they wanted, he would take their order and have it by the following day.

The tire shop a place where the most uncontrolled injection behaviors took place. Pope describes this:

> I take care of business as far as cleaning my works and all that stuff, but a lot of the people that were coming in there were disgusting. I tell you, the cookers are so filthy and people don't bother to wash them out before they use them. They'll just leave all that cut in it, and add more stuff to it. And many of them share works too. There's a lot of people that has AIDS or the virus and lend works and do not say anything. That is very fucked up.

Louie and Gus were major offenders in this regard. We often observed them practicing hazardous injection routines—sharing cookers, water, backloading, and so on—though never directly sharing syringes, the taboo magnet that drew stigma away from the other items in the injector's repertoire. Louie bragged on several occasions that he would inject more than 25 times per day inside the gallery and on several occasions professed not to care about his* or anyone else's HIV status:

> I was in the garage most of the day yesterday, from like 10 [AM] to 10 [PM] or 10 to 11. When I first went in, there was like 15 guys in there. Later, 30 or 35 showed up, in one room, in another room, in another room. I be getting off like crazy man with all kinds of guys, black, white, Spanish. Any of them. I know them all. I have a hell of a habit. Shit, I shot a storm man. I was gettin' busy yesterday. I'm telling you. I shot up 20 or 30 times or something. Every time was in the garage. Not one of those times was by myself, I was always getting tastes. Everybody goes to the garage. There's no other place in the neighborhood to go that I can think of. The garage is like Grand Central Station. It's like that. Everybody goes in there to get high.

Even though Louie shared drugs with a great many people who came into the garage, he never allowed others to inject him. But for those drug injectors who wanted assistance injecting themselves, the garage was the place to go, and Louie was always eager to be rewarded with a taste for accommodating such requests.

*Louie claimed that he never actually found out his HIV status until he went to Rikers Island (city jail) in late 1992. Though he was tested as part of the SFHR research in 1991, he never returned to the storefront to pick up his results. He later admitted that he had assumed that he must be positive and he was not terribly interested in confirming what he strongly suspected was bad news.

I shot up in my arm that time, but I had to go higher cause sometimes it's hard, you know. I always do it myself. I don't like nobody to hit me. Sometimes I hit other people in the neck. I hit Gus, I hit Mano, I hit Pete, I hit a couple of females, all yesterday. Yeah, I'm good at hitting people in the neck. For that, they give me a taste.

As the biggest magnet for injectors in the neighborhood, the tire shop became a familiar stopover for police and emergency medical technicians. It lasted for about a year before it was finally closed down. Before this ultimatum which finally sent drug injectors looking for more convenient quarters, the tire shop had been hotly contested ground. Police loathed going into the gallery and generally did not do so unless they were searching for a specific person. Many officers conveniently avoided it because it was located on the borderline between two police precincts. Sitting in a no-man's-land that neither precinct wanted to claim as its own, many injectors who were caught injecting drugs on the street by the police in one precinct (and whose arrest would have been too much hassle for officers) were told to "go across Flushing Avenue" to the tire shop where they would be in the jurisdiction of another precinct. When the underground needle exchange began in Bushwick during the summer of 1991, they too were often told by police officers to take their activities behind the tire shop where they would be "out of sight, out of mind."

Eventually, however, the tire shop became too obvious and the police began to pressure the landlord to do something about his property. The landlord realized that if he continued to plug the holes in the walls with cinderblocks, injectors would simply smash them and regain entrance to the building. The landlord attempted to solve the problem by welding large, half-inch-thick iron plates to the outside of the building. For one day, Louie and Gus were stumped and many injectors looking for a place to inject now crowded into the backyard, which had also been fenced off at the same time but ineffectively so. Louie solved their problem of access to the gallery by climbing to the top of the building, shimmying down a rope through a hole in the ceiling and starting a fire inside the tire shop. When the Fire Department arrived to put out the blaze, they ripped off the metal plates that had been welded up the previous day. The small fire did no further damage to the building (though it did retain a strong smell after that) and Louie, Gus, and the other injectors happily returned to their enclave. After having this scenario repeat itself on at least three subsequent occasions over the next 2 months, the landlord finally took additional steps, including a threat to shoot trespassers, to make his property inaccessible to injectors. Rather than risk being shot, Louie and Gus began searching for another location to start a gallery.

Within a week of being displaced from the tire shop, in mid-October 1991, Louie and Gus found a storage lot next to a factory building where piles of wooden pallets provided them with ample building materials. Thrown together with wood, nails, rope, and plastic sheeting, their new gallery was clearly not as sturdy as the brick and mortar of the tire shop, but as shacks went, it looked fairly sturdy. But once it was built along the east wall of the factory, the new gallery was not as spacious as their previous digs (5–6 people was its capacity) and it lacked the kind of protections afforded by the first. So, even though it was somewhat closer to the major drug selling blocks than the tire shop, it was not nearly as successful as its predecessor. As a result, several core network members who had come to depend on a steady rate of traffic through the gallery to "get straight" through the day were no longer able to sustain such large consumption routines. Within a month, several of them broke through the brick wall to the factory, which they discovered was actually a storage facility for a lamp wholesaler. For the next several days, before the hole in the wall was discovered by employees, hundred of lamps were sold on the streets of Bushwick. The police came immediately upon notification, and after two drug injectors were arrested, the gallery was demolished, the yard was cleaned of debris, and a sturdy fence with a locked gate and topped with razor ribbon was quickly erected.

For the next few weeks there were no large public or taste galleries in the neighborhood that offered unrestricted access. For core network members, finding a place to inject was not much of a problem, but lacking a place for outsiders to visit put a serious crimp in their ability to secure tastes:

> Since the garage closed, some of the customers have been doing it [injecting] outside the building in the back there by the corner. Then some people go by the gasoline station on Flushing where all the pallets are stacked up. But that got burned out two times already. There's no new places, so people are goin' back to the street like to Jefferson [Street] by the factory. The cops have been around hassling people but not me. I happen to be unfortunate not to have no money to be bothered. Since the galleries have closed, I haven't been able to make money. Nothing.

Over the duration of the winter, many core network members used the subway station and the park bathroom (mostly for women) as injection locations. Less accessible to many injectors were two crack houses (Chantel's and Pop's) where injectors were tolerated only if they did their business somewhat discreetly and the owner of the apartment was paid in crack. Missy and Earl, both African Americans, had apartments in the area where injectors who were close friends, were capable of respecting the place as a living space, and who were willing to share their drugs could find a place to inject. But these places and several others like them never drew much of a crowd. During the winter, secure and warm indoor spots remained at a premium and many core network members, like Bruce, who used the tops of stairwells in nearby factory buildings, kept good spots to themselves.

Shortly before Thanksgiving 1991, a house burned down on the major crack-selling street in Bushwick. By next May, Louie and his girlfriend had salvaged an upstairs bedroom and turned it into the busiest shooting gallery in the area. The story of that house and its occupants, both before and after the fire, is instructive.

The House on Crack Row

Maria and five of her children lived in the only single-family house on crack row. There were several small apartment buildings at the other end of the short block, but her house sat by itself, set back from the street, with a garage in front and flanked by overgrown garbage-strewn lots. Directly across the street from her frontyard was an empty lot between two factory buildings where makeshift shacks were constantly popping up to shelter street-level crack dealers and drug users of every variety. Maria's house, a city-owned building, was sandwiched between the two "businesses" that controlled the block. "White tops" crack controlled the corner, and "yellow tops" crack controlled the middle of the block and was run by another group of Dominicans from one of the small apartment buildings at the other end of the block. While Maria had little to do with either party, and they generally did not bother her, her relationships with many of the drug users in the neighborhood, including her own children, was complex.

At one time, her son Roger's girlfriend, Celia, lived in Maria's house, but after her breakup with Roger and the onset of her problems with crack and heroin, Celia was forced to live with her maternal uncle who lived in a nearby public housing project. Celia was not close with him and she rarely stayed in the apartment. Most of her time was spent directly in front of Maria's house: selling and smoking crack, sniffing and eventually shooting heroin, performing sex work, eating, sleeping, hustling, getting beaten up, getting arresting, and crying—all in view of the children (including her own) who played in the frontyard. Even though Roger despised Celia, Maria maintained a relationship with her. She felt sorry for Celia and occasionally took her in, fed her, gave her fresh clothes, let her sleep for a day or two, and generally provided emergency relief when she was desperate. Celia, for her part, would occasionally contribute food, baby clothing, and other necessities whenever she had extra money or when Maria was in dire need.

In June 1990, Celia was arrested and charged with possession with intent to sell 91 vials of crack. Of course, Celia was unable to raise bail and was sent to the Women's House of Detention at Riker's Island. In some ways, Maria still saw Celia as her daughter and continued to reach out to help her. After hearing from Celia in jail, Maria put together a care package and we drove her to Rikers Island at 7 AM on a Sunday morning. The package included four pairs of new denim pants, two new T-shirts, two pair of slippers, two pairs of socks, shampoo and creme rinse, four bars of soap, and a comb.

Carmen, Maria's 21-year-old daughter, occasionally contributed money to Maria's household, and she made money by selling crack around the corner late at night hoping to avoid the police by working off-hours. Maria worried that Carmen was selling heroin at the nearby heroin supermarket a couple of blocks away, but Carmen ridiculed this suggestion and insisted that she "would never be stupid enough to sell heroin." According to her, she "only sells crack." (Among street-level drug dealers and users, heroin distribution was thought to be much more dangerous than selling crack.) Even so, her heroin use got worse. She realized that after 2 years of sniffing heroin, she was beginning to develop a problem. She was also on probation, having been caught selling crack once before, and she knew that it was getting more difficult to lie to her probation officer, especially once she began missing her biweekly appointments without an alibi. By summer 1991, after several months of searching, Carmen was finally able to enroll in a methadone program located in a distant neighborhood. The methadone program was a good solution to some of her problems. It sent a message to her probation officer that she was (though she really wasn't) actively seeking help for her drug problem. It also gave her a ready excuse—the sedating effects of the methadone—for not seeking legitimate employment or job training, thereby retaining the welfare benefits that Maria depended on to feed and clothe Carmen's kids. Finally, it allowed her to sleep most of the day and run all night.

But while methadone might have been a solution to some of Carmen's problems, it compounded Maria's. Maria found that the methadone made Carmen drowsy and she had developed an annoying habit of lighting a cigarette right before lying down in bed. After only 2 months in the program, Carmen had burned holes in all of the household's sheets and several blankets and a grapefruit-sized hole in her mattress. While the methadone program allowed Carmen to make money and pursue her night life—selling crack, buying gold and outfits, "vogueing" (posing) for the boys—it did nothing for her standing in the household. Just after Thanksgiving 1991, Carmen lit a cigarette, lay down in bed, and burned down the house in the middle of the night.

Maria took her family to the emergency assistance unit (EAU), which temporarily placed them in an apartment until they could find another house. They lived in the EAU housing unit for almost 6 months before the city found another house for them on Euclid Avenue in East New York, Brooklyn. For Maria, the fire had been a blessing. It allowed her to move into a larger and better house, to get a fresh start with housing authorities, and to put real distance between her children and grandchildren and the biggest street-level drug market in Brooklyn. Even though drugs were readily available in East New York, their markets were much less blatant than was the case in Bushwick, and neither Carmen nor Roger knew or had histories with any of the local drug market participants.

When the house burned, Carmen's bedroom was almost completely demolished before the fire department put out the fire. The nearest fire house was only about three or four blocks away, but given that it was an old wooden house, it was surprising that it did not burn to the ground. The front of the house was both burned and ripped off by firefighters, giving the appearance of a large doll house. Downstairs, furniture and appliances were demolished by falling debris and waterlogged by hoses and pipes that had burst in the house. Within 2 weeks, when winter began to really set in, everything downstairs froze, including the small pool of water in the front yard, and the house remained virtually inaccessible to anyone until the spring thaw.

But while the house was severely damaged by the fire, the garage was unscathed. Within days after the fire, Celia searched the premises for personal possessions and any valuables she might salvage to sell. Celia was the first to realize the potential of the garage as a spot where she could live, work (selling crack for the white tops organization on the corner), and make money or drugs (charging people to use the premises). Because she was seen as related to the former tenant of the house, no one contested her claim to the garage when it became obvious that this was evolving into a spot where people could go and use drugs. Celia had also converted the garage into a living space, and she put up pictures of her children which she had found in an upstairs bedroom of the house. Celia had essentially been homeless ever since her mother died in 1989, and the garage was the first place of her own.

> I took over the place; now people pay me anytime they go in there. I've been in there for at least 2 weeks and I hooked it up real nice. I got candles for now. But see, we don't know how to take light from the light pole, we will do it, but I don't want to bother with that. When I'm not there, Shoty looks after the place? He's 14 and only smokes crack. People don't try and take us off. I mean they know we're running the place, but they've know us for a long time. Nobody has come to get it. Right now, the people who go there are me, Ruben, India, Linda, all the girls, and everybody goes in there with their dates. To use the place they either give me half a bottle of crack or give me half of their dope, or they give it to the others, you know, like that, whatever works. If they're going to shoot up, they bring their own works, but I've got the cookers there. A lot of people are coming there. Of the girls who were in there before I came here, one gave me a half bag of dope and India gave me crack.

At first, because the block had a reputation for crack sales and use, crack users dominated the garage. But within a month of opening, injectors began to flock there in larger numbers. And whenever Dominican crack managers searched for workers who had run off with their product, the garage was the first place they visited, brandishing weapons. The police were never far behind.

> Just before I came over to see you the cops took us out of there. A big stupid black cop that thinks he's bad. He was beating up on everybody. Well, he came and told us open up the door. I was about to shoot up, and when I seen his face I threw the works up in the air, and I threw the cooker away. I said, "Ah man, now he messed up my whole thing." I threw away the dope and everything and this girl had given me half a bag. At the time, me and this other female were inside the place. She had come there to shoot up a bag of dope. She gave me half, but she got to do hers. I was about to do mine, that's when he came in, and I had to throw the cooker and everything with the dope away. When the cop came, he started yelling, "Open the door, open door." Then, he started kicking the door and kicking the door and kicking the door. We got confused and we stood in the middle, and he kept on kicking the door and kicking the door. And then we said, "Wait, wait, wait, we will open it, it's open, you just have to slide it." So when I slided it open, that's when he goes, "What the fuck is wrong with you guys? What are you doing? You all

doing drugs, right?" He was standing there and the other girls say, "no, I don't do drugs." He goes, "Who the fuck you think you fooling bitch." He went by and smacked her and then he threw us out.

Between the police and crack managers, the front and back doors to the garage were quickly demolished, the building mysteriously caught fire a few times, and the usable space steadily shrunk until the building was virtually reduced to rubble by the end of February. In March, the partially burned house at the back of the lot, a place which had looked entirely inhospitable during the winter when it was frozen over in visible ice, began to attract the attention of several injectors who were eager to get another large gallery going.

THE SETTING—LOUIE AND CARMEN'S GALLERY

After being displaced from their gallery on the side of the lamp factory just when the weather was getting cold, Louie and Gus's fragile partnership quickly dissolved, and they both spent the winter making money from a wide variety of hustles and injecting in most of the places scattered around the neighborhood, including Celia's garage. When the cold weather began to moderate, Louie was one of the first drug injectors to venture into Maria's old house with the intention of finding a space that might be transformed into a new gallery. He and Carmen, now his girlfriend, spent several days cleaning out a bedroom on the second floor of the house, throwing all the waterlogged and/or burned refuse either out the windows or into adjacent rooms. Access to the second floor was limited to a wooden stairway at the back of the building and to get to it, caution was required to step through the maze of rubble and charred beams on the ground floor without incident. Though they were able to create a reasonable amount of space in the remaining bedroom and sometimes it even looked relatively clean, they could not get rid of the smoky, fire smell that seemed to cling to anyone who spent any amount of time there. In addition to the acrid aroma caused by the fire, there was a considerable amount of rotting material (food, wet clothing, and so on) inside the house that lent a pungent overlay to the fire smell. This nasty stew of offending odors was completed by drug users who regularly used the downstairs portion of the house as a bathroom. It was really necessary to be cautious in approaching the stairs! Of course, this mess attracted all manner of flying and crawling insects. Getting to the back stairs usually involved delicate footwork and flailing arms to slice through the veils of flies. Despite these drawbacks and the lack of many amenities desired by drug injectors, by spring 1992, Louie and Carmen's gallery was the busiest spot in the neighborhood.

We don't have many supplies in the house 'cause it's really all messed up. You see we haven't cleaned it. But we got a couple of kits stashed around, you know. Mostly everybody comes with their own water, their own shit, you know.

The Setup—Bleach, Water, Cookers, and Works

Farthest away from the stairs, along the far wall, a board across a few items of furniture served as a place to keep communal injection equipment like bottles of water and bleach, cookers, and pieces of cotton. Usually, the board was a jumble of materials, but in the early morning hours when core network members waited for working injectors to stop by, the materials were often carefully lined up with everything neatly arranged in a row, much like a popular pizzeria will line up their jars of spices at the beginning of the day. Some of the bottles were capped soda bottles but most were small plastic water bottles from the 50 bleach kits that were dropped off at least once a week by AIDS outreach workers. To make them last until the next delivery, the bleach kits were kept in a plastic milk crate and stuck under the bed, out of view of the public. The most coveted items in the bleach kits were the alcohol preps, with water bottles and cookers next in popularity. Bleach use itself was not strongly advocated by either the gallery owners or many of the core network members who visited there. During most of the injection events that we observed, it was not used. In fact, it was not unusual to see an injector open a bleach kit and pitch the bottle of bleach from the second floor window into the front yard. So many bleach bottles had been thrown from the second floor that on one occasion, a core network member who had injected cocaine and was feeling particularly energetic filled a paper shopping bag with several hundred filled bleach bottles after searching the overgrown frontyard for approximately 15 minutes. Thinking that he was doing a favor by returning the unused bottles to the research storefront, he succeeded only in impressing staff with the magnitude of the challenge of trying to change injection practices.

Cookers were indiscriminately used and there were many of them lying about the gallery. As long as they contained no rust, they were considered serviceable. While syringes had considerable stigma attached to them and were almost never visibly shared, injectors typically shared cookers, cottons, and water with almost no reluctance. On several occasions, injectors were seen collecting used cookers to scrape residue from the bottom in hopes of producing a tiny injection. The extent to which such residues can transmit HIV is not known. Some evidence suggests that large amounts of the virus can survive in syringes for 4 or more weeks after they are used, however (Heimer et al., 1996).

Diabetic syringes dominated the gallery. The needles at their tips could not be removed. Blue-tip syringes, with a removable needle, were much less common. Most injectors did not like blue-tips because their needle was thicker and longer. A thicker needle was more painful, especially after it became dulled through repeated use; and if it was too long, it was much easier to poke it all the way through a vein and into surrounding muscle, thereby resulting in the bane of all injectors, a "miss." Nearly everyone requested diabetic syringes and there were several places to get them in the neighborhood. Syringe salesmen usually milled around busy buying spots, peddling "sealed works" for $2 apiece. One salesman, Booker, an African-American long-term injector and member of the core network who came to the neighborhood early every morning, typically bought a box of 100 syringes for $30 each day. Booker would easily get his $2 from outsiders, but could only get $1 from other core network members. Selling syringes was not terribly lucrative; to make money required purchases by many customers (since few people bought more than a few at a time), and thus long hours. Booker rationalized his strategy by noting that the work was slow but steady. Best of all, he was largely out of harm's way because he did not risk becoming indebted to the vicious and punitive drug selling organizations that controlled the local market and he was not a primary target of law enforcement officers on their way to arrest dealers on nearby corners.

While there were several regular syringe sellers in the neighborhood like Booker, they faced competition from other sources. Other injectors occasionally repackaged used syringes in their original plastic wrapping to make them look sterile and sold them as new. Several injectors were adept at this repackaging scheme, but since it was a universally despised by all injectors, it generally occurred only when injectors were "sick" and needed to "get straight."

Syringes were also available in galleries and it was usually the prerogative of the owner to sell them. But in busy galleries, it was nearly impossible to maintain a steady supply of sterile syringes, so many used syringes were sold to sick injectors. In Louie's gallery, several hundred injections took place daily. He himself accounted for about 20–30 per day, so he could not sustain a supply of new syringes. When a needle exchange program began operating in the neighborhood on Wednesdays and Saturdays during the summer of 1991, Louie was one of the first to take advantage of it. Though each time he returned to the exchange he had 20–30 syringes, they were not the ones they had given him. (Syringes from the exchange were clearly marked with red nail polish). Typically, he sold the exchange's syringes within 24 hours, and then a day before the exchange showed up again collected syringes inside the gallery to trade them in for another bunch.

"Getting Straight" in the Gallery

Injecting took place around the clock in shooting galleries that did little to restrict access, but the busiest time of day was often early in the morning when injectors with jobs stopped by to "get straight" before going to work. The most popular shooting galleries often had more than a dozen people injecting and more often than not sharing drugs during this time. Drug sharing was more observable by the ethnographic team during this period than other times of the day because injectors frequently seemed to be in a rush: working injectors usually had little time to purchase drugs and inject before having to be at work, and core network members were frequently "dope sick" upon waking up. Though there were always street-level distributors working on Troutman or Jefferson Streets at this time of the morning, there were far fewer of them, and given the limited choices for buyers, the likelihood of buying a "beat" bag of heroin was much greater than in the afternoon or evening (a "beat" bag is one that fraudulently contains little or no heroin). To compensate for the time involved in searching for a good bag, many working drug injectors relied on a core network member (often a syringe seller with whom they had a previous working relationship) to make a recommendation of which bag to buy or to actually negotiate a purchase, since the threat of arrest was also much greater in early morning hours. A typical purchase of this kind would be two or three dime bags of heroin and two or three nickel bags of cocaine. Core network members preferred to be "paid" in bags, ideally one of each. At the very least, they expected to share some of the drugs bought by the working injector who they helped. Many working injectors insisted on accompanying core network members back to the shooting gallery and sharing drugs despite the threat of HIV and other diseases that core network members so obviously carried with them and the increased risk of arrest associated with those locations. This was often motivated by their need to "get straight" before going to work but not wanting to inject inside their cars and/or their desire to hold the core network members accountable for the quality of the drugs whose purchase they facilitated or made.

The Newcomer with a Habit—Carmen Goes First

One day, when she woke up at about 7:15, it was already hot and sticky outside and the swarm of flies that buzzed around inside the gallery made it almost impossible to sleep much beyond sunup. Even though Carmen had been injecting for less than a year and was still a relative newcomer to the scene, as Louie's companion she spent many hours inside the gallery sharing drugs with others. As a result, she had developed a habit of more than a "bundle" a day, larger than many other local injectors could sustain. When her eyes opened, she immediately felt "dope sick," and the queasiness in the pit of her stomach was compounded by her being 5 months pregnant. Louie had anticipated her discomfort upon waking and had set aside a single bag of heroin for her to "get straight." Just as many Americans wake up to a cup of coffee, many injectors need a "wake-up" bag to get them going in the morning. But while the single bag of heroin would have been enough to stave off withdrawal symptoms, which is why they call it "getting straight" rather than getting "high," it would not have satisfied Carmen or made her feel "nice" in any fashion. To achieve that feeling, more heroin and cocaine would have been required. Louie could have left more for her, but he knew that since she was managing the gallery for the better part of the day, Carmen would receive many tastes from gallery customers, and thus would have ample opportunity to get "high."

Louie had run the gallery throughout the night, so when Carmen woke, he quickly went out to "hustle," even though he had not slept the night before. He was dressed in a pair of second-hand pants and in dirty sneakers with no socks. As hot as it promised to be, he left his shirt behind. To fortify himself for the streets, Louie prepared a final speedball before leaving the gallery. He grabbed a cooker from the counter and dumped a bag of heroin and a $5 bag of cocaine into it. He pulled a bag of about a dozen loose syringes out of his pants pocket and selected one to use. Dipping the syringe into the water bottle, he filled it with water and forcefully squirted it out against the wall. He wanted to make sure that it was not clogged. He then measured 40 cc of water into the syringe and squirted it into the bottle cap, stirring the powdered drugs and water with the needle. Holding the metal bottle cap between his thumb and forefinger, he passed a flame underneath it so quickly that the bottlecap barely had time to heat up. The barely dissolved solution was then sucked up through a tiny cotton ball that he had placed in the cooker. He then wrapped a belt around his biceps to make a vein bulge out and was ready to inject. Louie nearly always hit himself in the same place—a vein on the underside of his forearm, near the elbow. He later explained that even though he had been injecting for many years, he had only recently become able to do it himself. Before that, he had always relied on others to inject him. Inexperience with self-injection probably accounted for his reluctance to search for veins elsewhere. In any case, the single, bulging vein in his forearm showed signs of being overworked. The protruding vein had nodules that bumped up just under the skin and the caked-on, dried blood that seemed to always cover it made it look even uglier. With the belt tightened, Louie cocked his arm and plunged the needle into it. A plume of red immediately wafted up the barrel of the needle, a sign that he had successfully reached the vein and that the needle had not missed or gone completely through it. He pressed the plunger and injected the speedball. Without "booting" (drawing blood back into the syringe and then reinjecting it, which is done both to make sure all the drug is used up and also because many users find it pleasurable) the solution as might be the case if he were injecting at a more leisurely pace, he pulled the needle out and stuck it back into the plastic bag containing the other ones. It was his intention to head out to the buying areas on Troutman Street and sell the contents of the plastic bag.

Carmen had a bag of heroin to get straight, but wanted more. At that moment, Patricia came into the gallery with a bag of cocaine and Carmen asked her if she wanted to "do an angle." This was precisely the reason why Patricia had come into the gallery. She had already gotten straight earlier in the morning and she had a bag of cocaine left over. Patricia often injected straight cocaine, but she did not like to inject it on the street because it made her too paranoid and she would imagine her physically abusive ex-boyfriend standing behind every lamppost and street sign. So, Patricia decided to visit the gallery in hopes of finding someone to "throw down" on a speedball with her. If no one was willing to "do an angle," at least she would be able to inject the cocaine in the relative security of the gallery, where the presence of others would partially offset the paranoia she knew that she would experience. When Carmen offered to share with her, it was a good deal: Carmen would contribute the heroin (double the value of Patricia's cocaine), which Patricia was confident was a good bag (since Louie would be unlikely to leave a "dummy" bag), and she would not have to "pay the house" for using the premises, since Carmen was the house. Patricia quickly turned over her bag of cocaine to Carmen. Of course, given the arrangements, Patricia would have to go second, but that did not bother her, since the etiquette shared by core network injectors dictated that among peers the person who was "dope sick" should go first.

Carmen picked up a cooker from the line of neatly arranged bottlecaps laying on the serving board and placed it directly in front of her. She then picked up the bag of "two-way" brand heroin and ripped off the heat-sealed plastic bag cover with her teeth. As she unfurled the glassine envelope, she plumped open the bag and tapped it with her index finger to loosen up any particles of heroin that might be stuck inside the bag. She poured the entire contents of the bag into the cooker. Then she picked up the bag of cocaine and ripped it open with her teeth. Slowly, she tapped about three quarters of the contents of the bag into the cooker. Neither she nor Patricia wanted the cocaine to dominate the speedball and Patricia wanted to keep enough cocaine for a second injection a little later. The pinch that remained in the bag was returned to Patricia and she quickly stuck it in her flannel shirt pocket. Carmen poured a little water from a soda bottle into the bottle cap in front of her. She dipped the diabetic syringe into the water and sucked up a full barrel. As she listened to Patricia gossip about Jeanette, another gallery owner's wife who owed her money, Carmen squirted the water forcefully against the blanket that hung as a shade and concealed the room from street view. After mindlessly dipping and squirting twice, the syringe was "clean" and Carmen carefully measured out 40 cc and shot it in a circular fashion into the cooker holding the heroin and cocaine. She stirred the mixture quickly with the tip of the needle, and after placing the needle on the board in front of her, pulled two matches from a book and struck them on the back of the cover. As she held the cooker between her thumb and index finger, her hand visibly shook as she passed the flame underneath the bottlecap. It was hard to tell how much of the shaking was due to anxiety, withdrawal symptoms, or the cooker being too hot, but Carmen managed to heat the speedball without spilling any. She blew out the matches and threw them on the table and then carefully placed the cooker in front of her. Picking up the syringe, she dipped it into the cooker, pulled 30 cc into the barrel, and then holding the syringe with the tip pointing skyward, she thwacked the barrel with a finger to get out the remaining air bubbles. The tiny bit that remained in the cooker, 10 cc, was left behind for Patricia, who said that it constituted a taste and was a little more than a "G-shot." Given that she had only contributed part of a bag of cocaine to the speedball, in her opinion, she still made out well.

Another reason why Carmen was eager to find an injection partner like Patricia was because she could not inject herself. Patricia was skilled at injecting other people and she had often benefitted from this arrangement with Carmen by "getting straight" when she might otherwise have been "dope sick." Carmen had been "hit" in many places by others—arms, legs, and neck—but she seemed to prefer a vein on the top of her hand. She handed Patricia the filled syringe and extended her hand. As Patricia tapped the top of her hand trying to raise a vein, Carmen turned her head, not wanting to watch herself being injected. When the needle punctured the skin, Carmen began to recoil and pull her hand back. Patricia tightened her grip on Carmen's hand and told her, "Don't run away from me." But Carmen, feeling the pinch of the needle, continued to pull her arm away from Patricia. Finally, with the needle fully into a vein in the top of Carmen's hand, Patricia released her and said, "You're a punk." Patricia went on to explain that Carmen's recoiling was not simply caused by pain, but was also psychological: once the needle had arrived at its destination and was fully inserted, it often caused a little bulge on the top of the hand, especially once the barrel was released and the weight of the dangling syringe put pressure on it. The sight of her vein bulging out made Carmen fear that the needle might cut through the skin and pop out. But if Carmen was frightened by the prospect of the needle cutting through her hand, she made no attempt to remove it. Indeed, as the rush of the speedball took hold, her whole disposition changed. She now played with the plunger and pulled it back to about three quarters length so that the syringe was almost entirely filled with blood. And there it dangled for the next 10 minutes. Carmen, no longer shaking but now rendered speechless, pulled out a cigarette and stuck it in her mouth. As she struck a match, the syringe that dangled off the back of her hand jerked back and forth like a lance on a bull's bloody back. She smoked the cigarette without speaking. Listening to Patricia rattle on about her problems, Carmen played with the glass crack stem that she had stuck under her pant leg. When she was finished with the cigarette, she plucked the syringe out of her hand, quickly wiped off any blood on her hand, and placed the syringe on the counter, apparently unconcerned with its fate after that.

The Old-Timer with a Need—Patricia Gets Straight

Patricia gingerly picked up the cooker with her thumb and forefinger. Sitting on the edge of the bed, she was in no rush to inject the taste and she spent several minutes making small talk while activity in the gallery swirled on around her. Barney came up the stairs and started searching for a paper bag that he had stashed in a spot underneath the bed. The bag had several vials of crack inside and he was eager to get out on the corner and sell enough of them to get straight. When he could not find the bag and began to get a worried look on his face, Patricia stopped her conversation and pointed to a different place. Barney spotted the bag there, grabbed it, and headed down the stairs.

Patricia resumed her conversation with whomever was interested in listening. She described how she had gotten a 3-inch gash on the heel of her left foot 3 weeks earlier. She had been walking on Jefferson Street when a lady who lived on the block (who was a crack smoker herself) came out of a building and threw a rusty pipe at her. Patricia did not fully explain why the woman was angry, but simply said that the woman objected to her walking on the block. The pipe had sliced a deep cut on the inside of the heel and clearly would have required stitches if Patricia had gone to the hospital. But with no Medicaid coverage, bad prior experiences with medical staff at local hospitals, and fearing withdrawal pains should she be admitted, Patricia decided to forgo medical treatment and hope that it would heal by itself. Within days, however, the cut became infected. When she began to see little white eggs in the liquid coming out of the infected cut—maggot eggs—she walked to the emergency room at Wyckoff Heights Hospital. For some time she had not had any feeling in her foot, so the cut did not cause her much pain but the smell was enough to turn her stomach. Another injector who had served time in the Army told Patricia that the smell was similar to a dead body's. When she finally showed up at the emergency room, Patricia said that none of the emergency room personnel wanted to deal with her disgusting foot. One of the on-duty nurses gave her a bottle of hydrogen peroxide and a box of Q-tips and sent her to the bathroom to clean out the wound before she saw the doctor. Patricia said, "I'm scared of those worms. And to see them coming out of my foot, I almost died." But she did clean out the cut. Once she had swabbed it clean with the Q-tips and the doctor had inspected it, he decided that there was little he could do at that point. They told her to keep the area clean and well-ventilated and it would heal by itself. At that point, Patricia pulled off her sock and showed her foot to anyone in the gallery who was interested in looking. The cut was wide and deep, but there was no more sign of infection. After everyone was sufficiently grossed out, she slipped her sock and shoe back on and turned her attention to the taste still in the cooker.

Carmen had left only 10 cc in the cooker for Patricia to inject and most of it was absorbed into the tiny cotton ball that served to filter the solution as it was being drawn into the syringe. With her syringe, Patricia sucked up any liquid that remained in the bottom of the cooker and then picked up the cotton ball with her left hand. She expertly placed the needle tip in the center of the cotton ball and deftly pulled the plunger back, drawing out all the remaining liquid. This was a delicate operation that required careful hand–eye coordination, but Patricia had done it so many times that it had become routine. While she continued to carry on a conversation, she successfully manipulated the syringe and the cotton ball without even looking at them. She dropped the cotton ball to the floor and placed the cooker back on the counter. Putting the syringe between her teeth, she rolled up one pants leg and began to search for a vein on her pock-marked calf.

Since Patricia had been abused as child, she had ugly scars on her forearms and back from scalding water. As a result, she always wore long-sleeved shirts, even on the hottest day of the summer. She also had great difficulty finding a vein anywhere on her arms. The veins in her hands had long since been burned out through overuse. The only places where she could still find veins were her neck, groin, and calves. One reason why Patricia had tried to avoid the hospital was that they usually wanted to give her an IV upon admission, but medical staff had great difficulty finding a vein. Patricia refused to tell them where they might locate one, since she feared that her few remaining veins would be damaged by the hospital IV, and thus would be unavailable for injecting drugs. Hospital personnel often wanted to perform a "cut down," where the chest is cut open and a vein is pulled out for an IV. Patricia said that cut downs were quite painful and she wanted to avoid them unless it was absolutely necessary.

With her pants leg rolled up and her legs crossed, Patricia began feeling for a vein in her calf muscle with her thumb. After several minutes, thinking that she might have found one, Patricia prepared to inject herself. First, she licked her thumb and spread saliva over the spot where she would stick in the needle. When she had alcohol preps, she used them, but preps were a popular item that disappeared quickly from the gallery. With the syringe in her right hand and resting on her ankle, she fully inserted the needle upward, toward the knee, in the lower portion of her calf. When there was no seepage of blood into the barrel of the syringe Patricia knew that she had not found the vein she thought that she had felt. When I commented, "you missed," she shot back correcting me, "a miss is when you inject drugs into the muscle, missing or going completely through a vein." But she was clearly annoyed that she had not found the vein on her first try. Patricia pulled the needle out almost to the tip to try again. Bending the syringe at a different angle, she pushed the needle almost three quarters of the way into the muscle, but again found nothing and pulled it almost entirely out. On her third attempt, at yet another angle, Patricia bobbed the needle in and out of the muscle, hoping to find a small vein along the way. When a small droplet of blood appeared near the end of the barrel, she knew that she was close and she began to probe the area for a good connection. Still searching after several minutes, Patricia's fishing expedition with the needle looked—and was—quite painful. Each time she got close to the vein, a small trail of blood flowed into the barrel. After several strikes on the vein, the barrel became so clouded with blood that it was difficult to tell whether the needle was in the proper position. When she finally thought that the vein was penetrated by the needle, she used her thumb to tightly clamp the syringe to her leg so that it would not move. With her other hand, she slowly pushed the plunger down to the bottom and then withdrew it about half way. After about a minute, she pushed in what remained in the barrel and then pulled the syringe out of her calf. She placed the syringe back into her shirt pocket and sat there speechless for a couple of minutes.

At that point, several other injectors came up the stairs to use the premises. Among them was Barney, a core network member who often sold "works" and drugs for different owners, accompanied by a couple of working drug injectors who were in a rush to get off before work. Barney already had his syringe out. As he searched around for a cooker and water to hook up an injection, he placed the syringe in his mouth. With a bandanna around his head and a look of anxiety in his eye, Barney looked like pillaging pirate with a sword in his mouth.

Splitting the Difference

As the owner of one of the only shooting galleries in the neighborhood, Louie was always keen to extract payment for the use of the premises. He often boasted that he was able to inject more than 30 times per day, an injection pace he could only sustain by collecting tastes from his many customers. More often than not, he would inject with the customer, occasionally sharing a syringe, but more often dipping two syringes into a shared cooker or dividing the drugs by sprinkling powder from the bags into separate cookers. But Louie was not always ready to inject when the customer "cooked up." In those instances, the easiest way for him to secure his taste was to allow them to prepare the solution (liquid is easier to measure and divide than powder) and then divide it according to some agreed upon split. Generally, there were two ways to divide a solution of drugs. Less experienced injectors (like Carmen) would carefully draw up an amount of water into the syringe (usually 60 cc) and squirt it into the cooker. After adding the drugs and cooking the solution, some agreed-upon portion of the liquid would be drawn up into the first syringe and the cooker would be passed on to Louie. He would then draw up the remainder into his syringe, place caps on both ends of the syringe so that it could not get accidentally discharged, and then stash the syringe in some safe place until he was ready to use it.

Injectors who were more experienced at splitting drugs, like Louie's sometimes hustling partner, Barney, generally dispensed with all of the steps described above in favor of a faster way of equally dividing drugs: backloading. Backloading involves squirting solution directly from one syringe into another. Though it sounds easy to do, it is a delicate operation that requires skill and is not generally attempted by inexperienced injectors (Grund et al., 1996). If done carelessly, it can easily result in spillage, a fate even worse than a "miss."

When Barney entered the gallery on this morning he was both "dope sick" and in a rush to get outside and sell crack for his Dominican managers. He had agreed to do an "angle" with Louie, but as he climbed the stairs, he noticed that the room was already crowded and that there was no place for him to sit and prepare his mixture. He grabbed a cooker from the table and stuck it in a pocket. Then he dipped his syringe into one of the open bottles resting on the table, sucked up a full barrel of water, and walked through the curtain into an adjacent room. This room had been hard hit by the fire 6 months earlier and Louie and others had made no attempt to salvage it as a usable space. Indeed, much garbage from the room that had been converted into a gallery had been tossed into this adjacent room. Barney thus found himself standing ankle deep in half-burnt refuse with no stable place to prepare his injection. He placed the syringe between his teeth and pulled a Marlboro out of a half empty pack of cigarettes. Using his fingernails, he ripped out a small portion of the filter and balled it up. Then, with the tiny ball still between his fingers, he took out the bags of heroin and cocaine and tore them open. Tapping the drugs into the cooker, he tossed the empty bags onto the growing pile of garbage, took the syringe out of his mouth, squirted the water into the cooker, and after placing the syringe back into his mouth and dropping the tiny filter ball into the liquid, he quickly passed a small flame from a Bic lighter under the bottlecap pinched between his thumb and forefinger. Barney put the lighter back into his front pocket and stirred the warm solution with the tip of the needle stuck through the filter ball. When he was satisfied that the drugs had been completely dissolved, Barney began to draw up the speedball into the syringe. When he had sucked up all the visible liquid, he stuck the needle into the filter ball and pulled it out of the cooker, placed the cooker back into his pocket, and used the syringe to suck out every remnant of solution from the ball. With a barrel full of speedball in his right hand, he pulled out a second syringe, and with one hand popped the covers back into his pocket. He then pulled out the plunger and holding the barrel of the second syringe nearly horizontal to the floor, squirted half of the solution from the first syringe into the second. As solution entered the barrel of the second syringe, he gradually tipped up its opening to prevent any of the mixture from dripping out. The transfer of liquid from one syringe to the other took about 2 seconds. When he finished splitting the injection, Barney placed the first syringe back into his mouth and quickly but cautiously began to refit the plunger into the back of the second syringe. As soon as the rubber stopper on the plunger was firmly in place, the needle was pointed skyward and, as the barrel was continuously thwacked by his index finger to dislodge any air bubbles, the plunger was slowly inserted until all the air was forced out. He then fished out the needle cover from his pocket, covered the exposed tip, and walked into the main gallery room and gave Louie his portion. Louie placed the half-filled syringe into his shirt pocket; he would inject it later. At that point, Barney wrapped a belt about his biceps and proceeded to inject in the "pit" of his elbow.

The practice of backloading, which has been found to be a risk factor for prevalent HIV infection (Jose et al., 1993; Stark et al., 1996) and incident human T-lymphotropic virus type 2 (HTLV-2) infection (Vlahov et al., 1995), is not thought of as a form of "sharing," since two syringes are used in the process. For example, Jose often injected outside on the loading dock near the major drug selling block. Below, he recounts one event when he "did an angle" with another injector.

> I made enough money selling works to do an angle. An angle is, if you got a $7.50 and he got a 7.50, you put it together and get a one and one. I angled this with this old guy. I did a angle with him before and he's the type of person that if you put less money—let's say I only got $5 and he's got $10—we put together for the angle, he'll still go half and half.

> We went right there on Troutman and we shot up. We didn't have to wait because he had his works, and I had my works. So we didn't have to wait. All we had to do was prepare everything. It really don't make no difference [who goes first] because what we do is we'll draw up the whole thing and we see what's in the syringe and then we say, "what you want to do?" What we usually do is see how much is in there. Then you pull the plunger out and put your half in your syringe. Then you put your plunger. But you got to know what you're doing because if you don't do it right, you could lose your whole shot. You lose your whole shot, you gonna cry. And you gonna stay sick. Some guys don't know how to do it. Some will try, and what happens they wind up losing they whole Goddamn shot.

For many drug injectors, the practice of backloading was risky. A "better" way of splitting drugs and one that may carry as much HIV risk as backloading was measuring an amount of drugs in a single syringe and squirting some agreed-upon portion of it back into a cooker for the second person to draw up into their syringe. Louie explains how he usually shared drugs with other injectors.

> At four o'clock in the morning I got off in this friend's house. Well, the old man with his wife. They got off too; I gave them enough. I did my half of coke, and gave them theirs in the cooker, you know. I measured a 60 and gave them 20 apiece. I put it back into my cooker and they picked it up with their needle. That's the way we always do it.

Banging in the Street: Patricia Takes a Chance

By 2 PM, Patricia was feeling "dope sick." Her last injection—a speedball— had been early in the morning in Louie's shooting gallery and its effects were rapidly fading. Walking up and down Irving Avenue in the wilting July sun with $8 in her pocket, Patricia was wondering how to scrape together another $7 to buy a "one and one" and tide herself over until the evening when she could get straight through her own hustling (either working the stroll or acting as a drug market functionary) or through the largess of another injector. The middle of the afternoon was a slow time for her: The commercial sex stroll was very slow, and she thought that her blackness and injection scars made her less competitive than the women who were full-time sex workers during daylight hours. Occasionally during afternoon hours she had an opportunity to accompany injectors with regular hustles like stealing cases of soda or "boosting" cosmetics from drug stores in other neighborhoods, but these chances were irregular and often involved being out of the neighborhood for extended periods of time. She also sometimes sold drugs for a variety of organizations, but today was not one of those occasions. Feeling nauseous, she hoped that if she patrolled the corner that served as the gateway to the main drug-selling area long enough, an opportunity to "get straight" would present itself.

While she was standing near the corner, several core network members ambled by, but none of them were in a position to help her. After about 20 minutes, she spotted Madeline hobbling down the street with her feet pinched into a pair of tight high heels. Madeline, a full-time Puerto Rican sex worker, had just come from a "date," and she was on her way to buy. Patricia met her potential meal ticket at the corner and they talked for a few minutes about what dope was "kickin' " on Troutman Street. Madeline's intention was to buy a few bags of heroin and cocaine and several vials of crack and then head to Tino's apartment to kick back and relax. Patricia, however, would receive a chilly reception from Tino, a 74-year-old Puerto Rican crack smoker who disliked black injectors, and today she could not afford to "pay" Tino for using his apartment to get off. If she was going to get straight this afternoon, it would have to be in the street. Patricia mentioned the $5 Madeline had borrowed several days earlier when she needed a hit of crack. Madeline pulled a wrinkled five dollar bill from inside her tiny pocketbook, handed it to Patricia, and continued down the street in search of the good bag.

Patricia now had $13, but needed $2 more to buy the components for a speedball. The cocaine she regularly bought was sold by Dominicans on Jefferson Street who were notorious for not "taking shorts" (accepting less than full payment). There was only one place where the competition and the large volume of business sometimes led distributors to take "shorts," especially when requested by core network members who might later return the favor by bringing by a lucrative customer. Patricia speculated that she could find a "pitcher" on Troutman who would sell her a bag of heroin for $9, but not $8. She needed one more dollar. Finally, after another 20 minutes of scuffing at the dirt on the corner, she spotted Jerry walking up the block from the subway. He had just finished his daily round of panhandling and selling newspapers on the L train and was on his way to cop. Patricia was one of Jerry's frequent injection partners and, knowing his routine, she immediately felt a sense of relief. She asked him if he wanted to "do an angle" and he agreed to meet her in the middle of the block on Jefferson Street in 5 minutes after both of them had bought their drugs.

Patricia bought a bag of heroin on Troutman Street while Jerry went to Knickerbocker to buy several nickel bags of cocaine and a bag of heroin. Patricia also picked up a small plastic juice bottle from the gutter, rinsed it out in a fire hydrant that was leaking water, filled the bottle with clean water, and walked down to Jefferson Street to set up the spot for Jerry. Many users injected openly on the sidewalk there because there was nothing but factories and pedestrian traffic was light. Yeti, a Puerto Rican injector who limped around the neighborhood with a flattened foot, often erected an outdoor shooting gallery made from discarded cardboard boxes on this block, but police officers customarily ran through it with their patrol cars, strewing injection materials all over the sidewalk and street. When Patricia walked onto Jefferson Street it was empty; the remnants of Yeti's gallery stretched half way down the block. She sat down in the middle of the block—the best spot to have maximum warning of anyone who might come around the corner while she was shooting up—and began to set up. Jerry arrived a few minutes later, sweating profusely from the heat, humidity, and anticipation.

Though she had asked him to do an angle, she realized that he did not need her to get straight and it was not necessary for her to share her bag of heroin with him. She put out separate cookers because she did not want to inject as much cocaine as he normally preferred (two bags of cocaine to one of heroin). They emptied the contents of their bags into their respective cookers and Jerry gave a half a bag of cocaine to Patricia to add to hers. After quickly waving a flame underneath each cooker, they each drew up into the separate syringes that they had carried with them. Patricia had brought a single syringe, but Jerry had more than a dozen stashed in a small pouch tied around his waist. Since Jerry had done her the favor of helping get her straight, Patricia knew that she was obliged to hit him first. She probably would have done it anyway, since that had often been their routine when they injected together. Jerry puffed out his cheeks and when the vein bulged out she plunged the needle into it. In two seconds it was over and she quickly pulled it out. Jerry immediately went into convulsions and writhed around on the sidewalk like an epileptic having a grand mal seizure. Patricia ignored him and went about her business. When they first became injection partners, his behavior alarmed her: She thought that he was overdosing and was going to die. But after witnessing his reaction to megadoses of cocaine on several occasions, she came to expect his rather bizarre reaction and was not so troubled by it. She quickly rolled up her right pants leg and searched for a vein. She was in a rush to find one, since Jerry's writhing might attract the attention of the police or other injectors. Fortunately, it did not take long, so she quickly poked the needle into place. As soon as she emptied the contents of the barrel, she pulled out the syringe and put it back into her pocket. Rolling down her pants leg, she looked up and down the block to see if anyone was watching her; she no longer felt "dope sick," but the cocaine had increased her paranoia. The police were now the least of her worries; she began to see her ex-boyfriend, Tommy, behind every lamppost and dumpster. She had to get out of there. Jerry was still flopping around on the sidewalk when she walked away in the direction of the park.

Hit Doctors and Hidden Spots

When injectors did not want to share drugs with others and/or wanted to inject at their own pace, which in the case of older injectors is often quite slow, they looked for secluded locations. Some had homes where this could be done. Others were homeless, lived far from the drug scene, or lived in circumstances where they could not use drugs at home. Unless they had access to a shack or other structure, such injectors usually looked for a private spot in an existing building. One such location was inside a three-story sheet metal factory located two blocks from the main drug-selling strip. Its single entrance was always open during the day. It led to a staircase separated from the factory floor by heavy steel doors. Drug injectors would walk up the stairs to a concrete landing just before the door to the roof. The concrete landing was big enough for two people to spread out their equipment. The factory was noisy, so injectors did not generally have to worry about making too much noise, but because workmen occasionally walked between the lower floors, it was impossible to have much traffic in the stairwell without risking discovery. Thus, the spot at the top of the stairs remained relatively private, and injectors who sometimes used the stairwell to inject knew that they were unlikely to be disturbed.

Around 11 AM one July morning, Patricia ran into Bruce near the corner of Starr Street and Irving Avenue. A day earlier, Bruce had been operating an outdoor shooting gallery in an empty lot surrounded by a chain link fence on Starr Street, directly across from the sheet metal factory. He and Mano, a dark-skinned Panamanian injector, had "owned" the gallery for about 2 months. It had become quite popular as a place where people could pop in for a quick injection. Not only was it conveniently located (between the buying spots and the subway), but there were usually injectors hanging out there who were proficient "hit doctors" and for a taste would quickly help others find a vein. But its popularity had attracted the attention of police. On several occasions during the previous month, officers had smashed up the hastily pieced together boxes and plastic canopies that sheltered participants from the elements and from view. The police finally became tired of seeing the gallery being easily reconstructed after they knocked it down. Mano reported that the cops woke him up after midnight and told him to get out of the lot. As he watched from the sidewalk, an officer poured gasoline on the gallery and struck a match. When the fire department came and doused the fire, their water destroyed everything that was not already ruined.

Bruce had become accustomed to a certain level of morning business (several tastes), so when that business suddenly disappeared, he felt sick. Patricia happened by, already aware of what had happened to his gallery. She had just come from hustling and had a "two and one" (two bags of heroin, one of cocaine), enough for both of them to get straight. Since Bruce was so obviously dope sick, she felt obliged to get him straight. And since she had such great difficulty hitting herself, she knew that he would be more than happy to hit her in the neck, something that he had done many times before.

Bruce and Patricia tried to look inconspicuous as they opened the factory door and crept up the stairs. When they reached the landing at the top of the stairwell they sat down, took things out of their pockets, and placed them on the cement among the existing clutter of empty heroin bags, crack vials, cookers, empty soda bottles, candy wrappers, and so on. They contributed even more to the growing pile. (This mess contradicted their long-term need for privacy, since it would eventually attract factory workers' attention.) When Patricia pulled the bags of drugs from her pockets, Bruce had a look of desperation in his eye. She let him prepare the mixture and go first. He carefully ripped open both bags of heroin and dumped them into the cooker followed by the bag of cocaine. Then he took a Newport cigarette from his pocket and ripped the filter from the end. Tearing the paper off of the filter, he pinched a small amount of the fibrous filter between his fingers, rolled it into a small ball and tossed it into the cooker. Next he took a syringe from his pocket, dipped it into the small water bottle that Patricia handed to him, and measured out about 60 cc of water. He squirted the water into the cooker and stirred the mixture with the tip of the needle. Patricia passed him a Bic lighter and he passed the flame under the cooker while holding it between his fingers. Placing the cooker on the cement, he measured out 30 cc into his syringe and immediately searched for a vein in his "pit" at the crook of the elbow. Bruce soon found a vein, and within a minute he had a much relieved look on his face. While he was hooking himself up, Patricia picked up the cooker and drew the rest of the liquid into her syringe through the filter. Then she held the syringe at eye level and tapped it with her index finger to be sure all the air bubbles were out of the barrel. Then she handed it to Bruce and prepared for him to hit her in the neck. Turning down her shirt collar slightly, she cocked her head to the side, placed her thumb in her mouth and blew as hard as she could. Her cheeks puffed out like Dizzy Gillespie blowing the trumpet and within seconds, a large vein on her neck bulged out. Needing to act before she ran out of air and the vein disappeared, Bruce stood up and with his hand resting on her jawline and the needle pointing down, he rapidly tapped it into her vein. Blood immediately surged into the barrel of the syringe and he quickly pushed down the plunger. In a matter of seconds the entire procedure was over. For Patricia, this method of administration was clearly superior to the painful and extensive poking and probing she endured when hitting herself.

AIDS TALK IN INJECTION SETTINGS

Conversations that took place at injection settings were remarkably uni-dimensional. Almost invariably, they were either directly related to injecting or about hustling money to buy more drugs. Seldom did we hear injectors talk about anything but those topics, and we never heard them talk about AIDS in these settings, except to comment that someone looked particularly bad (with the implication that they might not make the best injection partner) or in the process of urging someone to seek medical attention. Indeed, the lack of any other type of conversation in injection settings led several injectors to seek out the ethnographers and request another interview. At first, we thought they were looking to hustle us for a few dollars, but they explained that the interviews had been their first opportunity in years to have a "real conversation" about something other than using drugs or hustling money and they realized that this was a feature of "normal" life that they had sorely missed. (Of course, this "isolation" is true for only a minority of drug injectors, usually those most heavily immersed in the drug scene.) Such a drug injector's first ethnographic interview was often a great emotional release, so we kept a box of tissue on the desk. But while these interviews allowed them to momentarily revisit their former lives, the streets, shooting galleries, and other injection locales offered few opportunities for intimacy and honesty.

Shooting galleries were about using drugs, not scaring people away from them. It seemed to be an unwritten rule that AIDS risk would not be discussed unless someone was about to unwittingly use potentially infected equipment. Even then, most injectors we observed and talked with said that such warnings were seldom heeded. A few members of the core network, including Louie, admitted that they did not notify injection partners that they might be infected with the virus. Louie reasoned that he was not sure that he had the virus, so he felt no obligation to say anything. This may be one reason why he never picked up his SFHR test results: To know with certainty that he was HIV positive would cement his moral obligation and make it harder to live in silence.

Most injectors said that they had serious discussions about HIV/AIDS only in private, one-on-one settings. These sessions usually seemed more about commiserating than changing risk behaviors. In the following excerpt, Cathy talks about how and when she and Gus revealed their statuses to each other. Though the text of their conversation was filled with supportive language—and such conversations did reinforce them in some ways—and voiced knowledge of appropriate injection etiquette, the subtext was that they both knew that neither was going to change their behavior.

> We're both HIV positive. So we're using our own works. You see, everybody who's HIV positive feels like we can share each others' works cause we're all gonna die together. But I believe that we can also be harmful to each other like if one has a cold, and I don't, you can give me something that maybe I can't handle. So, you know, I'm not with that just 'cause we both are HIV positive we can, you know, do this. I think Gus thinks this way too; we've discussed it. When Gus found out he was HIV positive, he told me. He told me about 2 weeks after he found out. One day I saw him sittin' right on Irving and Troutman, on the steps, and he was sittin', you know, like just looking. And I said, "Gus what's up?" And he said, "Oh nothing." "Don't bullshit me. What's up?" And he said, "Blondie, I'm HIV positive." And I said, "Oh wow," and right away I said, "it's not the end of the world. Everything will be all right." He reacted just like I did. And he said, "I know, but wow." And we sat and we talked about it, and then 2 weeks later I came up HIV positive. So I went and told him, and he gave me the same line back. And I said, "Does this sound familiar." We kind of supported each other. Just the other day we had a talk about cleaning up and getting on the methadone program and start eating right, living right. And listening to me, he's saying, "You know, you're right." Shortly after that, he went into a detox and came out feeling great. He came out last week and he's already lookin' shriveled up a little. I told him, you know, I said, "It doesn't make any sense, you know." We had the talk like 2 or 3 days after he came out. And I said, "You're lookin' great, you're feelin' great. Stay like that, you know. This is how you're gonna live a long time." And he said, "Blondie, everything you're saying, take it to heart for yourself." And I said, "Damn, Gus, I should take my own advice." And that was the manner I started kickin' it with him. These are things I've learned that I

get from my mother. When somebody's feeling down, I learned how to make them laugh. And then he went to shoot a bag of coke. So my whole conversation went down the tubes.

Thus, as is also discussed quantitatively in later chapters, considerable high-risk behavior continues, particularly in the "core" of the drug scene. Looked at day by day, risk seems constant. Over the longer view, however, change has occurred. Syringe sharing takes place much less frequently now than it used to, for example. Drug injectors' norms now incorporate the value of not sharing syringes. Shortly after we told drug injectors in Bushwick that we were finding a relationship between backloading and HIV infection, the popularity of this practice waned.

The drug scene also seems to have changed in the way in which it initiates new members into injecting. There has been a marked decrease in the extent to which syringes and other injection equipment are shared "the very first time." This is the subject of the next chapter.

4

The Very First Hit

with *KATHERINE A. ATWOOD*

INTRODUCTION

As discussed in the previous chapter, there seems to have been a steep decline in the extent to which syringes are shared the first time a person injects. Little is known about how and why this has occurred, and this is the topic of the current chapter. In many ways, this chapter provides a transition for the volume. The previous two chapters discussed drug injectors' lives primarily using ethnographic data. In this chapter, we look at the beginning of their lives as drug injectors, with a strongly quantitative focus (although integrating in ethnographic data as well).

Despite extensive research on the relationship between drug injection practices and HIV transmission, remarkably little is known about the first injection event (Crofts, Louie, Rosenthal, & Jolley, 1996; Neaigus, Friedman, Stepherson, Jose, & Sufian, 1991; Rosenbaum, 1981). Qualitative research suggests that the first injection is a defining moment in a drug user's career, when he or she transitions from the social identity of a "drug user" to "drug addict" (Rosenbaum, 1981). The actual event, however, can sometimes be surprisingly unplanned (Friedman et al., 1989a). Friedman and co-workers suggest that new users tend not to have their own injection equipment and often borrow from a friend or relative at first injection.

Clearly, the first injection and early stages of an injection drug user's (IDU's) career present critical opportunities for intervention. Each new initiate is a potential AIDS case and potential transmitter of other blood-borne pathogens (Friedman, Doherty, Paone, & Jose, 1994b). Yet HIV prevention programs, such as syringe exchange, have difficulty reaching new users (Lart & Stimson, 1990; Lurie, Reingold, & Bowser, 1993). Interventions tend to reach moderate to long-term injectors, which can be after they have engaged in high-risk practices or become entrenched in high-risk networks. An informed understanding of the behaviors and network features of initiation could help to delay the transition to injection drug use or promote low-risk injection behaviors early in an IDU's career, when there is a greater likelihood of preventing HIV infection.

BACKGROUND AND SIGNIFICANCE

Before the AIDS epidemic, researchers documented the rise in parenterally acquired diseases (Cherubin, 1967; Minkin & Cohen, 1967). They acknowledged that these diseases were often caused by the sharing of nonsterile syringes, but few studies documented the prevalence and nature of these behaviors. To the extent that researchers studied drug initiations, they focused on the introduction to specific drugs rather than specific routes of drug administration. Many of these studies suggested gender power imbalances (Rosenbaum, 1979, 1981) and different trajectories for men and women from initiation, to addiction, and to subsequent recovery (Eldred & Washington, 1976; Rosenbaum, 1979, 1981). Women were reported to be introduced into illicit drugs by the opposite sex (Eldred & Washington, 1976; Freeland & Campbell, 1973; Prather & Fidell, 1978; Rosenbaum, 1979), particularly a sex partner (Binion, 1982), while men were generally initiated by male peers (Binion, 1982; Rosenbaum, 1979). Women, however, are not passive about their first use, often requesting it themselves (Hser, Anglin, & McGlothlin, 1987; Rosenbaum, 1979). Once addicted, many women lack the social and economic resources to move from addiction to subsequent recovery (Binion, 1982; Ellinwood, Smith, & Vaillant, 1966; Freeman, Rodriguez, & French, 1994).

Recent studies of trends in routes of drug administration (De la Fuente et al., 1996; Des Jarlais, Casriel, Friedman, & Rosenblum, 1992; Friedman, 1996; Griffiths, Gossop, Powis, & Strang, 1992; Griffiths, Gossop, Powis, & Strang, 1994; Hartgers, van den Hoek, Krijnen, van Brussel, & Coutinho, 1991; Neaigus et al., 1997; Strang, Des Jarlais, Griffiths, & Gossop, 1992a; Strang, Griffiths, Powis, & Gossop, 1992b) suggest that over time drug users shift back and forth from noninjection to injection drug use. Behavioral and structural factors affecting these shifts may include the impact of the AIDS epidemic on knowledge and behavior; the price and purity of street drugs; pharmacy laws restricting syringe access; and the need to reduce withdrawal effects (Strang et al., 1992a). Working with heroin sniffers to prevent the transition to drug injection, our research team found that having a close personal relationship with a current injector and the frequency of noninjection drug use were associated with subsequent injection (Des Jarlais et al., 1992).

A few studies describing the first injection event compare behaviors of recent initiates to the behaviors of those who initiated in the past. They found that the proportion who shared needles at first injection (Neaigus et al., 1991) or in the first 3 months of use (Vlahov, Anthony, Celentano, Solomon, & Chowdhury, 1991a) has declined over time.

This chapter offers further evidence of declining trends in high-risk injection practices at initiation but suggests that these declines began before the HIV/AIDS epidemic. Declines in high-risk behavior at first injection were evident as far back as the 1970. They may have occurred in response to non-HIV/AIDS injection-related morbidity and mortality. These declines continued and became more pronounced throughout the HIV/AIDS era. It is likely that they have been intensified by AIDS-related normative and behavior change.

To provide a historical context for these behavioral trends, we focus on three critical periods: before the emergence of HIV-1, during its rapid rise in seroprevalence, and during its subsequent stabilization. We document that parenterally acquired diseases were an object of study and concern by the medical community long before the HIV/AIDS epidemic. We propose that IDUs adopted safe injection practices in response to the devastating toll that injection drug use had on their lives. In this chapter, descriptive characteristics of the high-risk behaviors and network features of first injection are presented for each time period and placed within the context of what was known about injection-related diseases and the behaviors of drug injectors.

STUDY DESIGN

Two sources of data provide our information regarding the first injection. The primary source is a questionnaire administered to 767 participants of the Social Factors and HIV Risk Study (SFHR). (The methods of subject recruitment and a general description of the sociodemographic, behavioral, and other characteristics of this sample are presented later in Chapters 5 and 6). In a section on participants' first injection, the survey asks them to recall the drug setting, drug(s) injected, and the social, behavioral, and network characteristics of their first injection (described as injecting into a vein). Subjects were asked about other people present at first injection, including their demographic characteristics, injection behaviors, and social relationships to the initiate.

The supplementary source of data is in-depth interviews with 29 active injection drug users who both participated in the SFHR study and provided personal histories of their first injection experience. In this chapter we limit our analyses to the 738 IDUs who responded to questions about their first injection, including the year in which it occurred. We use the in-depth interviews to illustrate the dynamics of first injection and to add meaning and context to our statistical findings.

ANALYTIC METHODS

Quantitative data from this cross-sectional, retrospective study were collected from 1991 to 1993. The first injection event, however, could have occurred

Table 1. Calendar Periods of First Injection

Calender period of initiation	Sample population	
	Number	Percent
≤1968	138	19
1969–1974	161	21
1975–1978	78	11
1979–1983	118	16
1984–1987	105	14
1988–1992	138	19
Total	738	100

any time in the past. To account for this variation in calendar time, subjects were initially divided into six groups (≤ 1968; 1969–1974; 1975–1978; 1979–1983; 1984–1987; 1988–1992) (Table 1) by the year when they first injected drugs. Downward trends in high-risk behaviors at first injection were assessed and piecewise regression analysis was conducted to assess whether the rate of decline changed over specific calendar periods.

Based on the year of initiation, the data were then redivided into three broader time periods [pre-HIV (≤1974); HIV spread (1975–1983); HIV stabilization (1984–1992)]. As can been seen in Table 2, these periods correspond to the spread of injection-related diseases such as hepatitis in the early 1970s (≤1974); the emergence and rapid spread of HIV-1 among injection drug users (1975–1983); and its subsequent stabilization (Des Jarlais et al., 1989b) and (at the end of the period) beginning of decline (1984–1992) (Friedman et al., 1997b). The use of these three calendar periods both provides a useful historical context and also allows sufficient numbers for stratified statistical analysis. For each time period, the injection drug use research is discussed and descriptive statistics of initiation are presented. Quotations from IDUs who recalled initiating in each calendar period are included to contextualize research findings.

It is not enough, however, simply to look at overall trends in high-risk behaviors at initiation. Other things were going on that could confuse the issue. For example, the proportion in the sample who are women IDUs who first injected after 1983 (43%) is much greater than the proportion during the pre-HIV period (16% were women), and the proportion of initiates who are Latino also increased. Thus, to take such changes and others into account, we used stratified analysis and logistic regression techniques to identify significant predictors of high-risk injection practices at initiation, limiting the analysis to those who initiated in the company of other people. Those who initiated alone represented 7% of the study population (51/738). Of those 51 initiates, 5 responded that they had shared a

Table 2.   Calendar Periods and Parenterally Acquired Infection

Calendar period of initiation	Initiates during each calendar periods		Hepatitis and HIV infection rates in New York City
	Number	Percent	
≤1974	299	40	Pre-HIV: 70% of a sample of methadone maintenance clients had markers for hepatitis B[a]
1975–1983	196	27	HIV infection and rapid spread: 58–71% of drug treatment entrants testing positive for hepatitis B antibodies Suggested introduction of HIV-1 to IDUs in 1975 or 1976[b] First AIDS case diagnosed among IDUs (1981) Rapid spread of HIV infection [1978–1981 (< 20 to 50%)][b]
1984–1992	243	33	Stabilization and initial decline: No increase in observed seroprevalence form 1984 to 1987 in treatment samples[b] Stabilization of HIV-1 seroincidence between 55 and 60% (1984–1987)[b] 91% of a sample of methadone maintenance clients had markers for hepatitis B[c] Legal syringe exchange programs implemented in NYC (1991) Initial decline in HIV incidence (1991–1992)[d]

[a]Stimmel et al. (1973).
[b]Des Jarlais et al. (1989).
[c]Novick et al. (1990).
[d]Friedman et al. (1997b).

syringe with other people, perhaps because they had access to a used syringe and then injected with it when they were alone or considered themselves alone, although they were in a setting with other people. These 51 were excluded from the multivariate analysis. Likelihood ratio tests were conducted to assess goodness of fit (p value < 0.05) (Agresti, 1990).

RESULTS

Over time, there were substantial changes in the demographic characteristics of the study population at initiation. When stratifying by the six calendar periods, we found significant increases in the percentage of women and Latino initiates and

Percent

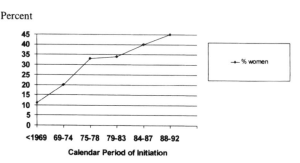

Calendar Period of Initiation

Figure 1. Percentage of initiates during each calendar period who were women.

significant declines in the percentage of African Americans (Figs. 1 and 2). Age of first injection also increased over time for both men (from 17 before 1969 to 26 for 1988–1992) and women (from 16 to 29), although shifts in age may be artifacts of the study design.*

In addition to changes in the demographic characteristics of first injection, we found significant downward trends over time in the receptive sharing of syringes, cookers, and cotton–rinse water at first injection [all $p < 0.001$; Mantel-Haenszel (MH) χ^2 test for trend]. As can been seen in Fig. 3, these high-risk behaviors began to decline before the first AIDS case was diagnosed in 1981. Receptive syringe sharing at initiation declined from about 70% before 1969 to 35% by 1978 to 10% by 1992. Downward trends in sharing are found in each racial–ethnic and age group (data not shown). Women, when compared to men, were less likely to share at initiation (Fig. 4).

The dominant drug of first injection was heroin (Fig. 5) in each calendar period. The drug that was injected, however, was not related to the probability of receptive syringe sharing (data not shown).

These data suggest that declining trends in receptive syringe sharing emerged long before the HIV/AIDS epidemic. Efforts to protect new users from other diseases might have been one reason why.

To further explore these behavioral trends, we recombined calendar periods into three broader time periods as outlined in Table 2 [pre-HIV (< 1975); HIV spread (1975–1983); and HIV stabilization (1984–1992)]. For each time period, we

*The cross-sectional retrospective design of this study may have made it less likely that those who were older and initiated in the past were included in the sample (since they might have been likely to have died before the start of the study). In addition, the eligibility criteria of the study prevented the inclusion of anyone < 18 years of age. Therefore, young initiates, who initiated in the more recent time period, would not be included in the study sample. The effects of these two factors may have created the appearance of an increase in the age of initiation over time.

Percent

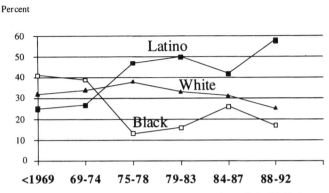

Figure 2.   Racial distribution during each calendar period of initiation.

describe the injection drug research, quantitative analysis from the survey and personal histories from in-depth interviews.

Pre-HIV (Calendar Period 1: 1955–1974)

Social and Behavioral Features of First Injection

During this pre-HIV era (1955–1974), tremendous attention was brought to bear on the emerging "drug epidemic" even before returning Vietnam veterans were found to have substantial heroin and opium addictions (Clayton & Voss, 1981; O'Donnell, 1965). By the mid-1960s, medical studies were documenting the rising morbidity and mortality associated with drug use (Cherubin, 1967; Cherubin & Sapira, 1993; Helpern & Rho, 1966; Ramsey, Gunnar, & Tobin, 1970; Thorton & Thorton, 1974). The sharing of nonsterile syringes often caused fatal medical

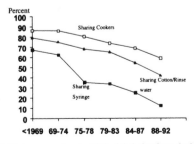

Figure 3.   Percentage of initiates engaging in high-risk behaviors during each calendar period of initiation.

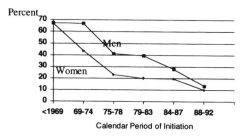

Figure 4.   Receptive syringe sharing at first injection, stratified by gender.

complications including tetanus, bacterial pneumonia, skin abscesses, cellulitis, and viral hepatitis (Cherubin, 1967; Louria, Hensle, & Rose, 1967; Minkin & Cohen, 1967). In response to these findings, researchers called for medical services to be integrated into drug treatment programs (Cherubin, 1967; Thorton & Thorton, 1974). By the 1970s, the prevalence of hepatitis B was used as an indicator of increases in injected heroin use (Rittenhouse, 1977) and needle sharing (White, 1973). Drug treatment studies found that up to 70% of heroin clients had markers for hepatitis B by 1970 (Stimmel, Vernace, & Heller, 1973). Although few studies measured the prevalence of syringe sharing before the AIDS era, a hepatitis-oriented study of drug treatment centers in Washington, DC, found that 70% of its IDU population shared syringes in 1974 (Seeff et al., 1975).

As described in earlier chapters, the Bushwick drug scene was much more clandestine during the pre-AIDS era than it was during the SFHR study period. Drug purchasing took place in specific indoor locations such as bars, bodegas, pool halls, and apartments and through personal connections to a drug dealer.

Quantitative Data on First Injection

During this period, our data reveal that initiations occurred within small networks of people (mean network size = 1.8) (Table 3). Initiates were overwhelmingly men (84%) who were "initiated" or helped to inject by male friends or

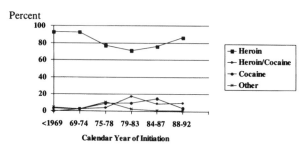

Figure 5.   Drug injected during each calendar period of initiation.

Table 3.   Social and Behavioral Features of the First Injection Sample, Stratified by Calendar Period of Initiation

	Pre- HIV ≤ 1974 (n = 299) n (%)	HIV-Spread 1975–83 (n = 196) n (%)	HIV stabilization 1984–1992 (n = 243) n (%)	Total (n = 738) n (%)
Male	252 (84)	130 (66)	139 (57)	521 (71)
Age of first injection in a vein	17 (15–19)[a]	20 (17–23)[a]	26 (22–29)[a]	21 (17–25)[a]
Population				
Men	17	20	25	20
Women	17	21	27	23
Race–ethnicity				
Latino	77 (26)	96 (49)	124 (51)	297 (40)
White	98 (33)	69 (35)	68 (28)	235 (32)
Black	119 (40)	29 (15)	50 (21)	198 (27)
Other	5 (1)	2 (1)	1 (0)	8 (1)
Total	299 (100)	196 (100)	.243 (100)	738 (100)
Egocentric network size	1.8 (1–2)[a]	1.5 (1–2)[a]	1.3 (1–2)[a]	1.6 (1–2)[a]
Population				
Men	1.8	1.6	1.2	1.6
Women	1.5	1.5	1.3	1.4
Social relationship with initiator[b]				
Men				
Male relative	22 (11)	10 (9)	17 (17)	49 (12)
Female lover/spouse	1 (−)	6 (5)	4 (4)	11 (3)
Male friend	156 (79)	76 (66)	59 (60)	291 (71)
Female friend	8 (4)	12 (10)	9 (9)	29 (7)
Other	11 (5)	11 (10)	9 (9)	31 (7)
Total	198 (100)	115 (100)	98 (100)	411 (100)
Women				
Male relative	2 (6)	2 (3)	2 (3)	6 (4)
Male lover/spouse	15 (42)	19 (32)	24 (35)	58 (35)
Male friend	7 (19)	16 (27)	13 (19)	36 (22)
Female friend	5 (14)	12 (20)	25 (36)	42 (26)
Other	7 (19)	10 (17)	5 (7)	22 (13)
Total	36 (100)	59 (100)	69 (100)	164 (100)
Feeling close/very close to initiator[b]				
Female initiator				
Men	9 (75)	17 (77)	9 (64)	35 (73)
Women	7 (88)	15 (83)	19 (73)	41 (79)
Male initiator				
Men	139 (75)	69 (74)	52 (62)	260 (71)
Female	23 (82)	28 (70)	32 (76)	83 (75)

[a]Interquartile range.
[b]Denominator is the number of men or women who helped/initiated the new user for each calendar period.

Table 4.   Drug Setting of the First Injection Sample,
Stratified by Calendar Period of Initiation

Drug setting of initiation	<1975 (n = 298) n (%)	1975–1983 (n = 196) n (%)	1984–1992 (n = 240) n (%)	Total (n = 733)[a] n (%)
Friend's home	131 (44)	75 (38)	75 (31)	281 (38)
Men	117 (47)	53 (41)	42 (31)	212 (41)
Women	14 (30)	22 (34)	33 (32)	69 (32)
Own home	52 (17)	43 (22)	82 (34)	177 (24)
Men	37 (15)	20 (15)	39 (28)	96 (19)
Women	15 (32)	23 (35)	43 (42)	81 (38)
Outdoor location/abandoned building	43 (14)	18 (9)	28 (12)	89 (12)
Men	39 (16)	16 (12)	22 (16)	77 (15)
Women	4 (9)	2 (3)	6 (6)	12 (6)
Shooting gallery	13 (4)	15 (8)	10 (4)	38 (5)
Men	10 (4)	9 (7)	5 (4)	24 (5)
Women	3 (6)	6 (9)	5 (5)	14 (7)
Other	59 (20)	45 (23)	45 (19)	149 (21)
Men	48 (19)	33 (26)	29 (21)	110 (21)
Women	11 (24)	12 (19)	16 (16)	39 (18)
Total	298 (100)	196 (100)	240 (100)	734 (100)
Men	251 (100)	131 (100)	137 (100)	519 (100)
Women	47 (100)	65 (100)	103 (100)	215 (100)

[a]Missing (n = 1).

relatives (Table 3). The mean age of first injection was 17, with half of this young, male population injecting in a friend's home (Table 4). The most common reason men offered for why they first injected was because their friends did (Table 5), concurrent with substance abuse research suggesting that peer influence plays a substantial role in young men's drug involvement (Binion, 1982; Kandel, 1973, 1985).

Approximately 70% of male initiates, yet only 50% of female initiates, receptively shared a syringe at first injection (Table 6). The sharing of cookers, cotton, and/or rinse water, which placed new initiates at additional risk for blood-borne infections, were even more widespread for both men and women (Table 6). Water was the primary method of cleaning syringes, presumably to unclog the syringe for the next injector (Table 6).

Qualitative Data on First Injection

Interviews with IDUs who initiated during this period reflect a male-dominated injection drug scene, with male peers involved in the initiation process.

Table 5. Reasons for Starting to Inject Drugs,
Stratified by Calendar Period of Initiation

Reasons mentioned for starting to inject[a]	<1975 (n = 298) n (%)	1975–1983 (n = 195) n (%)	1984–1992 (n = 238) n (%)	Total (n = 731)[a] n (%)
Curious to try	100 (34)	87 (45)	78 (33)	265 (36)
Men	84 (33)	64 (49)	47 (35)	195 (38)
Women	16 (34)	23 (35)	31 (30)	70 (32)
My friend(s) did it	126 (42)	63 (32)	53 (22)	242 (33)
Men	115 (46)	48 (37)	32 (24)	195 (38)
Women	11 (23)	15 (23)	21 (21)	47 (22)
To get a better high	66 (22)	48 (25)	105 (44)	219 (30)
Men	57 (23)	35 (27)	64 (47)	156 (30)
Women	9 (19)	13 (20)	41 (40)	63 (29)
Other	71 (24)	60 (31)	71 (30)	202 (28)
Men	54 (22)	36 (28)	41 (30)	131 (25)
Women	17 (36)	24 (37)	30 (29)	71 (33)
Total	298 (100)	195 (100)	238 (100)	731 (100)
Men	251 (100)	130 (100)	136 (100)	517 (100)
Women	47 (100)	65 (100)	102 (100)	214 (100)

[a]Respondents provided more than one response; therefore, percentages sum to more than 100%.

Table 6. Drug Injection Behaviors of the First Injection Sample,
Stratified by Calendar Period of Initiation

	< 1975 n (%)	1975–1983 n (%)	1984–1992 n (%)	Total n (%)
Sharing Needle (n = 702)	179 (65)	64 (34)	41 (17)	284 (40)
Men	158 (67)	51 (40)	27 (20)	236 (47)
Women	21 (50)	13 (21)	14 (14)	48 (23)
Sharing cooker (n = 708)	246 (86)	142 (76)	147 (63)	535 (76)
Men	212 (87)	96 (77)	79 (59)	387 (77)
Women	34 (81)	46 (74)	68 (67)	148 (72)
Sharing rinse water/cotton (n = 683)	215 (77)	115 (66)	106 (46)	436 (64)
Men	187 (78)	78 (67)	54 (42)	319 (66)
Women	28 (68)	37 (64)	52 (53)	117 (59)
Cleaning of needles/syringes (of those who shared a needle/syringe)				
Water	150 (84)	50 (78)	30 (73)	230 (81)
Alcohol	10 (6)	3 (5)	2 (5)	15 (5)
Other	1 —	— —	— —	1 —
Bleach	— —	1 (2)	3 (9)	4 (1)
Did not clean	18 (10)	10 (15)	6 (13)	34 (12)
Total	179 (100)	64 (100)	41 (100)	284 (100)

The interviews also suggest concerns about hepatitis and active efforts to reduce risk. A man who first injected in the early 1970s, recalls

> At that time, there was no AIDS, hepatitis was what we worried about. I had my own works. When me and the guy I lived with used it, we were always boiling water and using alcohol. And we would make sure there was nothing we could see. We had no microscope … but we had a boiling pot of water and we drew it up and squirted it, and drew it up and squirted it out and then filled the whole thing with alcohol and let it sit a while.

In-depth interviews suggest that first injection was part of a larger process of experimentation with injectable drugs that often began with skin popping (injection under the skin), followed by injecting into a vein (mainlining) with the help of others, and finally by independent injection. Transitions occurred when current routes of administration no longer sustained drug-induced euphoria. Two other men describe their initial (skin-popping) experiences in the late 1960s. One comments,

> The first time I injected, somebody had to do it to me because I didn't know how to do it. A friend did it for me. We were in a basement. It was just me and him. "You know," he asked me, "you sure you want to skin pop?" I told him "Uh huh, because I'm not feeling anything when I snort." He went first, then he hit me. I didn't skin pop very long before I mainlined, maybe about 2 months later. I went to mainlining because I wasn't feeling nothing from the skin pop. This was way before all the AIDS stuff. People didn't know about it at that time. People used to share works and everything because the sickness wasn't out.

The other, who initiated in 1969, recalls,

> The first time I did it, I hit myself. Most people don't do themselves the first time, but my friends had been shooting for many years before me. I had watched them before, so I wasn't afraid. I skin popped the first time before I mained, you know, about a week and then I mainlined.

HIV Spread (Calendar Period 2: 1975–1983)

Social and Behavioral Features of First Injection

As described in Chapter 1, HIV infection first entered the IDU community in New York during this period. By 1981, approximately half the IDUs were infected (Des Jarlais et al., 1989b). Needle sharing, shooting gallery use, and unprotected sex contributed to the rapid rise in seroprevalence (Des Jarlais et al., 1989a). Subjects from the SFHR study recalled that during the 1970s and 1980s, abandoned buildings in Bushwick were often taken over by IDUs and converted into living spaces and shooting galleries (see Chapter 3). Galleries were common settings for renting syringes, spreading HIV across otherwise-unlinked drug networks (Marmor et al., 1987).

In 1983, interviews with a convenience sample of 18 street IDUs in New York City indicated that all had heard about AIDS and believed it spread through sharing used needles (Des Jarlais et al., 1985). Street sellers of needles reported that "new" needle sales had increased over the last year. When asked if they had ever resold used needles as "new," 50% said they had. AIDS was incorporated into sales messages, with one seller saying "Get the good needles, don't get the bad AIDS" (Des Jarlais et al., 1985).

Quantitative Data on First Injection

During this period, there were greater proportions of Latino and women initiates than had been true during the pre-HIV time period (Table 3). Sixty percent of female initiates were helped to inject by a male spouse–lover or male friend and 20% were helped by a female friend (Table 3). As in other periods, most initiators, regardless of gender, were persons with whom the subject felt emotionally close or very close. The most common setting of initiation for both men and women remained a friend's home or the initiate's own home (Table 4). Shooting galleries were only rarely the sites for first injection (Table 4).

Men and women reported relatively similar reasons for initiation. Almost half said that they first injected because they were curious or because their friends injected (Table 5). Both men and women experienced substantial declines in receptive syringe sharing at initiation when compared to the pre-HIV period, suggesting that the initiate, initiator, or both might have been trying to prevent parenterally acquired infections (Table 6). The percentage of initiates who shared a cooker or cotton/rinse water also declined slightly (Table 6).

Qualitative Data on First Injection

Qualitative interviews suggest that if a new user did not rely on a friend, family member, or sex partner to navigate through the drug market or to help with the first hit, the initiation tended to involve some form of exchange. Interviews from this period reflect the growing presence of shooting galleries in the injection drug scene. In some cases, galleries are described as settings of first injection and in others as places for purchasing new needles.

Felicia, an African-American woman who initiated in 1976, points out that she knew people at the gallery where she first injected, so she did not have to pay.

> The first time I injected I was about 14 or 15 years old. I wanted to see what my father and his friends got out of it. I went out one day and went to a gallery in Harlem. I had asked somebody to mainline it for me. I didn't have to pay 'cause I knew people there.

Other interviews suggest that when an older friend helped navigate through the drug market, the first injection was perceived as more safe. One initiate recalls,

On that occasion it was just me, (my friend), and his wife. He was a little older than me. We did it in his house, but there were galleries all over the place. I went with them to Manhattan to the gallery on the Lower East Side and we all bought new works [needle and syringe]. Everybody had their own set.

HIV Stabilization and Initial Decline: Calendar Period 3: (1984–1992)

Social and Behavioral Features of First Injection

From 1984 to approximately 1990, HIV infection among IDUs in New York entered a phase of relative stability, with seroprevalence rates of 55 to 60% (Des Jarlais et al., 1989a). This seeming stability involved a balancing of several processes. Many IDUs became unavailable for study, whether through HIV-related death, overdose or other death, or stopping injecting. New initiates (mostly uninfected with HIV) began injection drug use, which also helped to prevent overall observed seroprevalence from rising. Risk reduction by drug injectors also contributed to the stability in seroprevalence (Des Jarlais et al., 1989a). In 1984, over half the IDUs in a methadone maintenance program in New York City reported that they had reduced high-risk injection practices (Friedman et al., 1987b). In the next several years, considerable evidence accrued that IDUs knew about the HIV risks associated with injection drug use and were changing their injection practices (Friedman et al., 1987b; Kleinman et al., 1990; Selwyn, Feiner, Cox, Lipshutz, & Cohen, 1987). Behavior change initiated by the drug users themselves was later bolstered by publicly funded outreach efforts in 1987 (Friedman et al., 1997b). The first sustained underground needle exchange program in New York City began in 1990. The increased purity of heroin and cocaine may have reduced the number of new drug injectors and contributed to long-term users shifting back to inhalant use. The expansion of syringe exchanges in New York City coincided with gradual declines in HIV seroprevalence from 1990 to 1992 (Des Jarlais et al., 1996, in press; Friedman et al., 1997b).

Quantitative Data on First Injection

During this period of HIV stabilization and initial decline, first-time users were older than was true earlier, initiating at the average age of 26 compared to 17 and 20 in the previous time periods (Table 3). Women were 43% of the initiate population. Greater percentages of female initiates were initiated by friends who were women, suggesting women's growing presence in the injection drug scene. The role of women as initiators, however, seemed limited to female initiations. The proportion of men who were initiated by women remained below 20% in each time period.

Reasons for starting to inject during this period seemed to shift from the curiosity or peer influence of previous time periods to a more utilitarian need to get a better high (perhaps due to the older age of this initiate population). There was a 20% increase in the number of men and women who reported that they first injected to get a better high when compared to the previous time period (Table 5). This period could be characterized as a time of high HIV prevalence rates, high purity of heroin and cocaine, and widespread risk reduction during which only 17% of initiates shared a needle or syringe at first injection (Table 6), with a 7% drop among women and a 20% drop among men. Nonetheless, substantial proportions (40–70%) of both men and women shared cookers or cotton and/or rinse water at initiation. Of the 41 subjects who shared a needle or syringe, less than 10% used bleach to clean the needle before injection (Table 6).

Qualitative Data on First Injection

The qualitative data are filled with reminders of morbidity associated with injection drug use. One woman recalls first injecting in 1985:

> There was a guy who lived right around the block. He ran a gallery up there in his apartment. My friend knew him, so we used to go up there. My friend did it first and then he hit me. I became good friends with this guy because I didn't know how to do it. One day I was there, he was in bed. He had abscessed and I don't know if he was shooting in his neck or something. He got paralyzed from the waist down. After that he said, "I'm not going to do it no more. You're gonna have to start doin' it yourself."

Interviews also suggest a gradual, growing fear of AIDS over time. A 20-year-old Puerto Rican women who initiated in the late 1980s highlights the protective role of the initiation network:

> I was at a friend's house, a guy and a girl … I didn't know what to do, so the guy hit me 'cause he knew more about it and he was older than she was. He was more into it. They threw the stuff into one big cooker and cooked it up. They said they didn't want to give me too much 'cause it was the first time. Then the girlfriend told him to do me next and then he did her. We were aware of the risk of AIDS so we didn't share syringes. Her mother was a diabetic so she got us new ones.

By 1989, concerns about AIDS seemed to pervade the first injection event with the initiate exerting greater control over injection practices. A man who was 26 at that time said,

> The first time I squeezed (injected) I was in my car. I requested to go first because it was a new syringe and I didn't know what he was about. By then we all knew about the threat of AIDS. The second time, I bought my own syringe and I got all my stuff together.

Rosie, a Dominican woman who initiated in the late 1980s, reveals this exchange component of initiation. She emphasizes that although her initiator hung out in a gallery, the needle she used was new:

> The first time somebody else hit me—a guy. He wasn't a friend, he was one of those guys who stays up in the gallery. I gave him a taste to hit me 'cause I didn't know how to

fix the stuff. He had the needle and he tied me off and hit me. Then he used the same syringe. It was new when he hit me. Then he cleaned it with water and used it second.

FURTHER STATISTICAL ANALYSIS

We used multivariate logistic regression to assess whether declines in high-risk injection practices persisted when controlling for the changing social and demographic features of first injection. Controlling for age, network size, gender, and drug setting of initiation, the relative odds of receptive syringe sharing at initiation fell steadily from the pre-AIDS era to the 1988–1992 period, when these odds were only one tenth what they were before 1979 (Table 7). In this same equation, syringe sharing was significantly less likely among women than men and among those who injected with only one other person rather than in larger groups.

Table 7. Multivariate Analysis of Factors Associated with Receptively Sharing a Needle/Syringe at First Injection (n = 621)[a]

	Total	Percent sharing	Crude			Model 1[b]		
			Odds ratio	95% CI	p value	Odds ratio	95% CI	p value
Women	178	25	0.3	0.2–0.4	0.0001	0.5	0.3–0.8	0.002
Men	443	51	1.0			1.0		
Age at initiation[c]			0.4	0.3–0.6	0.0001	0.9	0.7–1.3	0.614
> 25	120	19						
18–25	274	42						
< 18	227	59						
Own home	139	28	0.4	0.3–0.6	0.0001	0.6	0.4–1.0	0.051
All others	482	48	1.0			1.0		
Network size								
≥ 2	255	56	2.2	1.6–3.1	0.0001	1.6	1.1–2.3	0.016
1	366	36	1.0			1.0		
Calendar period								
≤ 1968	119	69	1.0			1.0		
1969–1974	136	65	0.9	0.5–1.4	0.557	0.9	0.5–1.6	0.824
1975–1978	71	37	0.3	0.1–0.5	0.0001	0.3	0.2–0.6	0.0003
1979–1983	104	35	0.2	0.1–0.4	0.0001	0.3	0.2–0.6	0.0002
1984–1987	87	28	0.2	0.1–0.3	0.0001	0.2	0.1–0.5	0.0002
1988–1992	104	14[d]	0.1	0.0–0.1	0.0001	0.1	0.1–0.2	0.0001

[a]Eliminated from the analysis: those who initiated alone; those who did not provide calendar year of initiation; and missings on any of the variables.
[b]Calendar period treated as categorical dummy variables.
[c]Age at initiation treated as a scored variable.
[d]$p < 0.0001$ (Mantel–Haenzel χ^2 test for trend).

Table 8. Multivariate Analysis of Factors Associated
with Sharing a Cooker at First Injection ($n = 628$)[a]

			Crude			Model 1[b]		
	Total	Percent sharing	Odds ratio	95% CI	p value	Odds ratio	95% CI	p value
Women	179	77	0.8	0.5–1.2	0.19	1.1	0.7–1.8	0.656
Men	449	81	1.0			1.0		
Age at initiation[c]			0.6	0.5–0.8	0.001	1.0	0.7–1.4	0.957
> 25	118	72						
18–25	277	77						
< 18	233	87						
Own home	146	71	0.5	0.3–0.8	0.003	0.6	0.4–1.0	0.052
All others	482	83	1.0			1.0		
Ego network size								
≥ 2	255	85	1.7	1.1–2.6	0.014	1.4	0.9–2.1	0.154
1	373	77	1.0			1.0		
Race–ethnicity								
Latino	252	83	1.3	0.9–1.9	0.182	1.8	1.2–2.8	0.008
All others	376	78	1.0			1.0		
Calendar period								
≤ 1968	120	87	1.0			1.0		
1969–1974	143	89	1.2	0.6–2.3	0.597	1.2	0.5–2.4	0.705
1975–1978	69	84	0.8	0.4–1.8	0.622	0.7	0.3–1.7	0.422
1979–1983	106	76	0.5	0.2–0.9	0.033	0.4	0.2–0.9	0.036
1984–1987	86	73	0.4	0.2–0.9	0.017	0.4	0.2–0.9	0.038
1988–1992	104	67[d]	0.3	0.2–0.6	0.001	0.3	0.1–0.7	0.005

[a]Eliminated from the analysis: those who initiated alone; did not provide calendar year of initiation; and missings on any of the variables in the model.
[b]Calendar time treated as categorical dummy variables.
[c]Age at initiation treated as a scored variable.
[d]$p < 0.0001$ (Mantel–Haenzel χ^2 test for trend).

Multivariate analyses also revealed declines over time in the probability of sharing a cooker or cotton/rinse water at initiation. However, these behaviors only became statistically significant in the later calendar periods when AIDS and its effects began to become visible (Tables 8 and 9). Few other variables were associated with the sharing of cookers or cotton–rinse water at initiation in multivariate models. Latinos were more likely to share a cooker than other racial–ethnic groups, while initiating in one's own home was slightly protective. The only marginally significant factors associated with sharing cotton filters and/or rinse water were younger age and being Latino.

Table 9. Multivariate Analysis of Factors Associated
with Sharing Cotton/Rinse Water at First Injection ($n = 604$)[a]

			Crude			Model 1[b]		
	Total	Percent sharing	Odds ratio	95% CI	p value	Odds ratio	95% CI	p value
Women	171	62	0.7	0.5–1.1	0.085	1.1	0.7–1.6	0.746
Men	433	69	1.0			1.0		
Age at initiation[c]			0.5	0.4–0.6	0.001	0.7	0.5–1.0	0.064
> 25	115	49						
18–25	266	65						
< 18	223	79						
Own home	142	57	0.6	0.4–0.8	0.003	0.7	0.5–1.1	0.123
All others	462	70	1.0			1.0		
Network size								
≥ 2	245	69	1.1	0.8–1.6	0.446	0.9	0.6–1.3	0.435
1	359	66	1.0			1.0		
Race–ethnicity								
Latino	244	68	1.1	0.8–1.6	0.598	1.4	0.9–2.0	0.099
All others	360	66	1.0			1.0		
Calendar period								
≤ 1968	119	79	1.0			1.0		
1969–1974	139	78	0.9	0.5–1.7	0.802	0.9	0.5–1.7	0.845
1975–1978	62	73	0.7	0.3–1.4	0.334	0.7	0.3–1.5	0.346
1979–1983	101	66	0.5	0.3–1.0	0.036	0.6	0.3–1.1	0.102
1984–1987	82	57	0.4	0.2–0.7	0.001	0.5	0.2–0.9	0.037
1988–1992	101	44[d]	0.2	0.1–0.4	0.001	0.3	0.1–0.6	0.001

[a]Eliminated from the analysis: those who initiated alone; did not provide calendar year of initiation; or missings for any of the variables in the model.
[b]Calendar period treated as categorical dummy variables.
[c]Age at initiation treated as a scored variable.
[d]$p < 0.0001$ (Mantel–Haenzel $\chi 2$ test for trend).

LIMITATIONS

In addition to the scientific limitations of the SFHR study (which are discussed elsewhere in this volume and include the nonrandom nature of the sample, the use of self-report data, and the difficulties of assessing causality using cross-sectional data), there are other limitations specific to these analyses of the first injection event. No assessment of the reliability or validity of questions about the first injection event in this study has been conducted. Because initiations in many cases occurred many years ago, the recalled network size may underestimate its true size (Wasserman & Faust, 1994). Interviewed subjects also may have under-reported the number of people who were present at first injection to shorten the length of the interview. They may also underreport high-risk injection practices to avoid admitting stigmatized behavior (Samuels, Vlahov, Anthony, & Chaisson, 1992). However, Vlahov et al. (1991b) provide data from Baltimore that suggest that retrospective data on initiation are not seriously affected by socially desirable responding.

Assessing the downward trend in high-risk injection practices at initiation may suffer from differential attrition. This study was cross-sectional, relying on IDUs who retrospectively recalled their first injection. Therefore, IDUs who died, stopped injecting, or otherwise left the study population were not included in the sample. If the study had included these initiates, observed trends in sharing at initiation may have been different from what we found. Through a modeling exercise described elsewhere (Atwood, 1998), we compared our declining trend estimates to estimates when taking differential attrition into account. Applying a series of hypothetical assumptions, we assumed that those who shared a syringe at initiation left the sampling frame at a faster rate than those who did not share (presumably because they continued to engage in high-risk behaviors and subsequently died from AIDS-related disease or other injection-related infection). Under this assumption, sampling bias would result in conservative estimates of declining trends in high-risk behaviors. In other words, if we had included those who left the population due to injection-related infection or AIDS-related disease, we would have observed a steeper decline in sharing at initiation than what we found in the cross-sectional retrospective sample.

DISCUSSION AND CONCLUSIONS

Receptive sharing of syringes at initiation seems to have declined sharply. This also has been reported for another New York study by Neaigus et al. (1991) and by Vlahov et al. (1991b) for Baltimore. This behavior began to change before the first AIDS cases were diagnosed in 1981.

It is possible that during these early time periods, IDUs began drawing a link between non-HIV injection-related infections and the widespread sharing of needles. Parenterally acquired infections were an object of study by the research community as early as 1966. Personal histories of IDUs attest to early concerns of hepatitis and a growing fear of AIDS over time.

Using piece-wise regression analysis, we assessed whether specific calendar years were points at which the downward slope in receptive syringe sharing over time became markedly more pronounced. No calendar year of initiation was found to significantly affect the observed slope, providing evidence that the decline in receptive sharing was a long-term trend in risk reduction.

In contrast, the sharing of cookers and cotton/rinse water began to significantly decline only in the more recent calendar periods, although this occurred at least by 1984–1987 (Tables 8 and 9), prior to programs of AIDS education for IDUs. A hierarchy of risk may have been developed by IDUs, with syringe sharing viewed as the primary risk factor followed by the sharing of cookers and cotton/rinse water. The quantitative data also indicate that many first injection events occur in emotionally close dyadic relationships between the initiate and initiator. Men were primarily initiated by male friends, but women's initiators included persons in a more diverse set of social relationships, including female and male friends and sex partners. Although we assumed there would be substantial gender power imbalances operating at first injection, women were significantly less likely to share a syringe at first injection, even with time trends and other confounders controlled. Initiating in a smaller network provided a protective effect against receptive syringe sharing, perhaps because there were fewer people to compete for limited resources or because safety can more easily be disregarded in multiperson interactions. Initiating in one's home also provided a slightly protective effect against the sharing of syringes or cookers, perhaps because initiates had greater control or authority there. Future research should identify the precise mechanisms that lead some initiations to be safer than others. We also need to know whether the events at initiation predict future risk behaviors, network characteristics, or infection.

Ethnographic data suggest that law enforcement began closing down shooting galleries in the early 1990s (see Chapter 3). Initiation, however, primarily took place in safer locations—a friend's home or one's own home—even in the period when shooting galleries were quite common. The private nature of these settings, while presenting a problem for outreach and intervention efforts, may postpone entrance into a more varied and perhaps high-risk drug network. These settings may also provide the opportunity for less hurried and less high-risk first injections.

IDUs provided vivid accounts of their first injection. Their personal histories suggest an awareness of the morbidity associated with injection drug use both before and during the AIDS epidemic. The first injection was described as part of a larger process of experimentation with injectable drugs, with IDUs transitioning from skin popping or intranasal use, to mainline injection, and finally to independent injection. Financial transaction or exchange was a common component of drug initiations, and IDUs emphasized when they began to inject independently. The interviews also point to widespread differences in the age or experience of the initiate and initiator, suggesting that attention has to be paid to status differences in initiator–initiate dyads.

In conclusion, reductions in risk behaviors at initiation are welcome news. Yet if AIDS incidence declines and fears of seroconversion subside, efforts may be needed to sustain low-risk behaviors. Outreach efforts should view active injectors as potential initiators of other users. Older IDUs could use the leverage of the initiate–initiator dyad to model safe injection behavior. But to support such efforts, policy-level changes must allow for safe and affordable access to sterile syringes. Although prevention of the initiation event may not be possible, we can at least equip new and potential users with methods to protect themselves from HIV infection and other parenterally acquired diseases.

Network Concepts and Serosurvey Methods

In this chapter, we discuss several of the network concepts used in this volume. We then describe how questionnaire and serological data were gathered, with some emphasis on the network data, and describe the 767 subjects whose interviews were included in the analyses. As will be recalled, the ethnographic techniques used to gather the qualitative data were discussed in Chapter 2.

NETWORK CONCEPTS AND DATA

The use of network concepts in studies of infectious disease epidemiology is relatively new. For reasons of clarity, we will briefly present a few terms and their relationships to the data that were collected in the Social Factors and HIV Risk (SFHR) study and to the databases and variables used in the analysis.

Social networks can be defined as a pattern of social linkages among a group of people. A linkage is some type of social tie between two persons. Thus, thinking about social patterns in terms of networks involves building larger patterns of relationships out of dyadic linkages between two of the people involved. One way of doing that is to think of the pattern of linkages in which a given person—say, for example, Sam—is directly involved. We can find out about Sam's egocentric network by asking him about it. This could lead to a diagram like Fig. 1. Here, all of Sam's friends are indicated by lines that extend outward from the box labeled "Sam." In this figure, Sam has named five other persons. Only one of them, "another subject," is indicated as somebody who was also recruited for the study. Thus, Fig. 1 presents Sam's egocentric network. The members of this network consist of four persons who did not take part in the study and one person ("another subject") who did. The social relationships and shared behaviors between the subject and the five members of subject's egocentric network are indicated as lines between boxes in the figure. Thus, if we had asked Sam to name the people who are his closest friends, the figure would present information about Sam's friendships; but if we had asked him to name the people he had seen most often in the last 30 days, the figure would present data on whom Sam had seen.

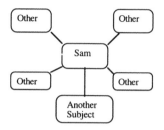

Figure 1. An egocentric network.

Some relationships go beyond the social in that they describe types of behaviors that could perhaps transmit HIV. As we have dealt with it for the SFHR study, the two key types of behaviors are injecting drugs together and having sex together. We have defined the set of relationships that can transmit HIV as a person's risk network. Thus, in Fig. 1, if we had asked Sam to name the people with whom he had injected drugs or had sex, the figure would be a description of Sam's egocentric risk network.

The distinction between a risk network and a social network can be made clearer. A risk network is a set of relationships that involve risk behaviors that can transmit HIV (or, for other purposes, other forms of risk). A social network is a set of social relationships, and is analytically distinguishable from a risk network in that it focuses on social interaction per se, which may or may not include behaviors that can transmit HIV. A social network is important because it can convey social influence, information, attitudes, and so forth, and thus can influence risk and protective behaviors or the use of services.

One final complication is that a risk network need not be a subset of a social network. Usually it is. People who have sex or who inject drugs together usually have at least a minimal social relationship, even if this consists primarily of the exchange of money for sex and perhaps 5 minutes of conversation during and after negotiations. On occasions, however, risk can occur without direct interaction having taken place. This can occur in a shooting gallery, even among people who have never met each other. For example, say Sam comes into the tire shop, finds a used syringe on the floor, and injects drugs with it. If we knew that the syringe had previously been used by Patricia, we could draw in a "risk linkage" between Sam and Patricia, even if they had never met each other. The issue of nonsocial risk linkages extends beyond shooting galleries, however. One large-scale example is blood banks. In the late 1970s and the first few years of the 1980s, thousands of people got infected with HIV by receiving transfusions with blood from a blood bank. Later on, the records of the blood banks were used to trace these linkages and figure out who had received infected blood. Thus, the blood banks used risk network data in tracing who might have become infected through such non–social-interactional linkages.

Analyses of egocentric network data can be conducted in either of two ways. First, the characteristics of a research participants' egocentric network can be treated as an individual attribute of that person. In this case, then, Sam could be described by his age, gender, and the fact that his egocentric network has five members (and, perhaps, by the fact that his egocentric network includes at least one person who has injected drugs for more than five years). Patricia's egocentric *risk* network includes at least two people who were mentioned in Chapter 3: Carmen, with whom she injected in the tire shop, and Jerry, with whom she injected in the street. Her social network (and perhaps her risk network) includes Barney, whose paper bag full of crack vials was hidden under a bed in the tire shop; Jeannette, the wife of a shooting gallery owner who owed Patricia money; and Madeline, who repaid her $5 but did not help her get straight. Thus, for Patricia, we could create variables indicating that her injection network includes both men and women; that her social network includes the wife of one shooting gallery owner and the partner (Carmen) of another; and that she herself injects in shooting galleries. In conducting analyses, then, egocentric network attributes can be analyzed just as can other attributes such as subject's gender or frequency of injection.

Another way to analyze egocentric network data is to consider the egocentric network as a set of relationships between the research participant and his or her network members. Thus, in Fig. 1, we can analyze five separate two-person relationships, each of which includes Sam as one of the people in it. These dyadic social relationships (indicated by connecting lines) between subjects and the members of their egocentric networks can be used as units of analysis. In the SFHR project, we created a "relationship database," which contains 3165 dyadic relationships as its component parts. The relationship database contains information about subjects and each of the (up to 10) members of their personal social network about whom they answered detailed questions. As is shown in Chapters 8 and 9, these relationship data have been used for analyses of the sexual relationships of subjects to study the extent of consistent condom use (Friedman et al., 1994c) and for analyses of drug-injecting networks to establish the extent of receptive syringe sharing. They have also been used to analyze relationship-specific predictors of syringe sharing at first injection (Chapter 3; Atwood, 1998).

So far, we have looked only at egocentric network-related variables, which look at the immediate social or risk contacts of a designated person. It is useful to take a broader view in many cases. Indeed, much of what we learned during the SFHR Project was based on our taking a view of the social and risk relationships among all the research participants in the study. To do this, we studied their sociometric networks. Sociometric networks consist of a set of people and the entire panoply of linkages between them. Figure 2 schematically presents one such network. It consists of one connected component of four members, another

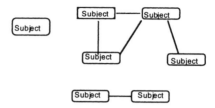

Figure 2.   Sociometric network.

component of two members, and an unlinked participant. (A connected component is a set of persons who all have direct or indirect links to each other, although these links may consist of paths through several other persons. Components are therefore separate if no members of either is linked to any member of the other.)

In the SFHR project, only 491 drug injectors were successfully linked to other research participants. This does not mean that the other 276 participants were in reality social isolates. Many of them named other people as part of their social networks, and indeed many of them named others as persons they had injected drugs within the last 30 days. In these cases, however, either we did not recruit these others for the project, or if we did, we were unable to determine that they were the person(s) nominated by the apparent "social isolates." Thus, the lines between subjects indicate that at least one of them named the other as part of their network of persons with whom they had injected drugs, had sex, or engaged in other noncasual interaction in the last 30 days. (Below and in Chapter 13, we describe how we actually went about determining which participants were linked to each other.)

As the reader can imagine, it is impossible to diagram the relationships we found among 491 drug injectors. As is discussed (in Chapter 10), when we analyzed data on the social linkages among these participants, we found 89 components. The sizes of the components varied between 2 members (dyads) and a large 277-member connected component. There were 214 participants who were members of 88 smaller components ranging in size from 2 to 7 members (2 components had 7 members, 4 had 5, 1 had 4, 14 had 3, and 67 had 2).

It is possible to present diagrams showing the relationships among some of our participants. In Figs. 3 and 4, we show data on the injection linkages and the sexual linkages among 40 members of an ethnographically defined ethnographic core. (The details of how this was defined also are presented in Chapter 10. Here, it suffices to say that many of the people the ethnographer spent most time with were members of this ethnographic core.) These 40 participants are a subset of the large connected component of 277 members. They are not typical, since they were chosen as members of a social core group of drug injectors whose activities are

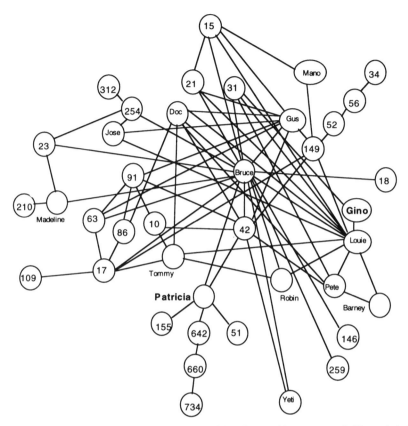

Figure 3. Injection links among the 40 members of the ethnographic core network. Names in bold indicate persons known to be deceased. An earlier version of this figure was published in Curtis et al., 1995.

central to the local Bushwick drug scene. Thus, they are more tightly interconnected with each other than would be true for most groups of 40 injectors chosen from this large connected component. Bruce, for example, clearly emerges as somebody who injects with many other people. Sexual linkages are much rarer within this core group, with only two pairs of its members ever having had sex together:

As should be evident, analyzing sociometric network data can be complicated. Part of these analyses relies on specialized network software. We used UCINET software to define connected components and other network variables. The input to these programs was a "sociometric database." This database contains

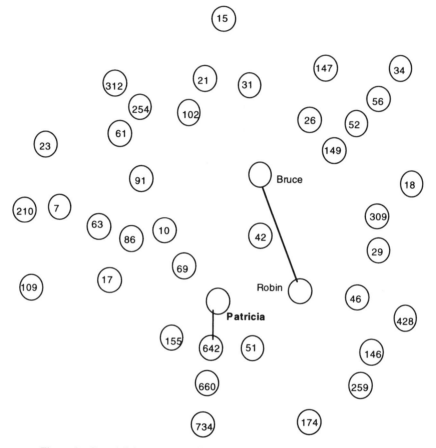

Figure 4. Sexual links among the 40 members of the ethnographic core network.

information about which participants were linked to each other, together with additional information that lets us analyze these data for specific kinds of linkages (such as injecting together in the last 30 days, syringe sharing, or sex). We can then analyze these data as a totality, as when we define the component structure for different kinds of linkages, or we can create individual-level variables that can then be used in analyses of individuals. For example, we can analyze whether members of the large connected component of 277 members are more likely than other research participants to be infected with HIV, or whether they are more likely to inject in shooting galleries.

Units of Analysis

These different databases provide the possibility of conducting studies based on different units of analysis. When we study the predictors of HIV infection or of risk behaviors as personal attributes, the unit of analysis is the *individual*. For such analyses, then, variables are used that describe the social network and risk network characteristics of individual subjects. Examples of this include variables that describe the egocentric networks of each individual, for example, does the subject have a drug injection contact who is 5 years or more older than the subject. Sociometric network location (e.g., being a member of the large connected component) is derived from the sociometric database that describes the relationships among linked research subjects, and is also an individual attribute.

Some risk behaviors (such as condom use and receptive syringe sharing) by a given subject differ depending on whom they engage in them with. Thus, many of our analyses of risk behaviors use the relationship database to study *relationships between subjects and their egocentric risk network members* as the unit of analysis. Individual attributes of research subjects are entered as aspects of the relationship, which means that in such analyses a subject's individual attributes appear as data for each of the relationships in which the subject is involved. Comparisons between a subject's individual attributes and those of his or her egocentric network members, such as their relative ages or whether they are of the same gender, are also used in some analyses. Individual sociometric network attributes described in the preceding paragraph, such as whether they are members of the periphery of the large connected component, can enter such analyses in the same fashion as any other individual attribute. [Since many of the members of the egocentric networks of our subjects (including all of their non–drug-injecting sex partners and friends) are not themselves members of our study population, and thus could not be sufficiently identified for incorporation as part of the sociometric database, the issue of directly incorporating higher-level network structures (from the sociometric data base) into studies of relationships between subjects and their egocentric network members does not arise. Higher-level network characteristics can only be incorporated into studies of these relationships in terms of the individual attributes of research subjects.]

A third level of analysis is the larger-than-dyadic *risk network*. This level of analysis looks at the structures of sociometric linkages among the different subjects who are part of the sociometric database. Connected components are one kind of sociometric structure. Further analyses can study network properties either of the entire set of sociometric relationships or of subsets of the database. One subset of particular interest is the relationships among the members of a large connected component (with over 200 members), which we found to exist among the drug injectors we studied. (This component and variation in the number of its members depending on whether we are studying *social* network ties or *risk* network ties are discussed in Chapter 10.)

SUBJECTS AND DATA

The data for this project were collected from July 1991 to January 1993. Drug injectors were recruited through ethnographically directed street outreach in areas of Bushwick with heavy drug use and through chain-referral by other subjects. To be eligible for the study, subjects had to have injected drugs within the prior year. Since drug abuse treatment status was not an eligibility criterion, the sample includes both in-treatment and out-of-treatment drug injectors.

Subjects were interviewed by project staff in the storefront that was set up as part of the SFHR project. HIV and other counseling and phlebotomy were provided by staff of the New York State Department of Health, which established a testing site for the Bushwick area in our storefront. Subjects were tested for HIV antibody [double enzyme-linked immunosorbent assay (ELISA) with Western blot confirmation] and hepatitis B core antibody.

Questionnaire

A face-to-face structured interview gathered data on subjects' sociodemographic and biographical background, drug and sexual risk behaviors during the prior 30 days and the prior 2 years, medical history, health beliefs, social roles in the drug scene, peer norms, and networks.

Network Information

Subjects were asked to provide information about up to 10 persons with whom they had injected drugs, had sex, or otherwise interacted in a noncasual way during the prior 30 days. They also provided information regarding how long they had known each network member, the nature of their relationship, the network member's risk behavior, and their risk behaviors together. These network data, together with the procedures to confirm that subjects were linked to each other, were the essential data for the network analyses presented in this volume. Thus, it is worth describing the questions through which these network data were collected in some detail.

Since the questions with which names are elicited is a key part of a network survey, it is important to understand exactly how we asked subjects about their network members. We developed our technique after much pretesting and soul-searching. Here, then, is the verbatim wording of the rather lengthy procedure used to ask about the names:

We are trying to find out more about how to prevent the spread of diseases like AIDS or hepatitis that can occur through close personal contact. Please think back over the last 30 days about the people you've *had more than casual contact with* (you've seen them or been in contact with them some other way, such as on the phone). Let's make a list of these people. Exclude people, such as counselors, that you only have contact with because you are in a program or were mandated by the court to have this kind of contact. Please, remember that all the information you give us is **confidential** and will only be used to help us learn how to prevent the spread of AIDS and hepatitis.

Please give me the first name and any street names of the people you've had more than casual contact with in the last 30 days, and tell me whether they were present when you first injected for the very first time.

First, lets start with the
* people who you *used drugs with* during the last 30 days
  (get list of these names before reading out the next naming stimulus)
Next the:
* people who you *had sex with* during the last 30 days
  (get list of these names before reading out the next naming stimulus)
Next the:
* people closest to you not mentioned before, seen in last 30 days
  (get list of these names before reading out the next naming stimulus)
Next the:
* people you *live with*
  (get list of these names before reading out the next naming stimulus)
Next the:
* any relatives you've been in contact with during the last 30 days
  (get list of these names before reading out the next naming stimulus)
Next the:
* people you've met socially or hung out with during the last 30 days
  (get list of these names before reading out the next naming stimulus)
Next the:
* people you know at work or who you hustle with
  (get list of these names before reading out the next naming stimulus)
Lastly:
* any other people who you had close contact with during the last 30 days.

The list on which these names were recorded had columns for the first name, two street names, and whether the person named was present at the subject's first injection or not. We recorded up to 20 names for each subject. However, because we then asked an extensive series of questions about nominees (including their gender, race–ethnicity, age, years of injection, risk behaviors, and other personal attributes, as well as about the relationship between the nominator and the nominee, such as how long they knew each other, did they talk about AIDS with each other, and risk behaviors they engaged in together) and we were concerned both about subjects' willingness to stay through the entire questionnaire and ability to recall accurate answers during an overly long session, we only asked questions about the first 10 network members named. (In actual fact, only 10% of the subjects named as many as 10 nominees, so little distortion results from this restriction.) Although we have no way to estimate the size of the problem, we are convinced

that the biggest problem with these data is the extent to which subjects under-
reported names either in order to shorten the interview or to maintain secrecy about
some contacts.

DEFINING LINKAGES

Data from these questionnaires were combined with ethnographic and other
data gathered during the project to define the sociometric linkages among research
participants. Such linkages were operationalized as follows. First, one or both of
the subjects must name the other as someone with whom he or she had (in the 30
days prior to the interview) injected drugs, had sex, or otherwise interacted on a
noncasual basis. Second, these linkages had to be supported by additional information that confirmed that the named other person was in fact the one we interviewed.
Specifically, a link was considered to be confirmed if two participants (1) engaged
in face-to-face contact with research staff at the same time, which could occur
when one of them brought the other in to be interviewed, or if they talked with
ethnographic staff in the field and identities were confirmed through further
contact with storefront staff, or (2) were observed together in public settings by
project ethnographic staff. An additional way in which links could be confirmed
(as is discussed in Chapter 13) was by matching selected characteristics reported by
index subject "A" (first name and/or street name, age within 5 years, race–
ethnicity, and gender) with the descriptors of "A" provided by another subject who
had nominated him or her.

Data Validity and Reliability

One issue that always needs to be considered in using questionnaire data is the
degree to which the information is accurate. There are many reasons for answers to
be imprecise. The participant may not remember the correct answer, or may choose
to present him- or herself in a particular light to the interviewer. Furthermore,
going through an interview is a mixture of fun (almost everybody enjoys talking
about her- or himself), toil, and boredom. Drug injectors may be motivated to finish
the interview, collect their $30 interview fee, and get back out into the streets,
particularly if the effects of their last injection are wearing off and they are worried
about withdrawal. Thus, one weakness we are fairly certain there is in the data is
that some of the participants probably deliberately reported on fewer network
contacts than they could have, since we asked about 50 questions about each listed
contact.

For some of the data that were provided, however, we were able to make
comparisons between the answers provided by different pairs of subjects who were
both in the study and who provided answers to questions about each other. These

comparisons indicate that the self-report data about personal characteristics and behaviors are of good reliability (Goldstein et al., 1995), that is, that by and large, the reports by different drug injectors about others' personal characteristics and risk behaviors, about the activities they engage in with each other, and about their relationship agreed with each other. There was 100% agreement, for example, between respondents and their contacts on the gender of the contact. There was 93% agreement on whether respondents had ever injected drugs together and 99% on whether they ever had sex together; the Pearson correlation coefficient for their estimates of the duration of these sexual relationships was $r = 0.89$ (whereas for duration of injection relationships r was only 0.71.)

In addition, the fact that many of our findings about risk factors for HIV find predicted relationships between social, behavioral, and network variables and HIV infection tends to provide construct validation for a number of these variables.

Limitations of These Data

Certain limitations of these data should be mentioned. First, as in all such studies, it is impossible to select a random sample of the population of drug injectors (Watters & Biernacki, 1989). Second, subjects may have underreported the number of persons with whom they had injected or had sex in the last 30 days as a way to shorten the interview or because they did not want to mention knowing certain other drug injectors or sex partners. Unknown biases may enter into the samples of egocentric dyadic relationships as a result. Since subjects recruited through snowball techniques had to be part of the list of subjects nominated by the index respondent, the sociometric database may also have limited representativeness. The use of such chain referral can result in possible selection bias reducing the generalizability of the study findings. Chain referral can also lead to clustering of data because participants may be more similar to each other (Samuels et al., 1992), resulting in less spread or variation in the data than if a simple random sample could have been selected (Sudman, 1976). In all these limitations, the SFHR data essentially share the problems of what is a developing area of research. In spite of these limitations, as has been discussed above, the data have provided us with the opportunity to make a number of important discoveries.

6

The Research Participants and Their Behaviors

Before going on to detailed examination of research participants' network involvement and relationships (in later chapters), it is worth looking at who they were in quantitative terms. Here, we present data on the 767 individuals who were interviewed with the SFHR project questionnaire. This interview was a fairly long one, often lasting for 1½ hour or more. It took place in our research storefront, which was located right in the middle of the Bushwick drug "supermarket." After participants were interviewed, they participated in HIV counseling and testing, which was conducted by staff of the New York State Department of Health AIDS Institute, which, in collaboration with this project, set up an alternative testing site for Bushwick in our storefront. Although participants did not have to agree to be tested to take part in the project, most did. For a few of these, difficulties in finding veins from which to take blood made this very painful. In some cases, they gave up and left without successfully having their blood taken. In spite of this, however, 90% of the participants provided blood samples that were then successfully tested for HIV.

A large majority of the participants were men (Table 1). This proportion is not unexpected. Most studies of drug injectors in the United States find similar proportions. As described in Chapter 4, participants who first injected more recently are more likely to be women.

The nature of the Bushwick drug scene as a drug supermarket is reflected in the data on race–ethnicity. Bushwick itself, in 1990, had a population that was 67% Latino and 29% African American according to census data (which may undercount Latino immigrants). Many whites, however, as well as other drug injectors come into Bushwick to get drugs. The racial–ethnic distribution of participants allowed us to conduct considerable research on differences among drug injectors' risk behaviors, risk networks, and HIV risk by race–ethnicity, some of which is included in this volume.

The sample included 24% "new injectors" who had begun injecting within the previous 6 years. We had hoped to recruit 400 new injectors. Fortunately for many high-risk youth, but unfortunately for our project, we began recruiting just as a strong trend toward noninjected heroin use became apparent (Neaigus et al.,

Table 1. Sociodemographic and Selected Other Characteristics of the Participants

Variable and category	Number of subjects	Percent
Number of subjects with behavioral data	767	
Gender		
Men	541	70
Women	226	30
Race–ethnicity		
African American (not Latino/a)	198	26
Latino/a (not black)	255	33
White (not Latino/a)	243	32
Black Latino/a	58	8
Other	13	2
Years of injection		
< 6	187	24
≥ 6	579	76
Homeless	153	20
With home	614	80
In drug abuse treatment	165	22
Not in drug abuse treatment	590	78
Ever in drug abuse treatment	529	69
Never in drug abuse treatment	238	31
Mean age (s.d.)	767	34.8 (7.0)
Mean years of injection (s.d.)	766	13.8 (9.0)
Mean monthly injections during previous 2 years (s.d.)	756	112 (139)
HIV[a]		
Negative	415	60
Positive	272	40
HBV core antibody[a]		
Negative	165	28
Positive	426	72

[a]HIV antibody test results were unavailable for 80 participants because they decided to forego testing or because of the difficulties phlebotomists had in drawing blood from the veins of drug injectors. Among those for whom sera were available, 96 specimens were unable to be tested for HBV core antibody because of insufficient quantity.

1997). This meant that we had to exert a lot of staff energy to locate and interview the 187 new injectors we found. Nonetheless, as is discussed in later chapters, we were able to learn much about new injectors and their risk for HIV.

The mean age of the participants was 34.8 years. This is similar to those found in other New York samples, but is much older than those found in other cities in the

World Health Organization Multicentre Study of Drug injectors and HIV/AIDS (Stimson et al., 1998). In that study, the mean ages of participants in 13 other cities was in the upper 20s, whereas that in New York was a little over 35 (similar to that found in SFHR). This reflects the fact that in New York, as in many other cities in the United States, there was a large number of recruits into drug injection in the early 1970s.

Homelessness is a major issue for drug injectors. It is also hard to define. One fifth of the participants reported that they were homeless (defined as currently residing in a shelter, welfare boarding home, the streets, an abandoned building, a car, van, or truck, or in a subway or train station).

Of our participants, 22% were in drug abuse treatment at the time we interviewed them. For some readers, it may seem strange that we let these treatment clients take part. After all, a large number of research projects that study "street" drug injectors exclude persons from eligibility if they are currently in drug abuse treatment. Sometimes, this may be justifiable, as when a project that is trying to evaluate an AIDS prevention intervention wants to restrict eligibility to out-of-treatment users. For them, this can be justified as a way to avoid complications (due to having some of the sample receiving both the intervention and treatment, which might interfere with each other or help each other in ways that would make analysis too complicated). Such justifications assume that future nonresearch prevention projects will also exclude people in treatment (which seems unlikely). Another justification for others to exclude those in treatment was perhaps a stronger one: Prior to the National AIDS Demonstration projects the National Institute on Drug Abuse started in 1987 (of which the Community AIDS Prevention Outreach Demonstration (CAPOD) project, which we conducted in Williamsburg, was part), very few researchers or interventionists had worked with drug injectors in street settings. Thus, excluding treatment clients from the projects may have been the only way to actually get attention paid to nontreatment samples.

For us, however, it seemed like it would be a mistake to omit drug injectors who are in treatment. First, for any epidemiological study of drug injectors, it has to be faced that many treatment clients continue to inject drugs and that many are "street users." They are part of the drug scene, so understanding this scene requires that we include them in the studies. This is particularly the case in a network study. After all, treatment clients inject with and in some cases have sex with nontreatment drug injectors. Thus, excluding them would artificially disrupt our ability to understand drug injectors' networks and their effects on risk behaviors and infection.

Fully 69% of the participants have been in drug abuse treatment of some kind at some time in their lives. Since the mean years of injection is 13.8, they have had plenty of time to learn the difficulties of life as a drug user and thereafter to negotiate treatment access and try out treatment. In some cases, they may have used treatment only as a way to moderate their habits and bring them more under control; in other cases, they may have tried to get off drugs altogether. In any case, those in our sample had not yet gotten off drugs. On average, during the preceding 2 years, they were injecting three or four times a day.

Unfortunately, 40% of this sample was infected with HIV. This reflects the history of the New York epidemic, as discussed elsewhere in this volume. For the participants in this study, of course, this is no mere statistic: It is, for many of them, a death sentence. Given the difficulties many drug injectors have had in getting access to up-to-date therapies, it continues to be so for many of the survivors, regardless of the success of therapy for others. Beyond that, as has been discussed in earlier chapters and will be discussed later, HIV infection among individuals and in the community has led many of the participants (and other drug injectors as well) to change their lives in innumerable ways.

Hepatitis B is another potentially fatal infection that drug injectors can be exposed to. We tested for hepatitis B core antibody, a marker of exposure to this virus; 72% of the sample had been exposed to hepatitis B. Data are not available on which participants had been exposed without developing core antibody.

RISK BEHAVIORS OF THE PARTICIPANTS IN THE 30 DAYS BEFORE THE INTERVIEW

The ethnographic materials described in earlier chapters present a vivid picture of life in the Bushwick drug scene. They also provided descriptions of a number of risk behaviors such as sharing syringes and backloading and of locations such as shooting galleries and outside spots where injecting occurs. They thus lay the basis for presenting quantitative survey data about some of the behaviors that have been described. Specifically, it is now possible to examine data on injection and sexual behaviors that were engaged in during the 30 days before participants were interviewed (see Table 2).

Many of the drug injectors in this study continued to engage in high-risk behaviors such as injecting with a syringe that was or may have been used by someone else (receptive syringe sharing), backloading, and injecting in high-risk settings such as shooting galleries and outdoor sites. There are few differences between men and women in these risk behaviors, although men are more likely to inject in shooting galleries and to inject cocaine or speedball, whereas women are more likely to engage in crack smoking and in sex for money or drugs. Blacks are less likely to share needles or to inject in outdoor settings, whites are less likely to inject in shooting galleries, and Latinos are less likely to inject cocaine or speedball. Sexual risk behaviors are also widespread. Approximately one third of the subjects had sex partners who inject drugs, and half of the subjects engaged in unprotected vaginal or anal sex. Women were more likely than men to be exposed

Table 2. Risk Behaviors during the 30 Days before the Interview

Behaviors in last 30 days	Gender				Race–ethnicity[a]			
	Total (767)[c]	Men (541)	Women (226)	p^b	Black (206)	Latino (309)	White (241)	p^b
Injected more than once a day	66%	68%	61%	0.090	63%	65%	68%	0.623
Injected with a needle or syringe after someone else injected with it OR that someone else may have used	38%	37%	39%	0.539	28%	41%	41%	0.006
"Got a taste" from someone else's syringe	22%	22%	22%	0.902	23%	24%	19%	0.420
Backloading (syringe-mediated drug sharing)	19%	19%	20%	0.946	20%	21%	16%	0.316
Shared cooker	58%	58%	57%	0.852	59%	61%	53%	0.159
Shared rinse water	42%	44%	38%	0.153	41%	43%	43%	0.945
Injected in shooting galleries	19%	21%	14%	0.015	20%	25%	11%	0.001
Injected in outside places	38%	39%	35%	0.274	30%	41%	39%	0.047
Injected cocaine or speedball	68%	72%	57%	0.001	76%	60%	71%	0.001
Crack use	45%	40%	57%	0.001	48%	40%	47%	0.168
Had a sex partner who is an IDU	32%	28%	42%	0.001	30%	31%	34%	0.548
Any unprotected vaginal or anal sex	54%	50%	66%	0.001	57%	57%	47%	0.068
Any sex for money or drugs	11%	1%	36%	0.001	8%	13%	11%	0.221

[a]Persons of other race–ethnicity are not included in this table because of their small number.
[b]Probabilities by χ^2.
[c]Number in parentheses are sample sizes. For some cells, the denominators vary from these due to missing data or, as for condom use, the exclusion of those who had no sex during the period from the table.

to both of these risks, and were also more likely to engage in sex for money or drugs.

In later chapters, we will examine the predictors and effects of these behaviors at some length.

INDIVIDUAL BEHAVIOR, BEHAVIOR IN NETWORKS, AND BEHAVIOR IN RELATIONSHIPS

The behaviors described in Table 2 are at the individual level. That is, they describe whether or not individuals engaged in specific behaviors, without regard to the fact that many such behaviors take place in relationships. It is possible to inject drugs alone; when one does so, this does not take place in a relationship with someone else (except perhaps in an indirect sort of way). Sharing syringes or having sex, however, are behaviors one engages in with someone else. Such relationships, as has been discussed, form the building blocks from which networks are defined. Furthermore, characteristics of both the other person(s) engaged in a relationship and of the relationship itself (such as its closeness, or how long it has lasted) affect the behaviors that take place in the relationship. Most of the remainder of the volume is devoted to examining the networks and relationships in which risk behaviors take place and the ways in which these patterns of networks and behaviors influence the HIV epidemic among drug injectors. Individuals have a number of such relationships; the pattern of relationships in egocentric networks is the subject of Chapter 7. Chapters 8 and 9 look at specific behaviors (syringe sharing, sexual risk) in the context of relationships rather than individuals.

Personal Risk Networks and High-Risk Injecting Settings of Drug Injectors

INTRODUCTION

Much of people's lives is defined and structured by their interactions with friends, colleagues, and relatives. This is true for injection drug users (IDUs) as well as for drug researchers, shopkeepers, or truck drivers. Current literature only partly reflects this. Thus, some commentators have viewed IDUs as having only acquaintances rather than friends, and as having little contact with relatives (Preble & Casey, 1969). In this viewpoint, drug injectors' social lives are seen as characterized by distrust, one-dimensionality (concern only or primarily with drugs), and loneliness.

Others have seen IDUs as having one prototypical type of relationship that transcends this loneliness and that offers many forms of support—the running partner (Agar, 1973; Preble & Casey, 1969). Running partners form two-person groups (dyads) who guard each others' backs in the many high-risk situations that drug injectors face (fights or other violence, overdoses, difficulties with police, problems finding the money to prevent withdrawal pains) and who also offer each other emotional support and friendship.

This chapter is primarily descriptive, although the description provided is quite different from the "loner" and "running-partner-oriented" views just described. It presents data on the immediate risk and social networks of the drug injectors in the Social Factors and HIV Risk (SFHR) project sample. Thus, it presents data on the number of persons drug injectors inject drugs with, the number they have sex with, the extent to which these network members would be expected to be at high risk of infection with HIV, how long and how well they know each other, and other questions. The extent of heterogeneity and homogeneity of drug injectors' personal networks is also described, for example, the extent to which they are mixed gender rather than composed only of women (or only of men).

We also describe the extent to which IDUs inject their drugs in high-risk settings such as shooting galleries and outdoor locations. IDUs who inject in these settings have been found to be at increased risk for HIV. In addition, these settings can perform an important linking function among friendship groups in which HIV or other infectious agents can be transferred from group to group through those group members who use these settings. Indeed, in shooting galleries where syringes are used by one person and then left around for others to use (Friedman et al., 1990), HIV can be transferred from one group to another without any member of the two groups ever meeting one another. In shooting galleries like the tire shop run by Louie and Gus (which was described in Chapter 3), there were times when two dozen or more people would be injecting in the same room, with a fair amount of coming and going by people who did not know one another. In these circumstances, if somebody injects with a used syringe or cooker that somebody else has left around, it is possible for HIV to be transmitted through "anonymous works" from one network to another even though the members of each network have not met those in the other (see Fig. 1).

Of course, drug injectors are different from one another in many ways. We thus also present data on whether drug injectors differ on these variables if they are of different race–ethnicities, genders, years of drug injecting experience, and if they have different roles in the drug scene (such as syringe seller, drug seller, commercial sex worker, or hit doctor). These data on roles are discussed in more detail in Friedman et al. (1998).

METHODS

The data used in this chapter, like those in the rest of the book, are from the SFHR project study sample. What is specific to this chapter is the focus on egocentric social and risk networks during the past 30 days and on the related issue of injecting in high-risk settings such as shooting galleries and outside settings.

RESULTS

Table 1 presents data on the egocentric networks of the sample members. The mean number of network members who were named by the subjects was a little over four. A few (8%) said that they had had no noncasual contacts during the last 30 days. Approximately two fifths (41%) nominated 1 to 3 network members and 38% gave more than 4 names.

On average, they named 2½ members each with whom they said, in response to a later question, they had ever injected drugs. (Remember, each of these is also someone with whom they had interacted in some way in the last 30 days.) Almost one fifth of the sample said they had no one in their 30-day network with whom they had ever injected drugs. The median number of members named as persons with whom they had ever injected was two.

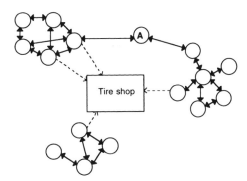

Figure 1. Two connected components. HIV can only be transmitted between them because some members of each component inject in the tire shop shooting gallery where they may unknowingly share "anonymous works." In addition, so long as person A stays uninfected, the only way for HIV to travel between the two halves of the large component is via the tire shop.

On average, they named 2.18 persons each with whom they said they had injected drugs in the prior 30 days. The median number provided was again 2. These data should not be confused with the number of persons with whom they had injected drugs during this period, since it is likely that many research participants did not include persons as network members if they shot drugs with them but did not know them. This can be exemplified by comparing data from the network section of the questionnaire with data provided in the "30-day behaviors" section of the questionnaire. Of the 181 subjects who, in the network section, said they had not injected with anyone in their network in the prior 30 days, 25 had previously said (in the behavioral section) that they had injected with other people in the past 30 days. Nine of these respondents had said they had injected with 1, one with 2, four with 4, five with 5, one with 8, one with 10, one with 18, and one with 75 persons. We have no way of telling whether these discrepancies are due to accurate and precise distinctions being made by the respondents as opposed to underreporting of contacts with whom they had injected. There were also some cases of clear inconsistency in the data, where the number of 30-day injection partners in the network section was greater than that in the behavioral section. For example, of the 177 respondents who said that they had one person in their network with whom they had injected in the last 30 days, 11 (6%) said that they had not injected with anyone in the last 30 days in the behavioral section of the questionnaire. Thus, as would be expected, these data contain a degree of inaccuracy. This finding is not at all surprising considering (1) the difficulty in remembering the number of persons with whom one has engaged in drug injection over a month-long period, particularly for unemployed street users for whom periods of time may have relatively few signposts to mark the passing of a 30-day period; (2) possible confusion about

Table 1. Characteristics of Participants' Networks and Injection Settings

	n	Percent
Number of nominated members of network		
0	64	8
1	115	15
2	86	11
3	114	15
4	101	13
5	74	10
6	43	6
7	46	6
8	25	3
9	20	3
10	79	10
Mean	4.11	
Standard deviation	3.00	
Number of network members subject has ever injected with		
0	146	19
1	176	23
2	118	15
3	119	16
4	91	12
5	38	5
6	30	4
7	12	2
8	10	1
9	10	1
10	17	2
Mean	2.51	
Standard deviation	2.31	
Number of network members subject has injected with in the last 30 days		
0	181	24
1	177	23
2	135	18
3	107	14
4	76	10
5	31	4
6	24	3
7	11	1
8	9	1
9	6	1
10	10	1
Mean	2.18	
Standard deviation	2.13	

Table 1. (*Continued*)

	n	Percent
Number of network members subject has shared syringes with in the last 30 days		
0	451	59
1	160	21
2	76	10
3	37	5
4	22	3
5	9	1
6	7	1
7	1	[a]
8	2	[a]
9	0	0
10	2	[a]
Mean	0.84	
Standard deviation	1.38	
Number of network members subject has ever had sex with		
0	327	43
1	329	43
2	70	9
3	25	3
4	11	1
5	1	[a]
6	2	[a]
7	1	[a]
8	1	[a]
Mean	0.81	
Standard deviation	0.97	
Number of members subject has ever had sex with who have ever injected drugs		
0	502	65
1	224	29
2	33	4
3	4	0.5
4	4	0.5
Mean	0.41	
Standard deviation	0.65	
Are any of the members IDUs who[b]:		
Are five or more years older than subject?	273	36
On average, inject drugs more than once a day?	391	51
Inject drugs in shooting galleries?	193	25
Subject has known for less than one year?	280	36

(*continued*)

Table 1.   (*Continued*)

	n	Percent
Duration and intensity of relationships with those 586 network members the subject had injected drugs with in the prior 30 days:		
Proportion of 30-day injection network whom subject had known for 1 year		
None	123	21
Some	153	26
All	310	53
Proportion of 30-day injection network whom subject sees daily		
None	177	30
Some	179	31
All	230	39
Proportion of 30-day injection network whom subject considers "very close"		
None	315	54
Some	173	29
All	98	17
Heterogeneity of 30-day injection networks:		
Proportion of 30-day injection network members who are of the different sex		
None	249	42
Some	222	38
All	115	20
Proportion of 30-day injection network members who are of a different race/ ethnicity		
None	354	60
Some	176	30
All	56	10
Proportion of 30-day injection network members who are at least five years older than the subject		
None	357	61
Some	156	27
All	73	12
Injection settings:		
Has subject injected in the prior 30 days in[b]:		
Shooting gallery?	146	19
Outside setting?	286	38

[a]Represents < 0.5%.
[b]The number and percent of a "yes" response.

what we really meant when we were asking about persons with whom one interacted more than casually in the network section; (3) a degree of anticipated
underreporting to reduce the length of the questionnaire; (4) possible increase in
willingness to report on injection contacts as subjects grew to trust us during the
course of taking the questionnaire; and (5) more accurate recall of injection events
and partners as successive sections of the questionnaire prompted the memory.
(Reasons 4 and 5 would lead to more injection partners being reported in the
network section, which was later in the questionnaire.)

A majority (59%) denied having shared syringes with any network members
in the last 30 days; 21% had shared with one; 10% with two; and 10% with more
than two. On average, they reported less than one (0.84) network member with
whom they had shared syringes in the last 30 days.

We also asked about sex with the members of the 30-day network. Approximately equal proportions—43% each—said that they had never had sex with any
members of their 30-day network and that they had had sex with one member. The
other 14% reported having had sex with two or more members at some time in their
lives (although most had done so with only two or three of their current network
members.) On average, they reported fewer than one (0.81) network member with
whom they had ever had sex.

Of the network members with whom they had ever had sex, only about half
were reported to have ever injected drugs. This amounted to a mean of 0.41 sex
partner network members who had ever injected drugs per subject. Almost two
thirds of the subjects (65%) reported that they did not have a sex partner in their 30-
day network who had ever injected drugs; and most of the other subjects (29%)
reported having only one such member.

High-Risk Network Members

Another way of thinking about egocentric networks is in terms of whether
they contain any "high-risk" injectors who might be particularly likely to be
infected with HIV or hepatitis. We used four indicators of such high risk:

1. Whether there were any drug-injecting network members who were 5 or
    more years older than the subject (and thus might have had more time to
    become infected). [We used the relative ages of network members, rather
    than whether any of them had been injecting 5 or more years longer than
    the subject, because these drug injectors' knowledge about how long
    their network members have been injecting is not very accurate (Golds-
    tein et al., 1995).] Over a third (36%) of the subjects reported having one
    or more drug injectors in their network who were 5 or more years older
    than they were.

2. About half reported having at least one member of their network who injects more than once a day. Drug injectors who inject more often are more likely than others to be HIV-infected (Marmor et al., 1987).

3. Drug injectors who inject in shooting galleries are also more likely to be infected (Marmor et al., 1987), and one quarter of the subjects reported having one or more such network members.

4. We reasoned that subjects whose networks showed evidence of "turn-over" might be more at risk of encountering an infected partner over the long run. We took special notice of a situation that we had suggested (Friedman et al., 1989a) could be important in some drug injectors' careers as users: That they and some friends might begin to inject at about the same time, but only inject with each other. Under these circumstances, if none had been infected through sex, and if none injected with anybody else, the group as a whole might be protected. However, if they began to inject with new people, this partial protection might be undone. Thus, we analyzed whether they had any drug injectors in their network whom they had known for less than one year. Over a third (36%) had at least one such newcomer in their egocentric network.

Duration and Intensity of Relationships

Another issue of some interest is the duration and intensity of relationships which drug injectors have with each other. As is shown in Chapters 8 and 9, these variables help predict whether syringes are shared within relationships and whether condoms are used by sex partners. (In general, the pattern is that drug injectors, like other people, engage in more risk behavior with those with whom they are close.)

Approximately half of the subjects reported that all of the network members with whom they had injected in the prior 30 days were persons whom they had known for at least a year. On the other hand, 21% report that none of their 30-day injection network members had been known for this long a time. About two fifths report that they see all of their 30-day injection network members on a daily basis, 31% seeing some of them daily, and 30% see none of them on a daily basis.

In spite of having known many of their network members a reasonable length of time (a year or more) and in many cases seeing them every day, relatively few of the 30-day injection networks seem to be oases of friendship. Only one sixth of the subjects report that all of the members of their 30-day injection networks are "very close" to them. Three fifths report that some are very close, but many—54%—of the subjects report that none of their 30-day injection network members are very close.

Heterogeneity

Heterogeneity of injection networks is an important consideration in the epidemiology of infections. If injection networks are totally homogeneous on a given characteristic such as gender, then HIV should not be transmitted (through injection) across this line. On the other hand, if networks are extremely hetero-geneous, the distinction will not serve as a barrier to viral transmission. A sizable proportion (42%) of subjects report that their 30-day injection networks are homogeneous by gender, a larger proportion (60%) report homoge-neity by race–ethnicity, and 61% report that no one in this network is 5 years or more older than they are. Elsewhere, one of the authors has carefully studied the impact of homogeneity and heterogeneity of networks by race–ethnicity in these data (Jose, 1996). He finds some evidence that the degree of racial–ethnic network homogeneity plays a part in the greater HIV seroprevalence of drug injectors of Puerto Rican race–ethnicity than of whites.

High-Risk Injection Settings

Not all injection-related HIV or hepatitis risk involves persons whom a drug injector knows. There are also injection settings that can pose the risk of injecting with "anonymous" syringes or with persons an injector does not know. These forms of risk, as was described at some length in Chapter 3, are particularly likely to occur in shooting galleries like the tire shop and when injecting in outdoor settings the way Patricia and Jerry did when they were "banging in the street." For example, on one occasion in summer 1991, Patricia spent several days hanging out with Danny, a 44-year-old white injector from Queens who had found a wallet lying in the street that contained several hundred dollars. Danny was a regular at the tire shop, but when he suddenly found himself in possession of a considerable amount of cash, he did not want to be put in the position of supporting the habits of the other injectors who were also regulars there. Instead, he teamed up with Patricia, a distant acquaintance who in many ways promised to be subordinate to and controllable by him as an injection partner, but one who was also familiar with the many spots in Bushwick where injectors could go to use drugs and the brand names of heroin that were potent on a daily basis. While the money lasted, Pat and Danny avoided the tire shop, but over the first 24-hour period, they injected numerous times in six different indoor and outdoor locations. Even as they tried to avoid other injectors who would drain their resources, however, they ended up sharing drugs with seven other people, including Yeti, a Puerto Rican injector who operated an "outdoor" shooting gallery on Jefferson Street, a "date" whom Patricia injected in the neck, and an anonymous African-American injector who stumbled across the pair as they sought privacy near a secluded section of railroad tracks. Injecting in shooting galleries (in the prior 30 days) was reported by 19% of the subjects, and injecting in outdoor settings (in the prior 30 days) by 38%.

VARIATION BY YEARS OF INJECTION, GENDER, RACE–ETHNICITY, AND DRUG SCENE ROLES

In this section, we briefly present data on how drug injectors' egocentric networks and use of high-risk injection settings differ by selected social characteristics. In presenting these data, we have chosen not to give the tables that show the numbers, since this would lead to an overwhelming number of tables. There are two exceptions to this: We have chosen to present the data on variation by years of injection and by race–ethnicity as illustrations of the complexity of the data. Elsewhere, we present the data in words. In most cases, there is little or no variation in egocentric networks or injection settings use by these characteristics of the research participants. Where differences are not only statistically significant but of large enough magnitude to be worth mentioning, we do so in the text.

Variation by Years of Drug Injection

In Table 2, data are presented on how networks and settings vary by how long a subject has been injecting drugs. There are few differences. New injectors are more likely to have older members of their networks, but this relationship is not strong. They also have somewhat fewer network members with whom they have ever injected drugs and fewer members in their 30-day injection networks. They tend to be more likely to have no members of their 30-day injection network whom they have known for as long as a year.

Variation by Gender

Men and women vary on a number of these variables. On the average, men named more network members with whom they had injected (2.62 vs. 2.24) and with whom they had injected in the last 30 days (2.30 vs. 2.18). Men (21%) are more likely than women (14%) to have injected in shooting galleries in the last 30 days. Women, on the other hand, are more likely to report injecting with someone who has been injecting drugs at least 5 years longer than they have (42% vs. 33%); and they report having had sex in the last 30 days with more drug injectors (0.55), on average, than men (0.36). Women's 30-day injection networks are also more likely to include only persons (1) with whom they are "very close" (24% vs. 14%); (2) who are of the opposite sex (54% of men's networks include only men, but only 14% of women's networks contain only women); and (3) who are of a different race–ethnicity (16% vs. 7%). Somewhat surprisingly, women's injection networks are more likely not to include persons who are 5 years or more older than they are (68% vs. 58%)

Variation by Race–Ethnicity

There are few significant differences in these network and other characteristics by race–ethnicity (Table 3). Blacks are least likely to report having injected in outside settings and to have drug injector network members whom they have known for less than a year, and are most likely to have known all of their 30-day injection network members for at least a year. Whites are least likely to report injecting in shooting galleries themselves and having network members who inject drugs in shooting galleries.

Variation by Roles in Drug Scene

There are 143 (19%) subjects who told us that they had sold drugs during the preceding 30 days. On average, they nominated more network members (4.9 vs. 3.9), more members with whom they had ever injected drugs (3.2 vs. 2.3), and with whom they had injected drugs in the last 30 days (2.8 vs. 2.0) than did other subjects. In addition, there is some evidence ($p < .07$) that they share syringes with more network members, have sex with more network members, and have sex with more drug-injecting network members than do other subjects. Drug sellers are more likely than other subjects to have named drug-injecting network members who inject at least daily (64% vs. 48%), who inject in shooting galleries (34% vs. 23%), and whom they have known for less than a year (45% vs. 35%), and perhaps (43% vs. 34%; $p < .06$) to have network members who had been injecting 5 or more years longer than they themselves had. They are also more likely than other subjects to inject in shooting galleries (29% vs. 17%) and outdoor settings (50% vs. 34%). Their 30-day injection networks do not vary significantly from other subjects' in terms of how close members are to the subject or in terms of heterogeneity.

There are 125 (17%) subjects who reported that they had *sold needles or syringes* during the preceding 30 days. On average, they named more network members (5.6 vs. 3.8), more members with whom they had injected drugs (4.0 vs. 2.2), more members with whom they had injected drugs in the last 30 days (3.5 vs. 1.9), and more network members with whom they had shared syringes in the prior 30 days (1.2 vs. 0.8) than other subjects. Their sexual networks, however, resembled those of other drug injectors. Syringe sellers are more likely than other subjects to have named drug-injecting network members who inject at least daily (75% vs. 46%), who inject in shooting galleries (40% vs. 22%), and whom they have known for less than a year (54% vs. 33%). They are also more likely than other subjects to inject in shooting galleries (34% vs. 16%) and outside settings

Table 2. Characteristics of Participants' Networks and Injection Settings, by Number of Years Participant Has Injected Drugs

	Years				p^a
	0–2	3–5	6–8	9+	
Number of subjects	90	97	83	496	
Are any of the members IDUs who:					
Are 5 or more years older than the subject?	42%	37%	53%	31%	0.014
On average, inject drugs more than once a day?	54%	45%	46%	52%	0.677
Inject drugs in shooting galleries?	28%	14%	28%	26%	0.362
Subject has known for less than 1 year?	41%	34%	45%	35%	0.328
Has subject injected in the prior 30 days in:					
Shooting gallery?	22%	16%	19%	19%	0.802
Outdoor setting?	34%	35%	43%	38%	0.666
Mean number of nominated members of network (p by linear regression on four-category injection years variable)	4.01	3.24	4.63	4.22	0.0805
Mean number of members subject has ever injected with (p by linear regression on four-category injection years variable)	2.24	1.98	2.61	2.65	0.0142
Mean number of members subject injected with in last 30 days	1.90	1.78	2.29	2.30	0.0213
Mean number of members subject shared syringes with in last 30 days (p by linear regression on four-category injection years variable)	0.70	0.70	0.98	0.86	0.2107
Mean number of members subject has ever had sex with (p by linear regression on four-category injection years variable)	0.79	0.99	0.89	0.76	0.2100
Mean number of members subject has ever had sex with who have ever injected drugs (p by linear regression on four-category injection years variable)	0.40	0.48	0.47	0.40	0.4739

Duration and intensity of relationships with those 586 network members the subject had injected drugs with in the prior 30 days:

					p[a]
Proportion of 30-day injection network whom subject had known for ≥1 year					0.001
None	51	27	13	16	
Some	17	25	40	26	
All	32	48	47	58	
Proportion of 30-day injection network whom subject sees daily					0.071
None	22	24	27	33	
Some	32	31	45	28	
All	46	45	28	39	
Proportion of 30-day injection network whom subject considers "very close"					0.407
None	59	51	43	55	
Some	29	34	40	27	
All	13	15	17	18	
Heterogeneity of 30-day injection networks:					
Proportion of 30-day injection network members who are of the different sex					0.259
None	38	33	38	45	
Some	37	40	38	38	
All	25	27	23	17	
Proportion of 30-day injection network members who are of a different race/ ethnicity					0.772
None	59	63	62	60	
Some	35	24	30	30	
All	6	13	8	10	
Proportion of 30-day injection network members who are at least five years older than the subject					0.001
None	76	72	80	54	
Some	13	19	18	31	
All	11	9	2	15	

[a]Probability by χ^2 test for trend.

Table 3. Characteristics of Participants' Networks and Injection Settings,
by Race–Ethnicity of Participant

	Black	Latino	White	p
Number of subjects	206	311	243	
Are any of the members IDUs who				
Are 5 or more years older than the subject?	33%	34%	40%	0.300
On average, inject drugs more than once a day?	49%	49%	56%	0.132
Inject drugs in shooting galleries?	28%	29%	18%	0.009
Subject has known for less than one year?	29%	38%	40%	0.039
Has subject injected in the prior 30 days in:				
Shooting gallery?	20%	25%	11%	0.001
Outside setting?	30%	41%	39%	0.047
Mean number of nominated members of network	4.29	3.98	4.12	0.507
(p by F test)				
Number of members subject has ever injected with	2.78	2.31	2.55	0.072
(p by F test)				
Mean number of members subject injected with in last 30	2.36	1.99	2.27	0.118
days (p by F test)				
Mean number of members subject shared syringes with in	0.73	0.85	0.91	0.385
last 30 days (p by F test)				
Mean number of members subject has ever had sex with	0.86	0.81	0.75	0.449
(p by F test)				
Mean number of members subject has ever had sex with	0.38	0.39	0.47	0.265
who have ever injected drugs (p by F test)				
Duration and intensity of relationships with those 586				
network members the subject had injected drugs with				
in the prior 30 days:				
Proportion of 30-day injection network whom subject had				0.001
known for ≥1 year				
None	12	28	21	
Some	21	26	30	
All	67	46	49	
Proportion of 30-day injection network whom subject				0.083
sees daily				
None	35	23	33	
Some	26	33	32	
All	39	44	36	
Proportion of 30-day injection network whom subject				0.902
considers "very close"				
None	52	53	56	
Some	31	29	29	
All	17	18	15	
Heterogeneity of 30-day injection networks:				
Proportion of 30-day injection network members who are				0.390
of the different sex				
None	44	44	40	
Some	41	34	40	
All	16	22	21	

Table 3. (*Continued*)

	Black	Latino	White	p
Proportion of 30-day injection network members who are of a different race–ethnicity				0.112
None	66	59	56	
Some	27	32	31	
All	7	8	14	
Proportion of 30-day injection network members who are at least 5 years older than the subject				0.490
None	60	65	58	
Some	27	25	27	
All	13	10	15	

(64% vs. 32%). Their 30-day injection networks are more likely than other subjects' to be categorized as "some" (i.e., some members of each kind) in terms of whether the subject was very close to the other members or not and in terms of whether the subject was of the same sex, age, and race–ethnicity as the members. This probably just reflects the greater size of their 30-day injection networks.

There are 51 (7%) subjects who told us that they had been paid by others to help them inject drugs during the preceding 30 days. Such persons are called *hit doctors*. On average, they named more network members (6.4 vs. 3.9), more members with whom they had injected drugs (4.9 vs. 2.3), more members of their 30-day injection network (4.4 vs. 2.0), and more network members with whom they had shared syringes in the prior 30 days (2.2 vs. 0.7) than other subjects. Indeed, their 30-day syringe-sharing networks were much larger (mean 2.25, as compared to 0.74) than those of other subjects. Their sexual networks, however, resembled those of other drug injectors. Hit doctors are more likely than other subjects to have named drug-injecting network members who are 5 or more years older than they are (55% vs. 34%), who inject at least daily (69% vs. 50%), who inject in shooting galleries (37% vs. 24%), and whom they have known for less than a year (63% vs. 35%). They are also considerably more likely than other subjects to inject in shooting galleries (35% vs. 18%) and outside settings (69% vs. 35%). As with syringe sellers, hit doctors' 30-day injection networks are more likely than other subjects' to be categorized as "some" (i.e., some members of each kind) in terms of whether the subject was close to the other members or not and in terms of whether the subject was of the same sex, age, and race–ethnicity as the members. This probably just reflects the greater size of their 30-day injection networks. The large extent to which other subjects' 30-day injection networks do not include members of other race–ethnicity or older injectors may also reflect the extent to which the job of being a hit doctor brings a drug injector into injecting with a wide variety of other drug injectors who need the service.

There are 87 (11%) subjects who told us that they had engaged in *commercial sex work* (i.e., traded sex for money or drugs) during the preceding 30 days. On average, they nominated more network members (5.0 vs. 4.0) and more members with whom they had ever injected drugs (3.1 vs. 2.4) than other subjects; and they shared syringes with more network members during the last 30 days (1.3 vs. 0.8). They have also had sex with more network members (1.2 vs. 0.8). Commercial sex workers are more likely than other subjects to have named drug-injecting network members who had been injecting 5 or more years longer than they themselves had (57% vs. 33%), who inject drugs more than once a day (64% vs. 50%), who inject in shooting galleries (38% vs. 24%), and whom they have known for less than a year (53% vs. 35%). They are also more likely than other subjects to inject in outdoor settings (60% vs. 35%) and perhaps in shooting galleries (26% vs. 18%; $p < .06$). As with syringe sellers and hit doctors, there is evidence that sex traders' 30-day injection networks are more likely than other subjects' to be categorized as "some" (i.e., some members of each kind) in terms of whether the subject was of the same sex and race–ethnicity as the members. This may just reflect the tendency to have 30-day injection networks, although this would not explain the finding that more sex workers than other IDUs have 30-day injection networks that contain only members of different race–ethnicity.

CONCLUSIONS

These data on egocentric networks have several implications. First, they suggest that the sizes of the networks of persons with whom the subjects interact in a noncasual way are fairly small (averaging 4.1 in size), or else that they are underreporting network size. The limited size of their sexual networks should disabuse us of any lingering fantasies that drug injectors' lives are filled with lots of sexual relationships. Indeed, 43% report having had no sexual network members in the last month, and approximately the same number reported having only one member of their sexual network.

The data on network characteristics by roles in the drug scene are, insofar as we know, unique. No one else has ever asked these questions. They suggest that sizable proportions of street drug injectors at least occasionally sell drugs or syringes, and that others, perhaps smaller in numbers, at least occasionally sell sex or sell their services as hit doctors. These role-holders have larger networks, have larger injection networks, share syringes with more network members, and are more likely to have high-risk injectors in their networks. As a consequence, they may be more likely to be infected with HIV. Their networks include persons of different race–ethnicities, genders, and ages, which means that *role-holders* might be important linkages in the spread of HIV or other infections across potential sociodemographic barriers. They also may be appropriate persons with whom to work to diffuse health-related messages to other drug injectors, both because their networks are large and diverse and also because they may be likely to have casual contact with other injectors in the course of doing business.

It is also of interest that the differences in network size, of the riskiness of injection network members, and in use of shooting galleries and outdoor settings over the course of an injector's career do not appear to be great. Perhaps of greatest interest, half (51%) of the subjects who have been injecting for fewer than 3 years report that *none* of their 30-day injection network members are people they have known for a year or more; and only 32% report that all of their 30-day injection risk network members are such "medium- to long-term" acquaintances. Thus, the first years of injection experience seem to involve considerable injecting with newcomers to one's network. This suggests [as do data from Baltimore showing that, among 216 people who had been injecting drugs for a year or less (Garfein, Vlahov, Galai, Doherty, & Nelson, 1996), 65% were infected with hepatitis C and 50% had been exposed to hepatitis B] that the limited immunity from infection that new injectors might have if they inject only within their preexisting peer group is limited indeed, and lasts long for only a minority at best.

8

Syringe Sharing and the Social Characteristics of Drug-Injecting Dyads

INTRODUCTION

Injecting with a syringe that has been used by another injector can lead to infection with HIV or other infectious agents (Des Jarlais et al., 1994; Friedman et al., 1995a; Metzger et al., 1993; Nicolosi et al., 1992). We refer to this behavior as "receptive syringe sharing." The risks for HIV infection through receptive syringe sharing have been known to both drug injectors and researchers since the early 1980s (Des Jarlais et al., 1985; Friedman et al., 1987a; Selwyn et al., 1987). However, substantial numbers of injection drug users (IDUs) continue to engage in this risk behavior. Lack of access to sterile injecting equipment is likely to be a major determinant of whether or not IDUs inject with other injectors' syringes (Des Jarlais & Friedman, 1992; Lurie et al., 1993; Normand, Vlahov, & Moses, 1995). However, since receptive syringe sharing often is a social behavior (since it usually requires the interaction of two or more persons), the characteristics of the social relationships among these persons may also influence whether syringes are shared.

In this chapter, we focus on how receptive syringe sharing is shaped by the social relationships between two injectors. Of course, other forces also affect syringe sharing. Dyads are made up of individuals who have their own particular attributes and drug use experience, and further they occur within the personal (or egocentric) social networks of the individuals involved. These personal networks may also be part of larger sociometric networks which have their own structural form and influence. Nevertheless, insofar as receptive syringe sharing, when it occurs directly between drug injectors, is an act involving two individuals, an analysis focusing heavily on the character of the dyadic relationship in which this risk behavior occurs may provide further understanding of the dynamics involved.

The community context in which the social factors and HIV risk (SFHR) study was conducted is discussed elsewhere in this volume. However, the ways in which this community context relates to receptive syringe sharing needs further discussion, since it sheds light on the structural constraints that affected the availability of sterile syringes and may have induced the sharing of syringes among Bushwick IDUs.

During the time in which the data were collected, between July 1991 and January 1993, approximately half of the IDUs in New York City had been infected with HIV. The syringe exchange programs that then existed were either "underground" programs, or, for programs in the latter part of the project, were covered by a waiver that exempted registered syringe exchange program participants from the New York State laws governing the illegal possession and use of syringes. Syringe exchanges were nonetheless neither widespread nor easily accessible. In Bushwick, a syringe exchange was established in 1991 (with the assistance of some project staff in their off-hours), but it operated only a few hours a week at various locations in the neighborhood. The laws against syringe possession were enforced by the New York City Police Department sporadically, with some police in Bushwick acting with particular vigor, involving the destruction of syringes by the police after they had been seized from drug injectors. Many IDUs in Bushwick were also homeless, which meant that they had problems in finding a secure place to store their supply of syringes. Thus, the context was such that even though many IDUs were very knowledgeable about the risks of sharing syringes, there were many structural impediments that sometimes prevented them from implementing such knowledge by only injecting with sterile syringes.

METHODS

In order to study the effect of the dyadic relationship on syringe sharing, the unit of analysis in this chapter is the *dyad*. These dyads comprise relationships, as described by interviewed subjects, between these subjects and those members of their networks whom they named in response to a naming stimulus. The analysis focuses on the subsample of dyads in which subjects injected with a network member in the prior 30 days. For example, if subject A nominated five people when asked to name the members of his or her social network with whom drugs were used in the prior 30 days, and three of these nominated people are people with whom A had injected, then A would have generated three injecting dyads. These three dyads are each considered separate units of analysis. Syringe sharing is examined as a function of the nature of the relationship, as described by A, in each of these dyads separately.

The dependent variable is thus receptive syringe sharing by the subject with an injecting partner whom the subject nominated as a social network member. Subjects were asked the question: "During the last 30 days how frequently have you injected with a needle/syringe after this person injected with it first?" Syringe sharing was validated by comparing the responses of 112 linked pairs of interviewed subjects who reported that they had injected with each other. These linked pairs generated 224 injector dyads. In 159 (71%) of these dyads there was agreement about whether or not subjects had engaged in receptive syringe sharing, that is, subjects' reports about whether or not they had injected with a syringe previously used by another interviewed subject were confirmed by these other subjects, who reported that they had (or had not) indeed passed on a syringe that they had used previously to these subjects. (Some cases of apparent nonagreement may have been the result of the two research participants' in a dyad having been interviewed at different times, and thus having accurately described what happened during different 30-day time periods.)

The independent variables of primary interest measured characteristics of the dyadic relationship. Such variables included the type of relationship of the network member to the subject (e.g., whether the network member was a spouse, friend, or other relative); indicators of the strength of ties between subjects and their injecting network members; whether or not there was homophily (i.e., "like with like") or, conversely, "heterophily" (i.e., heterogeneous categories within a dyad) by age, gender, and race–ethnicity between the subject and his or her injecting network members; and activities other than using drugs that subjects and their network members engaged in together.

The type of relationship was analyzed, since prior research has shown that IDUs tend to inject with or engage in drug risk behaviors with people whom they know, and specifically in certain kinds of family or friendship relationships (Barnard, 1993; Friedman, 1995; Latkin et al., 1995; Neaigus et al., 1994; Strathdee et al., 1997). This finding suggests that many of these injecting relationships are not casual relationships, but are characterized by strong social and emotional bonds, although other injecting relationships are more transient and casual.

Several measures of the strength of the tie between subjects and their injecting network members were used to characterize the dyads. These include measures of closeness, their frequency of injecting together, how long they have done so, and how long they have known each other.

Other research (e.g., Brunswick, Messeri, Dobkin, Flood, & Yang, 1995) has shown that mixing patterns among sex partners are assortative rather than random (Morris, 1991; Morris, 1993; Morris, Zavisca, & Dean, 1995b). Injecting partnerships have also been found to be structured along racial and ethnic lines (Jose, 1996) Thus, receptive syringe sharing may be structured by racial–ethnic sorting. We also examine the mix of gender and of age within the dyad. Because sociodemographic statuses are often tied to unequal access to social and economic resources, heterogeneity of such statuses within the dyad (i.e., dyads that are characterized by "heterophily") may reflect power imbalances that may influence whether or not IDUs engage in receptive syringe sharing.

The "multiplicity" of the dyadic relationship, that is, the degree to which dyads are characterized by two or more types of activities (and of types of relationships), is an indicator of the intensity of the dyad relationship (Scott, 1991).

In the ethnographic research that was conducted in the early part of this study (Neaigus et al., 1994), relationships among networks of injectors were found to be based on multiple types of activities. For example, some injectors had both a kinship and economic relationship with their injecting partners and many of these partnerships had lasted for several years. Injectors who are involved with one another in multiple types of activities may find that their behavior in one realm of activity with their dyad partner has consequences for other aspects of their relationship. Thus, drug injectors who are involved in "multiplex" ties with members of their networks may need to take into account the repercussions that their injecting behaviors will have on other aspects of their relationship and vice versa. We therefore examine whether the type of non–drug-using activities that subjects engage in with their injecting partners and the number of such activities have consequences for whether or not subjects engage in receptive syringe sharing with these partners.

Other independent variables were organized into domains of related variables. These domains were selected because prior research and/or theoretical interest suggest that they are connected with engaging in receptive syringe sharing. These domains included: (1) peer culture; (2) subject's economic resources; (3) subject's individual biography; (4) subject's contact with risk reduction organizations; (5) subject's drug behaviors; and (6) subject's sexual behavior. A complete list of these variables is given in Table 1.

Peer Culture

Variables measuring peer culture were included because peer culture provides "rules," or norms, about what are the appropriate ways of behaving. The questions used to create the variables asked respondents about the norms governing who injects first when syringes are shared and about appropriate behavior regarding the use of syringes.

Table 1.   List of Independent Variable Domains

Peer culture
[Mentioned in response to the question: "When people share a syringe, what usually determines who injects first with the syringe?"]
  The person who:
    Owns the syringe
    Paid for the syringe
    Paid for the drugs
    Paid the most for the drugs
    Paid the most for the syringe
    Whose place it is
    Who's sickest

Table 1. (*Continued*)

Peer culture (*continued*)
People rotate who goes first
A person who threatens/bullies other people
Nothing determines who goes first
Syringes are never shared
Other syringe use norms
[agree/disagree with the statements]
"A shooting partner who refuses to share a syringe with you is a true friend"
"A person should share works with a shooting partner who is drug sick"
"It is OK to use works someone has hidden somewhere"
"It is OK to use works your shooting partner has hidden somewhere"
Teaching bleach
"Has anyone else who uses drugs told you that you should use bleach to clean your works"
"Have you told anyone else they should use bleach to clean their works"
Talked about AIDS with a drug injector.
Subject's economic resources
Homeless
Regular work
Legal income
Income < $10,000
Sell drugs
Sell needles
Subject's individual biography
Injected 5 or more years
Age of first injection
Shared syringe at initiation
High school graduate
Ever in jail
Subject's contact with risk reduction organizations
Picked up HIV test results at last test
Ever tested for HIV
Ever counseled to prevent HIV infection
Currently in treatment
Ever in treatment
Received bleach
Received new syringes sealed in a sterile wrapper (in last 3 months)
Subject's drug behaviors (last 30 days)
Any crack use
Inject more than 1 time a day (total)
Inject cocaine more than 1 time a day
Inject heroin more than 1 time a day
Inject speedball more than 1 time a day
Subject's sexual behaviors (last 30 days)
Any unprotected sex
Any exchange of sex for money or drugs
Any anal sex
Any male–male sex
Any woman–woman sex

Subject's Economic Resources

There is a large market for syringes among IDUs. The acquisition of syringes, particularly in the absence of syringe exchange programs, is therefore governed by having the economic wherewithal to purchase such commodities. Furthermore, having the resources to live somewhere other than the streets or a shelter can make it possible to store syringes, and thus avoid having to borrow them, or provide an off-the-street setting in which to inject drugs less subject to pressures from others to share. (Such pressures have been described in Chapter 2.) Prior studies (e.g., Magura et al., 1989; Mandell, Vlahov, Latkin, Oziemkowska, & Cohn, 1994) have found variables that measure economic capacity to be significant predictors of engaging in syringe sharing. In this domain several measures of economic resources are considered which may have a bearing on whether or not IDUs share syringes.

Subject's Individual Biography

Past events in an injector's life may be predictive of later behaviors. In particular, early initiation into injecting and having shared syringes at initiation (see Chapter 4) may indicate a predilection for engaging in risk-taking behaviors and/or persisting structural constraints having to do with life circumstances that engender such behaviors (Neaigus et al., 1991; Rodríguez Arenas et al., 1996).

Subject's Contact with Risk Reduction Organizations

As discussed in Chapter 1, drug injectors were engaging in risk reduction even prior to the beginning of risk reduction interventions conducted by public health agencies. However, once such interventions were underway, drug injectors' efforts at risk reduction may have been initiated and/or reinforced by such contact. Typical interventions included providing information about the risks of engaging in syringe sharing and unprotected sex, HIV counseling and testing, and the provision of risk reduction materials, particularly condoms and in some cases bleach to clean used syringes. Some IDUs had also received sterile syringes from syringe exchange programs, although such programs were neither widespread nor easily accessible. Of 741 subjects (26 missing), 12% (86/741) reported that in the last 30 days they had obtained syringes (which they injected with) from a syringe distribution program; and in the prior 3 months, 31% (233/767) reported that they had received new syringe sealed in a sterile wrapper from outreach workers or organizations. Of the 593 subjects who nominated an injecting partner, 12% (72/593) reported that in the last 30 days they obtained syringes they injected with from a syringe distribution program, and 33% (196/593) reported that they had received new syringe sealed in a sterile wrapper from outreach workers or organizations. Barriers to syringe exchange access, such as not living near a syringe exchange, have been found to predict whether or not injectors use a syringe exchange (Rockwell, Des Jarlais, Friedman, Perlis, & Paone, manuscript submitted), which is likely to influence whether or not they engage in syringe sharing. Many injectors have also been in drug treatment, which may also have an impact on reducing HIV risk behaviors.

Subject's Drug Behaviors

The degree of dependency on drugs, as measured by frequency of injecting, has been found to be a predictor of HIV infection (D'Aquila et al., 1989; Dasgupta et al., 1995; Marmor et al., 1987) and of risk behavior change (Neaigus et al., 1990). As well as the overall frequency of drug use, the type and frequency of drugs used was also measured.

Subject's Sexual Behaviors

Variables measuring individual sexual behaviors that have been associated with HIV infection in prior studies were included in this domain. These sexual risk behaviors may also be associated with engaging in drug-related risk behaviors as part of a general set of risk-taking behaviors. They also may stem from similar kinds of social relationships, such as having a sex partner who is also a drug injector.

In addition to the domains of independent variables described above, subjects' sociodemographic statuses (i.e., age, race–ethnicity, and gender) and HIV serostatus are included as independent variables.

STATISTICAL ANALYSIS

The analysis first examines the univariate relationship between dyad characteristics and engaging in receptive sharing within the dyad. Those dyad characteristics that are significant are then combined with other variables in multiple logistic regression to determine independent significant predictors of receptive syringe sharing. In order to do this, however, we first have to decide which other variables should be included in the logistic model. As a first step, we analyze individual-level variables within each of the domains discussed above. Here, separate multiple logistic regressions are conducted within each domain (using stepwise with backward elimination) to determine which are independently and significantly associated with engaging in receptive syringe sharing. Finally, with the significant dyad characteristics variables forced into the equation, variables that were significant in the domain analyses of other independent variables, together with those from the univariate analysis of sociodemographic statuses (i.e., age, race–ethnicity, and gender) and HIV serostatus, were entered into a combined model (using forward stepwise analysis, which was then confirmed in a backward elimination model).

RESULTS

The number of injecting dyads used in the analysis was 1748. These dyads were generated by 593 subjects (77% of the total sample of 767). Those who nominated network members with whom they injected in the last 30 days, compared to those who did not, were less likely to be Latino (37% vs. 53%, $p < 0.001$), had injected for a longer period of time (14 years vs. 12.6 years, $p < 0.04$), and tended to be less likely to be in drug treatment (20% vs. 27%, $p < 0.07$). There were no significant differences by age, gender, and HIV serostatus.

The 593 participants who nominated injecting partner dyads were predominantly male (70%). Latinos comprised 37% of this analysis sample, whites 34%, and blacks 28%. The mean age was 35 and the mean years of injecting experience was 14. One fifth (20%, 119/585) were currently in drug abuse treatment. Thirty percent (176) of the 593 subjects nominated one injector dyad, 22% (132) two dyads, 18% (104) three dyads, and 30% (181) four or more dyads. Receptive syringe sharing by subjects was reported in 26% (457) of the 1748 dyads. Of the 417 subjects who nominated two or more injecting dyads, 15% reported that they shared syringes with all of their injecting partners, 28% with some, and 58% with none of their injecting partners.

The dyad characteristics associated with engaging in receptive syringe sharing in the univariate analysis are shown in Table 2. Respondents were more likely to engage in receptive syringe sharing in those dyads in which the injecting partner was a spouse or lover [odds ration (OR) = 4.35, as compared to dyads with an acquaintance, associate, or "get high" buddy]. The strength of the social tie was also associated with whether the respondent engaged in receptive syringe sharing in the dyad. Respondents were more likely to engage in receptive syringe sharing in those dyads in which they had daily or greater contact with the injecting partner (OR = 1.93), they had injected with the partner for more than 1 year (OR = 1.85), the respondent knew the injecting partner for more than 1 year (OR = 1.67), and the relationship with the injecting partner was reported by the respondent to be "very close" (OR = 2.12). Gender heterophily in the dyad was associated with respondents engaging in receptive syringe sharing in the dyad (OR = 1.58). Further, gender heterophily was significant for both male and female respondents (OR = 1.42, 95% CI = 1.05, 1.91, for dyads in which the respondent is male, and OR = 1.75, 95% CI = 1.15, 2.66, for dyads in which the respondent is female). Neither racial–ethnic heterophily nor age heterophily was associated with engaging in receptive syringe sharing in the dyad. The *activity* in the dyad that was most strongly associated with engaging in receptive syringe sharing by the respondent was in those dyads in which there was also a sexual relationship (OR = 2.67). Other dyad activities significantly associated with engaging in receptive syringe sharing in the dyad included stealing together (OR = 1.34), sharing a meal (OR = 1.63), and hanging out together (OR = 1.52). There was also a relationship between the number of activities engaged in together and receptive syringe sharing by the respondent. Receptive syringe sharing was more likely to occur in those dyads in which the respondents engaged in one compared to none non–drug-using activities with their injecting partners (OR = 1.41) and in two or more non–drug-using activities compared to none (OR = 1.91).

As shown in Table 3, there were 12 variables that were significant in the analysis of the (other) independent variable domains. Three variables were significant in the "peer culture" domain. In response to a question about the respondent's views and the views of the people he or she knows regarding syringe sharing, mentioning that "people rotate who goes first" and "the person who paid for the syringe goes first" were each significantly associated with the respondent engaging in receptive syringe sharing. Disagreeing with the statement that "a shooting partner who refuses to share a syringe with you is a true friend" was also significant. Having an income under $10,000 a year was significant in the "economic resources" domain. In the "individual biography" domain, younger age at first injection was associated with engaging in receptive syringe sharing. Three variables, all of which were protective, were significant in the "contact with risk reduction organizations" domain; these included ever having been counseled to prevent HIV infection, ever having been in drug treatment, and receiving new syringes in a sealed sterile wrapper in the last 3 months. In the "subject's drug behaviors" domain, injecting speedball more than one time a day was a risk factor for engaging in receptive syringe sharing, while injecting heroin more than one time a day was protective. In the sexual domain, engaging in unprotected sex and any exchange of sex for money or drugs were associated with engaging in receptive syringe sharing.

As Table 4 shows, women (OR = 1.30) were more likely and blacks less likely (OR = 0.70) to engage in receptive syringe sharing. Neither respondent's age nor respondent's HIV serostatus was significantly related to receptive syringe sharing.

In the multivariate logistic regression analysis, the same final equation was derived by both the forward selection and backward elimination models (see Table 5). Having a sexual relationship in the dyad was the dyad characteristic variable with the strongest association with engaging in receptive syringe sharing [adjusted odds ratio (AOR) = 2.39]. Three variables measuring the strength of the social tie in the dyad were also significantly associated with engaging in receptive syringe sharing. These included injecting together for more than 1 year (AOR = 1.78), having a "very close" relationship (AOR = 1.51), and having daily or greater contact (AOR = 1.38). Other variables significantly related to being more likely to engage in receptive syringe sharing were mentioning "people rotate who goes

Table 2.   The Relationship of Dyad Characteristics with Engaging
in Receptive Syringe Sharing within the Dyad (Bivariate Association)

	Number of dyads	Percent who engaged in receptive syringe sharing	Odds ratio	95% CI;
Type of relationship				
Acquaintance, associate, or "get high" buddy	347	21	(reference category)	
Spouse or lover	154	53	4.35	2.89, 6.55
Sibling	37	32	1.83	0.88, 3.83
Other relative	40	20	0.95	0.42, 2.16
Ex spouse or lover	19	26	1.36	0.48, 3.91
Friend	1148	24	1.22	0.91, 1.63
Strength of the social tie:				
Daily or greater contact				
Yes	894	32	1.93	1.55, 2.41
No	837	20		
Injecting together > 1 year				
Yes	934	31	1.85	1.48, 2.31
No	809	20		
Respondent knows injecting partner > 1 year				
Yes	1216	29	1.67	1.30, 2.14
No	522	20		
The relationship is "very close"				
Yes	377	39	2.12	1.71, 2.79
No	1336	23		
Dyad heterophily:				
Respondent and partner belong to different racial–ethnic groups				
No	1282	27	0.83	0.64, 1.07
Yes	433	24		
Respondent and partner are of different gender				
No	1203	23	1.58	1.26, 1.98
Yes	540	32		
Respondent's and partner's ages differ by > 5 years				
Yes	723	26	0.99	0.80, 1.23
No	976	26		
Non–drug-using activities that the respondent and injecting partner did together in the last 30 days:				
Had sex				
Yes	185	45	2.67	1.96, 3.65
No	1550	24		
Engaged in stealing				
Yes	273	31	1.34	1.01, 1.78
No	1446	25		

Table 2. (*Continued*)

	Number of dyads	Percent who engaged in receptive syringe sharing	Odds ratio	95% CI;
Shared a meal				
Yes	327	35	1.63	1.26, 2.11
No	1370	24		
Hung out together				
Yes	976	30	1.52	1.22, 1.90
No	724	22		
Talked about AIDS				
Yes	658	28	1.15	0.93, 1.44
No	1079	25		
Worked or ran a business				
Yes	26	27	1.03	0.43, 2.48
No	1705	26		
Did a legal "hustle"				
Yes	117	30	1.22	0.81, 1.84
No	1607	26		
Engaged in prostitution				
Yes	93	32	1.39	0.89, 2.17
No	1624	26		
Sold drugs or syringes				
Yes	191	29	1.19	0.85, 1.65
No	1537	26		
Played sports				
Yes	60	27	1.01	0.57, 1.81
No	1650	26		
Attended church				
Yes	18	39	1.79	0.69, 4.64
No	1680	26		
Went to parties				
Yes	69	20	0.93	0.41, 2.08
No	1630	27		
Went to social clubs				
Yes	32	25	0.70	0.39, 1.27
No	1665	26		
Went to movies, concerts and other cultural events				
Yes	199	30	1.20	0.87, 1.66
No	1500	26		
The number of non–drug-using events engaged in together in the last 30 days				
Two or more	620	32	1.91	1.46, 2.51
One	588	26	1.41	1.07, 1.87
None	535	20	(Reference category)	

Table 3. Variables Significant from Within-Domain Multiple Logistic Regression

	Adjusted odds ratio	95% CI
Peer culture		
[Mentioned in response to the question:		
"When people share a syringe, what usually determines who		
injects first with the syringe?"]		
People rotate who goes first	3.47	1.90, 6.31
The person who paid for the syringe goes first	1.52	1.03, 2.26
[Disagree with the statement]		
"A shooting partner who refuses to share a syringe with you	1.65	1.26, 2.17
is a true friend"		
Subject's economic resources		
Income < $10,000 per year	1.36	1.06, 1.75
Subject's individual biography		
Age at first injection	0.97	0.95, 0.99
Subject's contact with risk reduction organizations		
Ever counseled to prevent HIV infection	0.64	0.51, 0.80
Ever in drug treatment	0.79	0.63, 0.99
Received new syringes sealed in a sterile wrapper	0.77	0.61, 0.96
Subject's drug behaviors (last 30 days)		
Inject heroin > 1 time a day	0.76	0.61, 0.95
Inject speedball > 1 time a day	1.31	1.04, 1.64
Subject's sexual behaviors (last 30 days)		
Any unprotected sex	1.31	1.06, 1.63
Any exchange of sex for money or drugs	1.78	1.34, 2.36

first" in response to the question about what decides who injects first when syringes are shared; disagreeing with the statement "a shooting partner who refuses to share a syringe with you is a true friend"; injecting speedball more than one time a day; and any exchange of sex for money or drugs. Protective associations were found for age at first injection, ever being counseled to prevent HIV infection, ever in drug treatment, injecting heroin more than one time a day, and the respondent being of black race–ethnicity.

DISCUSSION

Receptive syringe sharing appears to be affected by the social relationships between injectors. Receptive syringe sharing is more likely to occur in those dyads in which there is a sexual relationship and in those dyads in which there are "strong" social ties, as characterized by having daily contact, injecting together for more than a year, and having a "very close" relationship.

Table 4. The Relationship of Respondents' Sociodemographic Status, and HIV Serostatus with Engaging in Receptive Syringe Sharing within the Dyad (Bivariate Association)

	Number of dyads	Percent who engaged in receptive syringe sharing	Odds ratio	95% CI
Sociodemographic status				
Gender				
Female	460	30	1.30	1.03, 1.65
Male	1288	25		
Age				
< 30	453	26	1.01	0.79, 1.28
≥ 30	1295	26		
Race–ethnicity				
Black (not Latino)	493	20	0.70	0.53, 0.94
Latino (not black)	525	29	1.13	0.87, 1.47
Latino (black)	129	32	1.27	0.84, 1.92
White	570	27		
HIV serostatus				
Positive	715	29	1.18	0.95, 1.48
Negative	871	25		

Peer culture is also important. Norms can mandate sharing syringes (rotating who "goes first") and can support and legitimate the refusal to give used syringes to other injectors (as a mark of "true friendship").

Certain drug use patterns are associated with whether or not respondents engaged in receptive syringe sharing. While injecting speedball more than once a day is a risk factor for engaging in receptive syringe sharing, injecting heroin more than once a day is protective. This may indicate that speedball, which requires combinations of heroin and cocaine, more often involves two or more drug injectors who share drugs, than does injecting only heroin, which may thus be a less "social" drug. In Chapter 3, for example, vignettes were given of the complex social interactions involved when Patricia injected speedball with Jerry and also with Bruce (although without engaging in syringe sharing in either instance). Those who exchange sex for money or drugs are also at higher risk of engaging in receptive syringe sharing.

Risk reduction interventions and drug treatment appear to be successful in reducing the probability of engaging in receptive syringe sharing. Those who began injecting drugs at an older age were also less likely to engage in receptive syringe sharing. Drug injectors of black racial–ethnic identity also are less likely to engage in receptive syringe sharing. In earlier research, we suggested that black drug injectors' greater aversion to receptive syringe sharing might reflect cultural

Table 5. Multivariate Logistic Regression
of Receptive Syringe Sharing in Drug Injector Dyads

	Adjusted odds ratio	95% CI
Social characteristics of dyads:		
Daily or greater contact	1.38	1.06, 1.78
Injecting together > 1 year	1.78	1.38, 2.31
"Very close" relationship	1.51	1.12, 2.03
Sexual relationship	2.39	1.63, 3.50
Other variables		
Risk factors:		
Subject reports that for self and peers		
"People rotate who goes first"	3.64	1.94, 6.83
"A shooting partner who *refuses* to share a syringe with you is a true friend" (Disagree)	1.88	1.39, 2.55
Inject speedball > 1 time a day	1.52	1.16, 1.99
Any exchange of sex for money or drugs	1.73	1.21, 2.47
Protective factors:		
Age at first injection	0.97	0.95, 0.99
Ever counseled to prevent HIV infection	0.64	0.50, 0.83
Ever in drug treatment	0.62	0.48, 0.81
Inject heroin > 1 time a day	0.69	0.53, 0.90
Black (not Latino) race–ethnicity	0.61	0.45, 0.81

[a]Receptive syringe sharing occurred in 400 (26%) of 1,510 injector dyads; model $\chi^2 = 173.85$; 13 df; $p < 0.0002$.

and social strengths developed during blacks' long history of struggle for rights and survival in this country (Friedman et al., 1987c).

Thus, dyad characteristics and individual attributes have a combined effect in determining whether or not receptive syringe sharing occurs. Interventions to reduce HIV risk behaviors that only target individuals, while having an effect on reducing syringe sharing, are only addressing part of the picture. While IDUs are less likely to share syringes with acquaintances and only very rarely with strangers, they may still share syringes with those with whom they have close friendships and/or love or sexual relationships. Therefore, there is a need to develop interventions that utilize strong social ties to reinforce norms against syringe sharing. These interventions should organize friendship groups of IDUs, as well as IDUs who are sexual partners and spouses (legally or informally), to assist each other in preventing the sharing of syringes as well as procuring sterile syringes. Such interventions should occur in tandem with increasing the availability of sterile syringes through the promotion of syringe exchange programs and other means (e.g., pharmacy sales) of legally distributing sterile syringes to IDUs.

9

Sexual Networks, Condom Use, and the Prospects for HIV Spread to Non-Injection Drug Users

INTRODUCTION

This chapter turns to an examination of sexual risk and condom use. Sexual transmission of HIV from drug injectors to other persons—both other injectors and partners who have never (or no longer) injected drugs—is quite widespread. In New York City during the time when data were being collected for this study, fully 89% of heterosexual transmission AIDS cases among noninjectors involved a drug injector as the source of infection (R. Quintyne, NYC Department of Health, personal communication, 20 September 1993). Condom use is important to understand as a potential barrier to the spread of HIV during sex (Centers for Disease Control and Prevention, 1993). Although there has been widespread drug-related risk reduction among drug users, sexual risk reduction has been more difficult to bring about (Friedman, 1994c; Malow et al., 1993).

In this chapter, we look at several issues related to sex and HIV among drug injectors. First, we describe the sexual behaviors of the participants in this study, including their involvement in commercial sex work. Then, we examine their condom use in some detail, with a primary focus on the relationship-specific and normative predictors of consistent condom use. Finally, we look at drug injectors' sexual behaviors with youth, and using data from a later study we conducted in Bushwick, we look at what Bushwick youth say about their sexual relationships with drug injectors.

DESCRIPTIVE DATA ON SEXUAL RELATIONSHIPS OF DRUG INJECTORS IN THIS STUDY

The sexual behavior of drug injectors in Bushwick is very different for men than for women. This is because a third or more of the women engage in trading sex for money, but almost none of the men report doing this. Thirty-five percent of women report commercial sex in the 30 days before their interview. Among men, only 6 of 538 (1.1%) report getting money for sex. (Data for the 2 years before the interview similarly show that 38.5% of women and 4% of men had engaged in sex for money or drugs.)

Given this, it should be no surprise that the mean frequency of sex for women is 40 per month and for men only 5.4 per month, and that women report a mean of 19 partners per month as compared with 1.1 for the men. These means are misleading, however, since they are greatly increased by a few persons who engage in commercial sex a large number of times with a large number of customers. Thus, for sexual frequency, although women report a mean of 40 events per month, 51% of them report having had sex four or fewer times in the last month; but 6% report sex twice a day, 5% report it about six times a day, and 7% report sex about ten times a day. Similarly, for women's numbers of partners, the mean may be 19 per month, but 61% report having zero or one partner per month. Five percent report 100 or more partners per month (including one participant who reported 500 and five others who reported 300). Women were also more likely ($p < 0.001$) than men to report having had sex with a drug injector in the prior 30 days. This was reported by 42% of the women and 28% of the men.

Drug injectors' sexual behaviors have consequences for their health. Twenty-six percent of the women (58/226) and 15% of the men (79/540) report having had a sexually transmitted disease (STD) during the prior 5 years. Although these figures are greater for women ($p < 0.001$), they are substantial for men, suggesting that women sex workers who become infected through unprotected sex with customers then pass the infection on to male drug injectors. (If they are lucky, the unprotected sex that transmits these STDs does not also transmit HIV.)

Images of drug injectors as sex fiends are not supported by the data in this study. Almost two fifths of the men (39%: 210/539) and almost one fourth of the women (22%: 49/224) report no sex during the prior 30 days. There is, of course, a sizable minority of women who have sex many times and/or with many partners, but this is commercial sex engaged in for the purposes of buying drugs and/or paying for other living expenses.

Some of the drug injectors report same-sex sex at least once during the last 5 years. This is reported by 3% of the men (16/540) and 16% of the women (37/225). As is discussed in Chapter 11, both the men who have sex with men and the women who have sex with women are more likely than other participants to be infected with HIV (and women who have sex with women are more likely to have been exposed to hepatitis B).

Both women and men began to have sex in their mid-teens. Median age for first vaginal sex was 15 for women and 14 for men. Three quarters of the women first had sex at age 14 or above, and three quarters of men at 13 or above. However, a minority of each sex (1.4% of women, and 7.2% of men) reported first sex at age ten or below. Unfortunately, we did not ask whether their first sex was the result of sex abuse, rape, or other coercion.

Much of the emphasis of public health efforts has been to urge drug injectors (and others) to engage in safer sex. Our findings on condom use are subsequently discussed. Here, however, it is useful to consider drug injectors' reports about their own and others' exposure to such messages, the passing on of such messages, and beliefs about sexual risk and safer sex. Almost half (43%) of the participants reported that they had been told by someone else to use condoms in the last 3 months, and 47% (44% of men and 55% of women; $p = 0.009$) reported having told someone else to use a condom in this time period. Women had received condoms on an average of seven occasions from outreach workers or other prevention programs in the prior 3 months, which was significantly more than the average of 3.3 for men (and may reflect the greater involvement of women in commercial sex). Women were more likely than men to report that the people they hang out with strongly *disagree* with the statements that using condoms (1) is embarrassing (63% of women vs. 49% of men report such strong disagreement); (2) interferes with sexual spontaneity (39% vs. 30%); and (3) is unnatural (45% vs. 29%). We are not sure whether these reports are really about the beliefs of participants' friends or about the beliefs of participants themselves. Interestingly, 43% of men but only 27% of women report that none of the men they know object if a woman wants to use a condom. This might reflect men's trying to appear more health-conscious than they are, but it might equally well reflect the experience of women drug injectors who engage in sex for money who find that some of their clients resist condom use.

We also asked subjects about what changes they had made in their sexual behaviors to protect themselves against AIDS. About two thirds of both men and women reported having made such changes. Twenty percent of men and 11% of women reported reducing their number of opposite-sex sex partners; about 27% of each sex reported using condoms more often (and 22% of women and 12% of men reported always using condoms). Ten percent of the participants reported having stopped having sex in order to protect themselves. Given the demands of street life and perhaps the effects of drugs on sexual desire, this may not have been as difficult as it may seem to the reader.

COMMERCIAL SEX WORK BY HIV-INFECTED AND -UNINFECTED WOMEN DRUG INJECTORS

Given the poverty of many drug injectors and the extent to which their poverty is aggravated both by their need to spend money on drugs and by the difficulties that their drug injecting creates for their ability to get employment, it is hardly surprising that many women drug injectors trade sex for money and/or for drugs.

Too few men trade sex for money or drugs for us to be able to analyze whether there are some categories of men who are more likely to do so or not. For women, however, such analyses are possible, since 35% report trading sex for money in the prior 30 days; 14% report trading sex for drugs in the prior 30 days; 36% report trading sex either for money or for drugs in the prior 30 days; and 39% report trading sex for money or drugs at least once in the previous 2 years. Since trading sex for money seems to dominate, and since few women reported trading sex in the 2-year period who did not also report doing so in the last 30 days, we will primarily focus here on which women engaged in sex for money in the last 30 days.

Women were more likely to trade sex for money if they were under 30 years of age. Fifty-five percent of these younger women had done so in the last 30 days, as compared to 25% of women 30 or older.

Much of the reason for sex trading seems to be economic. Homeless women were more likely to trade sex than those with homes (69% vs. 28%). Similarly, 64% of those who reported annual money incomes less than $10,000 in the prior year, as compared with 28% of women with $10,000 or more of income, traded sex for money in the 30 days before being interviewed. Sex trading was also more common among those with no legal income than among those with any legal income (59% vs. 25%).

Access to money or drugs through other roles in the drug scene had differing relationships to engaging in sex trading. We have analyzed such roles in more depth (Friedman et al., 1998). Drug sellers were more likely than non-drug-selling women to trade sex for money (55% vs. 31%), as were hit doctors (75% vs. 33%). Women who control space that other people pay money or drugs to inject in, however, appear to have less need to sell sex. Only 22% (of 60 such women) did so, as compared to 41% of 161 women who lacked this resource. Interestingly, syringe sellers were not significantly more likely to engage in sex for money, but were more likely to engage in sex for drugs (27% vs. 12%).

Crack use was associated with trading sex both for money and for drugs. The 127 (57%) women drug injectors who used crack in the last 30 days were more likely to have traded sex for money (50% vs. 15%) and for drugs (21% vs. 5%) in this period than were the 97 who did not use crack at all during it.

CONSISTENT CONDOM USE IN RELATIONSHIPS

In this section, which is based on but goes farther than that in Friedman et al. (1994c), we will describe the relationship-specific predictors of consistent condom use in relationships. The methodological and substantive logic of this analysis parallels that of our earlier analysis of receptive syringe sharing in Chapter 8.

Theoretical Background

To understand condom use during sex, we have to consider its epidemiological, personal, and social complexities. Epidemiologically, a large proportion of drug injectors in New York are infected with HIV but a large proportion are not. Most noninjector heterosexual sexual partners of drug injectors remain uninfected, although there has been considerable sexual transmission outward from drug injectors to crack smokers. Nonetheless, most crack smokers remain uninfected (Edlin, Irwin, & Faruque, 1994). Thus, condom use may have different meanings in sex between two drug injectors, depending on their beliefs about their infection statuses and also on the extent to which they engage in so much high-risk injecting together that they believe their sexual risks to be relatively less important. Sex between drug injectors and heterosexual partners who do not inject drugs (or smoke crack) almost always presents an asymmetrical pattern of risk, at least in the long term, in which the drug injector is much more likely to be or to become infected than his or her partner. Indeed, Ouellet, Rahimian, and Wiebel (in press) have suggested that the largest risk of infection for noninjector partners in Chicago may not be through sexual transmission, but instead through their becoming drug injectors themselves. This epidemiological pattern means that drug injectors' perspectives on condom use may well vary depending on whether they are infected with HIV or not. From the perspective of the uninfected, the issue is how to protect themselves from becoming infected. From the perspective of the infected, the issue is how to avoid infecting others.

In some ways, condom use can be looked at as a simple behavior. Thus, those people who do not like to use condoms, seeing it as less pleasurable and less intimate than sex without condoms, would be expected to be less likely to use condoms. However, neither sex nor condom use is a matter of unfettered choice. At one extreme, sex itself is not always fully consensual. Rape and sexual abuse do occur. Indeed, Miller, Paone, and Friedmann (1998) report that between 25 and 50% of women have undergone sexual abuse or rape, and in a study of a small probability sample of household-recruited 18- to 21-year-olds that we conducted in Bushwick after the conclusion of the SFHR project on which this volume is based, 30% of the women reported being coerced the first time they had sex. Even in adult relationships, including marriage, it has been suggested that physical retribution may occur if a partner insists on condom use (Auerbach, Wypijewska, & Brodie, 1994, pp. 96–97). Beyond that, if suggesting condom use causes the other partner to think that you have been having sex with other persons (or to think that you think that they have), or if it is in other ways seriously threatening to one or both of the partners, it can threaten the stability of relationships and marriages (Amaro, 1995). Furthermore, economic compulsion can restrict options about both having sex and using condoms when one does so.

Sex, then, is a behavior in which two people interact, and, at least to the extent that the sex is consensual, condom use in a relationship usually involves at least acquiescence on the part of both partners. (In commercial sex, it is sometimes possible for a woman to put a condom on a man without his realizing this has been done; but this is rarely feasible as a regular practice in a long-term relationship.)

Thus, condom use is a characteristic of relationships rather than simply of individuals (Sibthorpe, 1992).

In these regards, then, condom use is like receptive syringe sharing (as we discussed it in Chapter 8) in that relationship characteristics are likely to influence whether sexual partners do or do not use condoms. Thus, both in trying to study the condom use by drug injectors and in trying to develop programs to increase condom use, we should consider characteristics of the social relationship itself, characteristics of each participant in the relationship, and characteristics of the social environment of the relationship.

Relationship Characteristics

A number of studies of condom use among IDUs indicate that condoms are more widely used with casual partners than with primary partners (Morris, Pramualratana, Podhisita, & Wawer, 1995a; Paone, Caloir, Shi, & Des Jarlais, 1995a; van den Hoek et al., 1990; Watkins et al., 1993; White, Phillips, Mulleady, & Cupitt, 1993a). Furthermore, condoms are particularly likely to be used in those sexual relationships that are commercial in nature (Watkins et al., 1993; White et al., 1993a). Some studies have concluded that it will be very difficult to encourage widespread condom use in primary relationships. For example, Sibthorpe (1992), on the basis of a review of a number of studies on condom use by IDUs and her own research on sex practices of IDUs in Portland, Oregon, concludes that "the greatest gains in safer sex practices can be expected in those relationships that only minimally reaffirm social bonds," and that "the likelihood of a significant increase in safer sex practices within conjugal and paraconjugal relationships is not strong" (p. 267). However, there is some evidence that such pessimism may be overstated. For example, in a study of New York drug injectors' condom use at the last intercourse, which we conducted as part of a different research project, event-specific condom use with primary partners increased markedly (from 59 to 70%) from 1990/91 to 1994/95 (Friedman et al., 1996b). More precise specification of the characteristics of drug injectors' relationships that may affect condom use has not been reported [except in Friedman et al. (1994c), which was an earlier paper based on the SFHR project data]. Such relationship characteristics might include the form of the relationship (marriage; lovers; ex-spouses; friends; and so on); the length of time the partners have known each other; the length of time the partners have been having sex; how often they see each other; and the perceived closeness of the relationship.

Personal Characteristics

Personal characteristics of a drug injector can also affect whether condoms are used. Such characteristics include age, gender, race–ethnicity, homelessness, crack use, commercial sex work, prison experience, general behavior change to avoid AIDS, HIV status, frequency of carrying condoms, number of sex partners, frequency of sex, and health beliefs (Gossop, Griggiths, Powis, & Strang, 1993; Jose et al., 1996; Lewis & Watters, 1991; Nyamathi, Lewis, Leake, Flaskerud, & Bennett, 1995; Rhodes, 1996; Rietmeijer et al., 1996; Schilling et al., 1991; White, Phillips, Mulleady, & Cupitt, 1993b).

In addition, personal participation in some HIV prevention interventions has been found to be associated with increased condom use among IDUs (Corby & Wolitski, 1996; Jose et al., 1996; Rietmeijer et al., 1996). A number of studies have shown that drug injectors who know that they are HIV-positive are less likely to have unprotected sex than are HIV-negatives; they do this either by not having sex or by using condoms (Casadonte et al., 1990; Colón, Robles, Marrero, Reyes, & Sahai, 1996; van Ameijden, van den Hoek, & Coutinho, 1996; van den Hoek et al., 1990; Vanichseni et al., 1993; Watkins et al., 1993). On the other hand, Friedman et al. (1994c) have reported that, in the SFHR data, even seropositives who report that they have never (previously) been diagnosed as seropositive are more likely always to use condoms (and to do so, especially, with non-IDU partners) than are seronegatives. Furthermore, among drug injectors, having participated in conversations about HIV/AIDS with sex partners and/or friends has been found to be related to drug-injection-related risk reduction (Des Jarlais et al., 1995a) and (at least at the univariate level) with consistent condom use (Friedman et al., 1994c).

Personal characteristics of a drug injector's sexual or drug-using partner have also been found to be related to his or her HIV risk and protective behaviors. Deliberate efforts by drug injectors to reduce risk have been reported since early in the epidemic, and both drug-related and sexual risk reduction have been more common among those who reported that their friends had also tried to reduce their AIDS risks (Abdul-Quader et al., 1990; Friedman et al., 1987b). Consistent condom use by drug injectors is more common with noninjector partners (Friedman et al., 1994c; Lorvick, Estilo, & Watters, 1993).

If the partner is also a drug injector, whether or not the partner has these same individual characteristics would be expected to affect condom use. We might also expect the extent of condom use and the processes by which condoms come either to be used or not to be used to differ depending on whether the partner is or is not a drug injector. There are reasons to think that condoms are *more* likely to be used in relationships with partners who also inject drugs, but there are also other reasons to think that they are *less* likely to be used in relationships with partners who also inject drugs. In relationships of a drug injector with another drug injector, there is no need to hide the fact of drug use, and this means the couple may be more able to discuss AIDS risk and risk reduction [which has been linked to lower levels of risk behavior and to higher levels of deliberate risk reduction (Des Jarlais et al., 1995a; Neaigus et al., 1994)]. On the other hand, drug injectors may have been more likely to focus their efforts to reduce risk on preventing parenteral rather than sexual transmission.

In relationships between a drug injector and a noninjector, the fact that one of the couple injects drugs may not be known to the other; and if it is known, one or both of them may try not to think about this knowledge. In either case, communication about condom use as a way to prevent HIV transmission is less likely to occur. On the other hand, the drug-injecting member of the couple will ordinarily realize that the primary risk of HIV infection for his or her partner is through the drug injector's transmitting it sexually. This may engender a strong desire to prevent such transmission from occurring, and thus lead to condom use. Furthermore, if the partner does know his or her partner is a drug injector, he or she might instigate condom use.

Social Environment

Social environments are major determinants of risk behaviors (Friedman, Des Jarlais, & Ward, 1994a). These include such characteristics of the immediate social environment as acquaintances' norms (Friedman et al., 1994a; Magura, Shapiro, Siddiqi, & Lipton, 1990). Condom use and other sexual behaviors among drug injectors and other populations may also be affected by large-scale issues of socioeconomic structure (Farmer, 1992; Farmer, Connors, & Simmins, 1996; Zierler & Krieger, 1997) and historical change (Friedman, 1992; Friedman, 1998) that the data presented here cannot address.

THE STUDY

Data

The subjects for this analysis of condom use in relationships consist of a subset of the total data set: Those 317 IDUs who (1) provided information in the network section of the questionnaire about condom use during the prior 30 days with identified partners of the opposite sex, and (2) were successfully tested for HIV antibody (using double ELISA with Western blot confirmation).

The *dependent variable*, consistent condom use, is specific to the relationship. It describes whether an IDU subject and an identified opposite-sex network member with whom the subject reports having had sex in the prior 30 days used a condom every time the pair had sex during this time period.

The *unit of analysis* is the relationship. The 317 subjects reported on 421 heterosexual relationships in the last 30 days. Of the 421 relationships, 202 (48%) were with sexual partners who injected drugs and 219 (52%) were with noninjectors.

Validation

Data in which one subject (ego) described another subject (alter), their mutual behaviors, or characteristics of their social relationship were linked to and compared with data provided by alter about ego. When the reports by subjects who were in linked pairs were compared regarding the proportion of condom use during sex in the last 30 days, 32 of 38 (84%) linked pairs agreed on the proportion of sex acts in which they used condoms (Goldstein et al., 1995).

Limitations of the Data

As was discussed in Chapter 5, the sample of IDUs is not a random sample of any definable universe. Data about many variables are based on self-report; although condom use is validated through cross-checking of linked pairs of IDUs, subjects' reports on condom use with non-IDUs could not be validated. Furthermore, the relationships that are studied are not a random sample of the relationships of the subjects, since the questions asking for names of network members prioritize relationships with IDUs. Subjects (especially commercial sex workers) may underreport their number of relationships in order to shorten the interviews. Data on a number of theoretically relevant variables, particularly those relating to individual characteristics such as self-efficacy, response efficacy, and communication skills, are quite limited due to the demands of a long questionnaire that also collected extensive data about respondents' social networks and risk histories. Data were not collected on respondents' levels of general or partner-specific altruism/solidarity, nor on the extent to which partners had pressured for condom use, since the importance of these variables only became clear after the data had been collected.

Statistical analyses use χ^2 and multiple logistic regression techniques. The applicability of these inferential statistics is limited in two ways: (1) The sample of relationships is not random, and (2) the inclusion of more than one relationship for some subjects limits the independence of the relationships. (The degree of such clustering, however, is quite moderate: 60% of the relationships were reported by subjects who mentioned only one relationship; 29% by those with two or three relationships; and only 11% by those with four or more relationships.)

Results

Of the 317 respondents who reported sex in the prior 30 days with network members and who had HIV results available, 68% were men; 44% Latino(a), 32% white, and 24% black; and 34% were HIV-seropositive. Their mean age was 34.3 (SD = 6.9), and mean years of injection 13.3 (SD = 8.9). Fourteen percent had engaged in sex for money or drugs in the prior 2 years. Seventy percent reported that they had ever been in drug abuse treatment, and 23.5% were enrolled in drug abuse treatment at the time of interview. Always using condoms is reported in 33.5% (141/421) of relationships.

Consistent condom use is less common in more intimate relationships (see Table 1). Thus, consistent condom use is less likely with sex partners who are spouses, ex-spouses, or lovers than with friends or acquaintances (26% vs. 53%);

Table 1.   Selected Bivariate Analyses of Consistent Condom Use
in Relationships in the Last 30 days

	n	Percent "always used condom"	Odds ratio	p
Relationship characteristics				
Spouse, lover, ex-spouse	304	26	0.31	0.001
Friend, acquaintance, other	117	53	1.00	
Very close	203	24	0.42	0.001
Other	205	43	1.00	
Daily contact	246	27	0.48	0.001
Less contact	174	43	1.00	
Duration of sexual relationship				
≤ 12 months	158	42	1.00	0.002
> 12 months	262	28	0.52	
Subject				
HIV−	274	27	1.00	0.001
HIV+	147	46	2.37	
Male	295	34	1.00	0.79
Female	126	33	0.94	
Age				
< 30	133	45	2.10	0.001
≥ 30	288	28	1.00	
Race−ethnicity				0.042
White (non-Latino/a)	122	28	1.00	
Black (non-Latino/a)	96	28	1.01	
Latino/a (nonblack)	151	38	1.57	
Black Latino/a	44	48	2.36	
Has home	350	36	1.00	0.007
Homeless	71	20	0.43	
Feels "very likely" to develop AIDS	103	47	2.09	0.001
Does not	312	29	1.00	
No prior HIV test	166	28	1.00	0.069
Prior HIV test	255	37	1.4	
Talked with > 1 person about condoms and AIDS in last 30 days	155	43	1.96	0.001
Did not	265	28	1.00	
Crack use (30 days)				
None	215	34	1.00	0.84
Any	206	33	0.96	
Engaged in sex for money or drugs (2 years)				
None	331	28	1.00	0 .001
Any	71	58	3.49	

Table 1. (*Continued*)

	n	Percent "always used condom"	Odds ratio	p
Subject's health beliefs				
People can have sex and protect themselves from the virus that causes aids if they				
Only have sex with a condom	404	34	3.41	0.09
Not mentioned	15	13	1.00	
Avoid sex with other people who may be at risk	17	12	0.25	0.051
Not mentioned	402	35	1.00	
Avoid sex with gay–bisexual men	12	58	1.00	0.066
Not mentioned	407	33	2.85	
Partner				
not IDU	219	44	2.72	0.001
IDU	202	22	1.00	
Age < 25	63	56	2.96	0.001
Age ⩾ 25	357	30	1.00	
HIV+ subject with non-IDU partner	78	68	6.14	0.001
Other relationships	343	26	1.00	
Race–ethnicity				0.116
Black	109	29	0.97	
Latino	167	40	1.52	
White	140	30	1.00	
Subject's reports of peers' views on condom use				
Means you sleep around a lot				
Agree	36	17	1.00	.022
Neutral, disagree	374	36	2.76	
Prevents you from getting AIDS				
Agree	22	34	1.00	0.802
Neutral, disagree	388	36	1.12	
Prevents you from giving AIDS				
Agree	389	35	3.23	0.051
Neutral, disagree	21	14	1.00	
Interferes with sexual spontaneity				
Strongly agree	181	29	1.00	0.059
Other	223	38	1.50	
How many of the men you know object if a woman wants to use a condom?				
⩽ Half	341	37	1.00	0.001
> Half	54	13	0.25	
How many of the women you know object if a man wants to use a condom?				
⩽ Half	370	35	1.00	0.301
> Half	28	25	0.63	
Peers believe that "it is okay to refuse to use a condom with your wife or husband"				
Somewhat or strongly disagree	134	45	2.08	0.001
Neutral or agree	275	28	1.00	

(*continued*)

Table 1. (*Continued*)

Continuous variables	Mean values for		
	Consistent condom users	Others	p (t)
Number of months they have injected together	29.8	52.5	0.03
Sexual frequency in the last 30 days	7.4	10.9	0.042
Subject's monthly speedball injections	47	31	0.04
Subject's monthly injection frequency	130	90	0.0006

with sex partners with whom subjects feel very close than with other sex partners (24% vs. 43%); in relationships in which the partners are in daily contact (27% vs. 43%); and in relationships that have lasted a year or less (28% vs. 42%).

Subject characteristics also affect condom use. Seropositive subjects report always using condoms in 46% of relationships—significantly ($p < 0.001$) more than for seronegatives (27%). Knowledge of serostatus is not related to consistent condom use in seropositive subjects' relationships: Seropositive subjects who had previously been tested (regardless of whether or not they picked up their test results) report always using condoms in 47% of their relationships, whereas those who had not previously been tested report consistent condom use in 45% of their relationships ($p > 0.80$). This could be because some who had never been tested nonetheless believe themselves to be infected. In the relationships of seronegative subjects, however, those who had previously been tested (but who may or may not have picked up their test results) are significantly ($p < 0.002$) more likely to report consistent condom use (33%) than those who have not (15%). Subjects who feel they are very likely to develop AIDS are more likely to report consistent condom use than those who do not (47% vs. 29%).

Other subject characteristics significantly associated with consistent condom use include not being homeless, being Latino or black Latino, being less than 30 years old, engaging in commercial sex work, and talking to other people about condoms and AIDS. Health beliefs that indicate response efficacy were not significantly related to consistent condom use, although several were related to it at the $p < 0.10$ level. Neither crack use nor injecting cocaine was related to consistent condom use (data not shown).

Men and women do not differ in their level of consistent condom use; this might seem surprising, since commercial sex workers are more likely both to report consistent condom use and to be commercial sex workers (46% vs. 5%; $p < 0.001$). In the relationships of commercial sex workers, there is no significant variation in consistent condom use by gender (50% of men, 60% of women; $p < 0.52$); but in the relationships of other subjects, 33% of men but only 10% of women subjects report consistent condom use ($p < 0.001$). This is because the relationships of men who do not engage in commercial sex work are more likely to be with noninjectors than are the relationships of women who do not engage in commercial sex work (55% vs. 28%; $p < 0.001$). In other words, although women would be more likely to report consistent condom use due to being commercial sex workers, this is balanced out by their being more likely to have IDU sex partners.

Turning now to partner characteristics, consistent condom use is more common with younger partners, but partner's race–ethnicity is not related to consistent condom use. Condoms are used consistently in a smaller proportion (22%) of relationships with sex partners who are IDUs than in relationships with sex partners who have never injected drugs (44%; $p < 0.001$). Among a subsample of 74 IDUs who had both injecting and noninjecting sex partners, consistent condom use was less common with IDU sex partners (26%) than with non-IDU sex partners (51%; $p < 0.029$).

Consistent condom use is particularly widespread (68%) in relationships in which the drug-injecting respondent is seropositive and the sex partner of the respondent is reported not to be an IDU (see Table 2).

The social environments of drug injectors also affect condom use, as is shown by the relationship between consistent condom use and subjects' reports of the beliefs and activities of their peers (Table 1). Condom use is less likely if peers believe it is an indicator of sleeping around a lot, if male (but not female) peers object to condom use, or if peers see refusal to use condoms with a spouse as illegitimate.

Multiple Regression Analyses

From Tables 1 and 2, it is evident that many different variables are significantly related to consistent condom use. Stepwise multivariate logistic regression (with forward inclusion, given the large number of significant predictors at the

Table 2. Proportion of Relationships in which Condoms Were Always Used in the Prior 30 Days

	Does sex partner inject drugs?		
Respondent is	No	Yes	p
Seronegative	31%	23%	0.137
	(43/141)	(30/133)	
Seropositive	68%	22%	0.001
	(53/78)	(15/69)	
p	0.001	0.895	

Table 3. Multivariate Logistic Regression Analysis
of Consistent Condom Use in the Total Sample[a]

	Without interaction term		With interaction term	
	Odds ratio	95% CI	Odds ratio	95% CI
Interaction term				
Subject is HIV+, sex partner is not an IDU			5.47	1.73, 17.32
Subject characteristics				
Subject is HIV+	2.45	1.41, 4.24	0.903	.362, 2.25
Subject is homeless	0.244	0.097, 0.614	0.265	0.103, 0.680
Subject has engaged in sex for money or drugs in last 2 years	2.83	1.43, 5.59	2.72	1.35, 5.48
Sex partner characteristics				
Sex partner is not an IDU	2.40	1.39, 4.13	1.18	0.594, 2.34
Partner's age ≥ 25	None significant		0.467	0.222, 0.981
Relationship characteristics				
Sex partner is spouse, ex-spouse, or lover	0.486	0.258, 0.914	0.510	0.268, 0.970
Relationship is "very close"	0.507	0.284, 0.905	0.512	0.281, 0.933
Peer culture				
Peers' disagree that "it is okay to refuse to use a condom with your wife or husband"	3.36	1.91, 5.89	3.29	1.85, 5.85
More than half of the men that the respondent knows object if a woman wants to use a condom	0.197	0.067, 0.576	0.215	0.070, 0.657

[a]Number of relationships with consistent condom use is 118 out of 349.

bivariate level) was used to determine independent significant predictors, with and without including an interaction term to reflect the greater condom use in relationships between seropositive IDUs and non-IDUs (see Table 3). Significant predictors of consistent condom use include subject characteristics (positive serostatus, not being homeless, commercial sex work), partner characteristics [noninjector, age at least 25 (as a trend at $p < 0.06$ in the equation without the interaction term)], relationship characteristics (more distant relationship), and peer culture that is supportive of condom use.

Subset Analyses

Epidemiologic Subsets

Condom use by seropositives and by seronegatives have very different meanings. Condom use by seropositives can reduce the spread of HIV; indeed, in relationships with sex partners who do not themselves inject drugs, consistent condom use may greatly reduce the probability that sex partners may ever become infected. Condom use by seronegative IDUs is important as a self-protective measure, which may be counteracted, however, if the IDU engages in high-risk injecting behaviors. For example, Watkins et al. (1993) found that among subjects who know their serostatus, seronegatives who perceived their partners as likely to be infected were more likely to use condoms, but that seropositives' perceptions of partner serostatus were not related to condom use. Thus, we conducted separate analyses to determine the predictors of consistent condom use in the relationships of subjects who are (1) seropositive and (2) seronegative. Analyses are complicated by the fact that 49% of the seropositive subjects have and 51% have not been previously tested for HIV (and many of those who have been tested may not have picked up their results) and by the fact that many of the untested may nonetheless have accurate beliefs about their serostatus.

The *seropositive* IDUs report always using condoms in 46% of their relationships. Condoms are consistently used less with sex partners who are IDUs (22%) than with sex partners who have never injected drugs (68%; $p < 0.001$). Seropositives' consistent condom use with their non-IDU sex partners remains high (>57%), and the difference in condom use with sex partners who are IDUs and those who are not remains statistically significant among subsets of relationships in which (1) the subject is male, (2) the subject is female, (3) the subject describes the relationship as "very close," (4) the subject describes the relationship as not being "very close," (5) the subject describes the partner as a spouse or lover, (6) the subject describes the partner as a friend or acquaintance, (7) the subject has previously been tested for HIV, (8) the subject has not previously been tested for HIV, (9) the subject reports feeling that he or she is very likely to have been exposed to HIV, (10) the subject reports feeling that he or she is not "very likely" to have been exposed to HIV, (11) the subject has known the partner for 1 year or less, and (12) the subject has known the partner for more than 1 year.

Some of the seropositive subjects report having sexual partnerships with both IDUs and non-IDUs in the preceding 30 days. These subjects had 28 relationships: 18 with non-IDUs and 10 with IDUs. Condoms were always used during the prior 30 days in 72% (13) of the relationships with non-IDUs as compared to 30% (3) of the relationships with IDUs ($p < 0.05$, Fisher's exact test).

In multiple logistic regression analysis among the subset of relationships of seropositive subjects, consistent condom use is greater if (1) the sex partner is not a drug injector, (2) peer culture is supportive of condom use, (3) the relationship is less close, (4) the subject has not used crack in the prior 30 days, and (5) the subject is not homeless (Table 4).

Consistent condom use was reported in 27% (73/274) of the relationships of *seronegative* subjects. Multivariate predictors of consistent condom use in the relationships of seronegative subjects are a supportive peer culture, a relationship that is not "very close," and younger age (< 30 years) on the part of the subject.

Table 4.   Multivariate Logistic Regression Analysis
of Consistent Condom Use by Subject Serostatus

	Seropositive subjects		Seronegative subjects	
	Odds ratio	95% CI	Odds ratio	95% CI
Subject characteristics				
Subject is homeless	0.265	0.103, 0.680	0.218	0.050, 0.949
Subject used crack in prior 30 days	0.387	0.153, 0.978		
Sex partner characteristics			None significant	
Sex partner is not an IDU	6.52	2.48, 17.1		
Relationship characteristics				
Sex partner is spouse, ex-spouse, or lover	0.329	0.109, 0.992		
Relationship is "very close"	0.316	0.111, 0.900	0.402	0.208, 0.779
Peer culture				
Peers disagree that "it is okay to refuse to use a condom with your wife or husband"	4.72	1.72, 13.0	3.08	1.55, 6.12
More than half of the men that the respondent knows object if a woman wants to use a condom	0.099	0.011, 0.901		
Number of relationships with consistent condom use	64 of 132		59 of 233	

Relationship Subsets

There is considerable knowledge about the mechanisms of HIV transmission among drug injectors and sexual partners in New York City. Thus, we would expect that, in a sexual relationship between a drug injector and a non-IDU, sexual transmission might be seen as the primary risk for the non-IDU both by the IDU and, if the partner knows that the subject injects drugs, by the partner. In sexual relationships between IDUs, efforts to reduce risk might focus on parenteral transmission, sexual transmission, or both. Thus, we analyzed predictors of consistent condom use separately for relationships among IDUs and for relationships of IDUs with noninjectors (Table 5).

Relatively few (22%; 45/202) of the relationships among IDUs had consistent condom use. Significant independent predictors of consistent condom use are a relationship that is not "very close," a sexual relationship that had formed within the previous year, and the subject's engaging in commercial sex work.

In relationships between IDUs and noninjectors, consistent common use is more common (44%; 96/219). Significant independent predictors are subject's positive serostatus (odds ratio = 8.18), subject not being homeless, supportive peer norms, a sex partner who is younger, and a relationship that is not "very close."

Table 5. Multivariate Logistic Regression Analysis
of Consistent Condom Use by Whether or Not Sex Partner Injects Drugs

	Partner is IDU		Partner is non-IDU	
	Odds ratio	95% CI	Odds ratio	95% CI
Subject characteristics				
Subject is HIV+			8.18	3.81, 17.6
Subject is homeless			0.131	0.025, 0.680
Subject has engaged in sex for money or drugs in last 2 years	5.01	1.81, 14.1		
Sex partner characteristics	None significant			
Partner's age ≥ 25			0.334	0.131, 0.853
Relationship characteristics				
Relationship is "very close"	0.367	0.156, 0.864	0.347	0.163, 0.739
Sexual relationship has lasted ≥ 1 year	0.439	0.195, 0.986		
Peer culture	None significant			
Peers disagree that "it is okay to refuse to use a condom with your wife or husband'			4.96	2.29, 10.7
Number of relationships with consistent condom use	37 of 161		86 of 191	

Implications of the Analysis of Consistent Condom Use in Relationships

These findings, of course, are limited by the quality of the data. These limitations were described above, and include the fact that the relationships studied cannot be considered a random sample of drug injectors' relationships; the inherent weakness of any study based on self-reports (although a degree of validation was available through comparison of subjects' reports with those of others about them); and the relative weakness of our measures of psychosocial variables and the lack of data on subjects' altruism/solidarity and on their partners' pressures to encourage condom use.

To the extent that they were measured in this study, personal characteristics that are the primary focus of such theories as the health belief model (Becker & Joseph, 1974, 1988), social learning theory (Bandura, 1977, 1993), the theory of reasoned action (Ajzen & Fishbein, 1980; Ajzen & Timko, 1986; Fishbein & Ajzen, 1975; Fishbein & Middlestadt, 1987), or the AIDS risk reduction model (Catania et al., 1990) were not significant predictors of consistent condom use in the multivariate model and the subset analyses. Instead, the personal characteristics that predict consistent condom use are measures of subjects' conditions or situations rather than of their cognitive or emotional traits: HIV serostatus, homelessness, and occupation (since commercial sex workers are more likely to report consistent condom use in their sexual relationships, including their relationships with other drug injectors.) The prevention implications of these findings are that counseling and testing programs and programs to provide stable living conditions for drug injectors may be more effective in promoting condom use than psychosocial interventions of the kind that have been the major focus of most of the National Institute on Drug Abuse community outreach projects. (Readers should be aware, however, that our ability to measure the variables that are the focus of the health belief and AIDS risk reduction models was limited by the amount of time spent on other variables, so this may not be a "fair" test of these models.)

Characteristics of the subject's partner are an important determinant of consistent condom use for seropositive (but not for seronegative) subjects. Contrary to the suggestion by Malow et al. (1993) that drug injectors might use condoms more with high-risk partners than with low-risk partners, consistent condom use in high-seroprevalence New York City is more common in IDUs' relationships with persons who do not inject drugs than in relationships among IDUs. This suggests either or both that:

1. Drug injectors may be more concerned about preventing their noninjecting partners from becoming infected by sexual transmission than they are about themselves becoming infected through sexual transmission. (Their lack of concern about themselves becoming infected via sexual transmission may result from their focusing on drug-injection-related behaviors as their main concern in trying to protect themselves.)
2. The partners of seropositive drug users may exert pressure for them to use condoms. This assumes that these partners know or suspect that their partners use drugs in ways that have (or are likely to have) gotten them infected with HIV or other infectious agents.

Consistent condom use among *seronegative* subjects is not a function of whether or not the partner is a drug injector. On the other hand, *infected* subjects are less likely to engage in unprotected sex with partners who are not themselves drug injectors. This suggests that infected drug injectors may be protecting partners who are at little other risk for HIV infection as a result of altruism, solidarity, and/or love, and perhaps because of pressure by partners who want to protect themselves.

The large extent of consistent condom use in relationships between seropositive IDUs and noninjecting partners has implications both for epidemiology and for prevention programs. Epidemiologically, condom use may be particularly high (at least in a high-seroprevalence area like New York) in precisely those relationships that are most likely to transfer HIV from injectors to non-injectors (Friedman et al., 1994c). For prevention, it suggests that there may have been too much pessimism about our inability to encourage safer sex in steady or close relationships. Watkins et al. (1993, p. 723), for example, suggest that "current interventions are not effectively changing behavior among steady partners" of IDUs and that "it is their non-IDU steady partners who are likely to be most at risk of infection from unprotected intercourse." Similarly, Sibthorpe (1992) doubted that condom use would become widespread in IDUs' conjugal and paraconjugal relationships. Our data, however, suggest a modification of this conclusion. Even in very close or long-term sexual relationships and in relationships with spouses, ex-spouses, and lovers, seropositive IDUs report high levels of consistent condom use with their non-IDU partners. For this epidemiologically important subset of relationships, then, it may be more appropriate to approach changing sexual risk behaviors in steady relationships with a degree of optimism.

Further, since altruism–solidarity and/or partners' actions may contribute in important ways to consistent condom use, prevention programs should find ways to use altruism–solidarity and partners' actions as resources to promote risk reduction among those who do not already practice safe sex, including among those who are seronegative and those relationships in which both partners are IDUs. In particular, such programs might be developed as part of HIV counseling and testing, as part of outreach protocols, in syringe exchanges, and in outreach or drop-in centers aimed at gay male IDUs.

Many of the predictors of consistent condom use are variables that measure characteristics of the social relationships of IDUs. In the relationships of drug injectors with other drug injectors, for example, relationship closeness and duration were both (negative) predictors of consistent condom use. Thus, risk behavior and risk reduction are clearly affected by the social relationships in which behaviors occur. We need to develop a deeper understanding of how social relationships affect risk behaviors and risk reduction within these social relationships. To some extent, of course, these social relationships provide the context within which prevention efforts have to operate, which may suggest that different approaches should be developed to try to affect condom use in relatively casual, short-term relationships and in longer-term, more intimate or institutionalized relationships.

Subjects whose peers encourage condom use are more likely to have relationships in which they use condoms consistently. Peer culture was a significant predictor in the total sample and in every subset of relationships except those of IDUs with partners who are also IDUs. Peer influence has previously been shown to affect risk reduction by IDUs (Des Jarlais et al., 1995a; Friedman et al., 1987b; Latkin et al., 1995b; Magura et al., 1989, 1990; Neaigus et al., 1994), and interventions based on mobilizing peer influence to increase HIV risk reduction have been effective among gay men (Kelly et al., 1991, 1992) and IDUs (Friedman et al., 1991, 1992; Friedman, Wiebel, Jose, & Levin, 1993b; Jose et al., 1996; Latkin et al., 1996). Thus, the findings of this study also suggest that prevention efforts should attempt to change peer cultures as a way to develop self-sustaining long-term risk reduction. One way in which this has been done is to encourage the formation of drug users' organizations (Friedman & Wypijewska, 1995; Friedman, 1996; Friedman, de Jong, & Wodak, 1993a; Price, 1992).

Finally, this analysis suggests that condom use should be seen as a social process, shaped primarily by the situations in which the partners find themselves; the duration, intimacy, and institutionalization of the relationship itself; and the normative environment in which it is embedded. Efforts to promote risk reduction must understand that these social contexts cannot be ignored, and efforts to develop theories that can assist in health promotion and risk reduction within relationships must incorporate the characteristics and situations of the relationship and of the peer culture as core problematic foci rather than viewing them as peripheral to psychosocial variables.

NON-IDU YOUTHS AT RISK: SEXUAL RELATIONSHIPS BY SEROPOSITIVE AND SERONEGATIVE IDUs WITH NON-IDU YOUTHS*

The 767 IDUs studied in the SFHR project provided us with data about 617 of their sexual relationships. Almost half (299) of the sexual relationships reported by the IDUs in this study were with persons who do not inject drugs. Few (23) of these relationships were with non-IDUs who were 21 years old or younger, with the youngest non-IDU sex partners being three 16-year-olds. In 8 of these 23 relationships (including one long-standing relationship between two women), the drug injector was infected with HIV. One seropositive male IDU who was 24 years old had sexual relations with 5 different young women: a 17-year-old and an 18-year-old with each of whom he had been having sex for 2 years; a 19-year-old with whom he had been having sex for 6 years; and two 20-year-olds with whom he had been having sex for 1 and for 4 years. He reported that he always used condoms with four of these women; for the fifth woman, no data are available. Indeed, in 14 out of 21 (67%) of the relationships with young non-IDUs for which data are available about the HIV serostatus of the IDU, the drug injector who was the research participant reported that she or he always used condoms. There were no instances in which an HIV-infected IDU reported having unprotected sex with any of these noninjecting youth (nor with other noninjectors aged 25 years or less), although, as discussed above, there were instances of unprotected sex in relationships of HIV-positive IDUs with older noninjectors.

These data provide a number of reasons for optimism. Although data are not available about the HIV serostatuses of the non-IDU sex partners (since they were not themselves participants in the research), it is notable that few youthful (aged 21 or below) non-IDUs seem to be at high risk of HIV transmission from this group of almost 800 IDUs. That is, only 23 are reported to be having sex with these 767 IDUs (although this may well be an underestimate, since research subjects may

*This section of the chapter is adapted from a previous paper published in Sherr (1997).

have reported on fewer relationships than they really had in order to shorten their interviews). Although 36% of the non-IDU youth are having sex with HIV-infected IDUs, consistent condom use seems to be taking place in most if not all of these relationships.

Furthermore, this study also suggests that the average age at which people start to inject drugs has been increasing during the AIDS epidemic. For long-term injectors (those who began to inject 7 or more years before they were interviewed for the study), the average age of initiation was 19; but for new injectors, the average age of initiation has increased to 27. This may imply that, as time passes in an AIDS epidemic, fewer people begin to inject drugs and that they do so later in life. This in turn would probably decrease the number of adolescents who have sexual relations with IDUs.

PRELIMINARY VIEWS FROM THE OTHER SIDE: WHAT YOUTHS LIVING IN BUSHWICK HOUSEHOLDS REPORT ABOUT SEX WITH IDUs

Since sexual transmission of HIV had led to many infections in the United States and to much more widespread epidemics in Africa and Thailand, we became concerned about the extent to which the virus (and other infectious agents that are widespread among drug injectors, such as hepatitis B) might be spreading to youth in Bushwick. We thus decided to conduct a study of a representative household sample of Bushwick 18- to 21-year-olds. Although we were delayed by difficulties in obtaining funding for such a study, we have been able to collect data from a medium-sized sample. (The data presented here have previously been reported in Friedman et al., 1997a).

Specifically, a multistage probability sample of English-speaking 18- to 21-year-olds was recruited in Bushwick in 1994 to 1995 from 12 primary sampling units, each of which was a pair of adjacent face blocks. (A face block is the buildings along and across a street.) The primary sampling units were randomly selected from a listing of all such adjacent face blocks in Bushwick. All households in each of the 12 selected primary sampling units were screened to locate those containing age-eligible youths. In each household with any age-eligible youth, one youth was randomly selected to be interviewed and to give blood and urine specimens (with informed consent). The consent process included a full description of the questionnaire and of the tests for infectious agents. Participants were reimbursed with a small fee ($20) at completion of the interview and another $20 after pretest counseling, in recognition of their time and effort. From 129 selected youths, 111 (86%) were interviewed and 104 (81%) specimens were obtained. Failures to obtain interviews were due either to refusals or to inability to arrange a time for the interview before the study (which, as a pilot study, had very limited funding) had to cease field operations. Seven youths declined to provide specimens either after pretest counseling or after an unsuccessful attempt to draw blood by a field phlebotomist who needed additional training. The distribution on race–ethnicity and gender of these English-speaking youths (plus an additional 11 non-English-speaking youths who were interviewed with a short questionnaire in Spanish, but who are not included in these analyses because only a portion of the questionnaire was translated into Spanish due to shortages of funds) was similar to those from US Census data, which report that, of Bushwick youth aged 18 to 21, 29% are black, 67% Hispanic, and 52% are women; the sample proportions were essentially the same, 28%, 67%, and 51%, respectively.

Interviews and specimen collections were conducted in private settings either in participants' homes or in a project storefront. In no case were interviews conducted where anyone besides the interviewer and the participant would hear the questions and answers.

Sera were tested for HIV-1 [Genetic Systems ELISA; positive results were confirmed with Western blot (Bio-Rad Laboratories), hepatitis C antibody, hepatitis B core antibody, HTLV-I and HTLV-II (all using enzyme immunoassay tests, Abbott Laboratories)]. Subjects who were positive for hepatitis B core antibody were tested for surface antigen by neutralization (Abbott). Syphilis serology was determined by rapid plasma reagin (Becton-Dickinson) and confirmed by fluorescent antibody (FTA). All commercially available tests were performed in accordance with quality control procedures recommended by the manufacturer and licensing agencies. Herpes simplex type 2 serology was performed by Western blot as previously described (Ashley et al., 1988). Urines were tested for *Chlamydia* by Abbott ligase chain reaction (Bassiri et al., 1995; Chernesky et al., 1994). Eighty-seven remainder urines were tested for opiate and cocaine metabolites (EMIT, SYVA); these tests detect recent drug use. Since the decision to test remainder urines was reached after subject identifiers had been unlinked from the data, informed consent could not be obtained. When subjects returned for their test results, they were given appropriate counseling and referrals.

Results

Of 111 youths, 48% (53) were women; 65% (72) were Latino and 31% (34) African American; and 41% (46) were neither employed nor attending school. Subjects reported considerable sexual risk: 89% (99) had had sex in the last year, and 45% (50) had sex with two or more partners. Only 19% (19/99) of those who had had sex always used condoms. None reported that they had ever had sex with a drug injector, and only 2% (2/95) had ever had sex with a crack smoker. Five percent of men (3/58) reported homosexual orientation (being sexually attracted to men); but none of the 55 women reported being sexually attracted to women. None of the men or women reported having had sex with someone of the same gender in the prior 12 months. Fifty-eight percent (30/52) of the women have been pregnant. One woman (out of 47) had had sex with a crack smoker. Some sex was involuntary: 30% (14/47) of women report they were coerced the first time they had sex, and 23% (12/52) of women and 3% (2/58) of men report having been victims of sex abuse. (Note that a number of the youths did not answer all of the questions. This is why some totals add up to less than 111.)

Although 18% (20/109) have engaged in selling cocaine or heroin at some time in their lives, only 3 of 111 subjects (3%) reported ever using heroin and ten (9%) reported ever using cocaine. Only one subject reported having ever injected drugs or smoked crack; she had done both. An additional 2 youths reported having smoked "blunts," which are composed of a mixture of tobacco and crack. Some underreporting of recent drug use was documented: 2 of 85 "nonreporters" with available data had opiate-positive urines and 2 of 80 had cocaine-positive urines.

None of the youths showed serological evidence of infection with HIV-1, HTLV-II, or syphilis. Two percent (2/103) tested positive for HTLV-I and 3% (3/103) for hepatitis C; 3% (3/103) had indicators of prior infection with hepatitis B, and 50% (51/102) with herpes simplex, type 2. Twelve percent (8/64) were infected with *Chlamydia*. There is some reason to suspect that some or all of the three young adults who tested positive for hepatitis C (but who all deny that they have ever injected drugs) might in fact have engaged in drug injection.

Conclusions

The modest sample size in this study did not preclude the possibility that there may be substantial heroin use, drug injection, or HIV infection among household young adults in Bushwick. The 95% upper bound on HIV seroprevalence, for example, is almost 5%. Nevertheless, these data do indicate that sexual transmission of HIV to Bushwick household youths, so far, is well below the "disaster" stage. The findings here also do not preclude the possibility that heroin and cocaine use, drug injection, and HIV infection may increase among these subjects as they grow older, or that historical developments (for example, increased socioeconomic marginalization of youths in high-risk neighborhoods) might lead to increased drug use among youths of this age in the future.

The low rates of heroin and cocaine use and of drug injection may reflect a community response to the highly visible negative consequences of prior drug injection, crack smoking, and HIV/AIDS in this community (Musto, 1991), many of which are elsewhere described in this volume. The subjects also appear to be avoiding sexual relationships with known drug injectors and crack smokers who might be sources of HIV transmission. Nevertheless, most subjects are clearly sexually active, a majority of women have been pregnant, and less than a fifth report consistent condom use.

There is a clear disparity between the relatively low rates of heroin and cocaine use, drug injection, and hepatitis C and B virus and HIV infection, which may be important future health problems for these youth, and the high rates of chlamydia and herpes infection, which are clearly already substantial health problems. The herpes simplex, type 2 rates are higher than those among youths in a high-risk San Francisco neighborhood with fewer drug injectors (Robert Fullilove, personal communication, August 9, 1995), where 16% of 20- to 24-year-olds and 24% of 25- to 29-year-olds were infected (Siegel et al., 1992).

Furthermore, these data tend to confirm the findings of the SFHR project data about the rarity of sexual liaisons between drug injectors in the neighborhood and Bushwick youths. The network data on drug injectors found few such relationships (and, of these, some may have been with non-Bushwick youths); and, in this smaller household sample of youths, no such relationships were found. This lack of sexual network linkage with drug injectors may explain why HIV is not present in the youth sample. As discussed, however, the high prevalence of herpes simplex, type 2 suggests the possibility that HIV could spread rapidly among Bushwick youths through sexual transmission if sexual linkages with HIV-infected drug injectors (or crack smokers) should form in any number.

Sociometric Networks among Bushwick Drug Injectors

Most of our attention so far in this volume has been on the individual and her or his immediate social environment. As we discussed in Chapter 5, however, networks can be conceived of in wider terms. Specifically, they can be used to study the structure of social and/or risk relationships in a community of drug injectors (or other persons).

Sociologists have developed "sociograms" as ways to diagram the relationships in social networks. In these diagrams, relationships are shown as lines among individuals. The patterns formed by these relationships can vary within communities of a given number of members. Figure 1 provides an example of two groups with the same number of people. Assume first that Fig. 1 depicts a risk network in which each link represents a high-risk behavior such as sharing syringes. Then, looking at social network Fig. 1A, if person "a" becomes infected with HIV, the virus can be transmitted by "a" directly to "d" (as well as to "b"), and to all the others thereafter by "d." Epidemiologically, as Klovdahl (1985) has pointed out, HIV would take longer to spread through a pattern like that in Fig. 1B, since it would take five steps to go from "a" to "f." Furthermore, there is no pathway through which the virus could spread from the larger component (a, b, c, d, e, and f) to the smaller dyad composed of "g" and "h."

Figure 1 can also be used to consider *social* networks rather than *risk* networks. Here, the lines would be thought of as social interactions, such as friendships, that can spread messages and social influence. Looked at in terms of prevention, a message can flow from "a" to the others more directly in Fig. 1A than in Fig. 1B. Looked at in terms of social influence, "d" in Fig. 1A has the social potential to be a very influential person, since she or he has relationships with all the others (and thus is likely both to know what is going on in their lives and also to be able to exert influence on them). In Fig. 1B, however, no individual stands out as likely to be particularly influential.

As discussed in Chapter 5, some areas of networks may be particularly likely to serve as centers where high-risk behaviors can become concentrated and/or where messages and influence may be transmitted more effectively. These are typically social regions where the patterns of interaction are denser, in some sense,

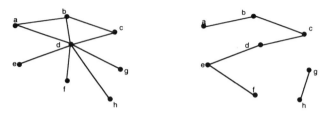

Figure 1. Schematic diagrams of sociometric networks.

than in other regions. In Fig. 1A, but not in Fig. 1B, the individuals a, b, c, and d seem to form such a region; each of them has a relationship with at least two of the others; and half of them (b and d) have relationships with all three of the others. One measure of such a region is the "Seidman k-core," defined as a subset of a social or risk network in which every member of the subset is connected to at least k of the other members. In Fig. 1A, a, b, c, and d form a two-core; and there is no three-core since there is no subset in which each member is connected to at least three of the other members. (If "a" and "c" were linked, on the other hand, [a, b, c, d] would also be a three-core). In Fig. 1B, however, there are no k-cores where k is greater than one. On the other hand, Fig. 1B does contain two different "connected components," where a connected component is a subset of persons with paths that can connect every subset member with every other subset member.

These patterns are easy to define and talk about in the context of Fig. 1, where there are only eight individuals (a through h). In our study of Bushwick, however, there were 767 drug injectors and a single large component with over 200 members. With this number of individuals and lines, little meaning can be obtained from a diagram of all the relationships in the largest connected component (see Fig. 2). Indeed, as was discussed in Chapter 5 (and in Chapter 13), it was a major task involving the efforts of several staff members over many months simply to try to figure out which of the network members whom respondents had named were persons who were interviewed (and thus could be linked with the namer). In addition, hundreds of such "nominees" were never linked to other research participants. We have no way to know which of them were nonetheless in the study. Such nominees who were in fact nominated but never linked can be thought of as having "missing links," which are not hominoids are but a form of missing data that lends some inaccuracy to our analyses. (The fact that we find relationships in spite of these inaccuracies probably speaks to the underlying strength of the relationships we are studying rather than to "false findings." This is because the errors in finding the links are unlikely to be correlated with the dependent variables in these analyses.)

In spite of the size and complexity of network data on 767 drug injectors,

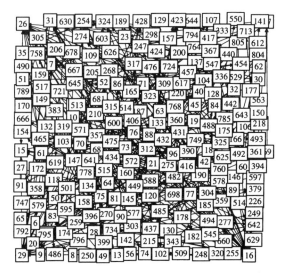

Figure 2. Diagram of connections among 230 members of the large connected component. Note well how crowded this diagram is.

there are many ways to describe or measure their risk networks and social networks. Most of our attention will focus on the measure we have called "sociometric network location," which seems to capture important epidemiological and social patterns. However, other measures, such as various measures of "centrality" or "clique membership," can also be defined (Needle, Coyle, Genser, & Trotter, 1995; Scott, 1991).

Sociometric risk network location is defined in terms of the categories described above using data on risk linkages. (A linkage here can be in either direction, i.e., even if a respondent "x" does not name "y," they may be linked if "y" names "x." In fact, there were a number of shooting gallery operators who were named by many of their customers whom they did not name as part of their risk or social networks.) Sociometric risk network location, then, uses linkage data to define four "locations" as follows. First, the "unlinked" subjects are those for whom there is the least evidence of risk linkage with other drug injectors. There were 299 of these subjects, defined as those who were not linked to other IDUs in the study. Most of these 299 unlinked drug injectors do seem to have other drug injectors (who either were not in the study or who could not be identified as linked to them) in their risk networks. Thus, 187 of them reported having interacted in the last 30 days with another IDU with whom at some time in their lives they have either injected drugs or had sex.

As a second step in defining sociometric risk network location, we used

UCINET software to look at the pattern of components among those respondents whom we had linked to somebody else in the study. Ninety connected components were identified. Sixty-nine of them were dyads with two members, 14 had 3 members each, 2 had 4 members, 3 had 5 members, and 1 had 7 members. There was also a large 258-member connected component. Within the large component, the Seidman *k*-core routine of UCINET was used to detect one two-core with 125 members.

Four structural categories were then defined that operationalize the concept of sociometric risk network location:

1. A two-core within the large component (all 125 of whose members are linked to two or more other members of the two-core).
2. The periphery of the large component, composed of its other 133 members.
3. Members (*n* = 210) of the other 89 connected components.
4. Unlinked IDUs (*n* = 299).

These categories, then, form a scale of decreasing high-risk social connection to other IDUs.

THREE MEASURES OF NETWORK LOCATION

Sociometric risk network location is used below to analyze how sociometric structure is related to the personal characteristics, egocentric network characteristics, risk behaviors, and infection probabilities of individual drug injectors. Before turning to these analyses, however, it is worth considering two other methods we have used to define network location during this project (Curtis et al., 1995; Friedman et al., 1997b). These are sociometric *social* network location and ethnographic social network location.

Defining Sociometric Social Network Location

Sociometric social network location is defined using procedures identical to those used to define sociometric risk network location with one exception: Instead of restricting the linkages being considered to those that involve the potential for engaging in behaviors that can transmit HIV (i.e., relationships in which the members have injected drugs together or had sex, regardless of whether they actually engaged in particularly high-risk behaviors such as sharing syringes or unprotected anal sex), all linkages are included. The major weakness of this measure is that we did not do a very complete job of ascertaining those social relationships of respondents that did not involve injecting drugs together or having sex. When we interviewed respondents about their networks, we asked them to prioritize naming the people with whom they had injected drugs during the prior 30 days and those with whom they had had sex. Other relationships, whether with friends or relatives, were essentially treated as residuals, and thus were undercounted. Furthermore, since only drug injectors were included as participants in the study, linkages can only be formed (and sociometric network analyses conducted) with drug injectors who took part. Thus, relationships with persons who do not inject drugs are excluded from these analyses.

When we analyzed these data on *social* linkages, 89 components were detected. The sizes of the components varied between 2 members (dyads) and a large 277-member connected component. The *k*-core routine of UCINET was used to detect a two-core within the large 277-member component.

Four structural categories were defined on the bases of these analyses:

1. A core (all of whose members are linked as social contacts of two or more other members) of 131 drug injectors within the 277-member linked component.
2. The periphery of this component, comprised of its other 146 members.
3. 214 IDUs who are members of 88 components ranging in size from 2 to 7 members (there are 2 with 7 members, 4 with 5, 1 with 4, 14 with 3, and 67 with 2).
4. 276 unlinked IDUs.

These categories form a scale of decreasing social connection to other IDUs.

Ethnographic social network location was defined using a combination of two data-gathering techniques. The first is ethnography and the second is the data on social (not risk) network linkages. Ethnography was used to define a 40-member *ethnographic core*. Noncore respondents who said they had injected drugs (during the prior 30 days) with members of the ethnographic core, or who were reported by an ethnographic core member as someone with whom the core member had injected drugs during the 30 days prior to the core member's interview, were defined as members of an *inner periphery* of 95 members; the 632 drug injectors who were not linked to the ethnographic core were defined as members of an *outer periphery*.

Defining the Ethnographic Core Network

The most important criterion for inclusion in the ethnographic core network was validation by other core network members. Ethnographic core members often talked about other network members as regulars in the neighborhood or as being "from around the way." To gain this validation by other core network members, drug users interact with other drug market participants in a manner that is characteristic of ethnographic core network members. For example, one of the most important norms shared by all ethnographic core network members was *sharing drugs* with each other. While the most important people in defining membership in

the ethnographic core network were the members themselves, other market participants, like drug distributors, also contributed to the definition of ethnographic core
network members. In the study area, on any given day, there were 15 to 20 brand
names of heroin sold within a two-block radius. The quality of brand names often
changed dramatically from day to day. To attract customers, business owners
would give out free samples whenever they introduced a new brand name or when
they wanted to revitalize sales of a successful brand name whose sales had begun to
stagnate. The most efficient way of promoting sales was to give samples to
influential customers—an indicator of ethnographic core network membership.
Many organizations targeted ethnographic core network members by regularly
visiting shooting galleries and giving several bags of heroin to each member. If
particularly influential network members were not immediately found by visiting
injection locations, distributors would often set aside a few bags, confident that
they would soon meet. By observing which IDUs were sought out by business
managers, the ethnographic staff was able to gain a clearer picture of ethnographic
core network membership as well as of the relative status of individuals within the
network.

The market behavior of drug injectors who did not seem to be members of the
ethnographic core was another variable that helped identify members of the ethnographic core network. Other drug injectors often sought the assistance of ethnographic core network members to help them buy drugs (especially heroin) as well
as to gain access to local places where they could use drugs. By observing whom
other drug injectors sought out to help them do these things, the identification of
ethnographic core network members was further facilitated.

The membership of the ethnographic core network was constantly changing.
Members would often disappear for extended periods of time for reasons such as
incarceration, drug rehabilitation, the avoidance of drug distributors bent on
exacting punishment for transgressions of market etiquette, or finding a reliable
source of income large enough to support a habit. Upon returning to the neighborhood and participating in activities that were characteristic of ethnographic core
network members, however, former members were immediately accepted back by
all market participants. Since presence in the neighborhood and/or status as a
member of the ethnographic core changed over time, we added two other criteria
for ethnographic core membership: (1) that they were present in the neighborhood
for at least half of the research period and (2) that they completed structured
questionnaires at the research storefront that were able to be flagged for further
analysis and comparison with the remainder of the structured questionnaire
database. By using the methods and parameters outlined above, the ethnographic
staff was able to identify 40 of the 767 drug injectors in the sample as being
members of the ethnographic core.

Figure 3 provides a sociometric diagram of the drug-injecting linkages among
members of the ethnographic core. Each line connects persons at least one of

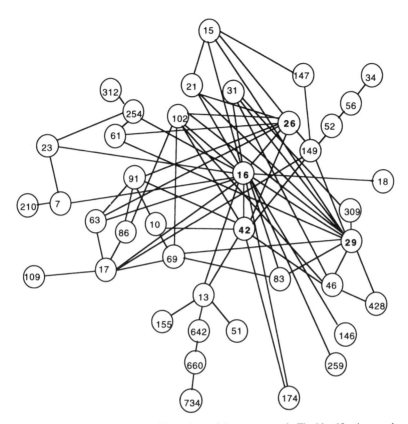

Figure 3.   Injection links among the 40 members of the core network. The identification number of each node is the respondent identification number assigned to the subject at the time she or he was interviewed and offered the opportunity for HIV and hepatitis B testing. From Curtis et al., 1995.

whom reported that they had injected drugs with the other in the previous 30 days. This figure shows that, even within the ethnographic core, there is a hierarchy of degree of linkage with other drug injectors. A review of the ethnographic data revealed that the four IDUs in this figure with the greatest number of connecting lines (numbers 16, 26, 29, and 42) were shooting gallery operators.

COMPARING THE THREE MEASURES OF NETWORK LOCATION

Clearly, one interesting question is whether the members of the core as defined by one measure of network location are core members by the other definitions as well. Comparing the data on sociometric social network and on sociometric risk network, of the 767 participants in the study, 732 (95%) are categorized identically by the two measures (125 as two-core members, 129 as peripheral members of a large component, 202 as members of smaller components, and 276 as unlinked). As would be expected (since all risk links were also included as social links), there are no cases of individuals who are categorized as "more tightly connected" in terms of risk network location than in terms of social network location. Thus, there are 35 participants whose social network category is "more connected" than their risk network location. Twenty-three of these 35 are persons who reported no injection or sex partners in the prior 30 days (and also were not linked to alters who reported injecting or having sex with them in the 30 days before the alter's interview) but who did report social links (12 of these were categorized as being in small social network components, 10 as in the periphery of the large sociometric social network, and one in the social network two-core). Seven members of small risk network components were in the periphery of the large social network component (and one in its core). Finally, four members of the periphery of the large risk network component fall into the two-core of the large social network component. In sum, there is little difference between the sociometric social and risk network measures; however, had we not prioritized measuring drug injection and sexual links, this difference might have been larger.

It is more difficult to approach the comparison of the ethnographic categorization with either the sociometric risk network location or the sociometric social network location. To help clarify these issues, Table 1 is a cross-tabulation of sociometric risk network location by ethnographic social network location. (Given the close relationship of sociometric risk and social networks, only the sociometric risk network will be discussed here.) All but one of the members of the ethnographic core were members of the large component of the sociometric risk network. Many members of the sociometric risk network two-core, however, were classified as in the inner periphery and even more as in the outer periphery of the ethnographic classification. This suggests that ethnographic techniques may some-

Table 1. Cross-Tabulation of Sociometric Risk Network Location by Ethnographic Social Network Location

Sociometric risk network location	Ethnographic social network location		
	Core	Inner periphery	Outer periphery
Two-core of large component	32	39	54
Periphery of large component	7	46	80
Smaller component	1	3	206
Unlinked	0	7	292

times only capture a portion of the high-risk drug injector population—most likely, those who have visible roles like needle or drug dealing. Thus, of the 40 members of the ethnographic core, 32 report having engaged during the prior 30 days in selling needles, selling drugs, commercial sex work, or being paid to be a hit doctor. Conversely, 47% (59/125) of the drug injectors in the two-core of the sociometric risk network are not within the ethnographic core or engaging in these drug scene roles, which suggests that snowball techniques of recruitment may be useful both for research on street injectors and for AIDS outreach and other public health work among them.

WHO IS IN WHAT SOCIOMETRIC RISK NETWORK LOCATION

For the remainder of this chapter, we will discuss only one of these measures: sociometric risk network location. We will focus on this because in many ways it seems like the "cleanest" of our variables, and because, since it is based on risk linkages, it seems to be the one with the most intuitive relationship to HIV. However, we have conducted similar analyses to those below using each of the other measures. Ethnographic social network location is analyzed in Curtis et al. (1995) and sociometric social network location in Friedman et al. (1997b).

First, let us consider which sociometric risk network locations are populated by various kinds of drug injectors. These data are presented in Table 2. [Parallel data using a slightly different version of this typology are presented and discussed in Friedman et al. (1997a). That paper uses a five-category typology (rather than the four-category typology used here) in which the "unlinked" are divided into (1) those who nominated other IDUs as persons with whom they had injected or had sex in the prior 30 days, without, however, any of these nominees being interviewed by our project and linked to them; and (2) those who did not make such nominations.] As can be seen, women are equally present in each category.

Race–ethnicity, however, tends to vary by risk network location. White drug injectors are particularly unlikely to be unlinked, which may reflect the difficulty for a white person to function as a drug injector in a minority neighborhood. In particular, friends are needed to assure that drug dealers will sell you "good dope" rather than "beating you" by selling you very low purity goods. (As discussed in earlier chapters, when many drug injectors were driven to Bushwick by the increasing gentrification of Williamsburg and its accompanying increased police pressure and hostility from neighbors, they initially had to establish ties to local users in order to buy quality drugs.) The nature of Bushwick as a drug supermarket that attracted buyers from outside meant that many (primarily white) drug users came into the neighborhood to buy their drugs. They established ephemeral, weak ties to local users (often core members) by trading a taste of drugs or a small amount of money for the service of buying them the drugs. The dynamics of this

Table 2. Relationships between Sociometric Risk Network Location and the Background, Social Marginalization, and Roles of Drug Injectors ($N = 767$)[a]

	Large connected component		Small components ($n = 210$)	Unlinked ($n = 299$)	p[b]
	Two-core ($n = 125$)	Periphery ($n = 133$)			
Background					
Female	28%	30%	32%	28%	0.928
Race–ethnicity[c]					0.130
White	37%	40%	37%	22%	
Black/African American	30%	29%	27%	25%	
Latino/a	31%	32%	38%	51%	
Age ⩾35	55%	51%	51%	52%	0.758
Percent new injectors (< 6 years)	17%	14%	20%	25%	0.014
Social marginalization/integration					
Homeless	29%	22%	18%	17%	0.006
No legal income in prior 6 months	38%	23%	19%	23%	0.005
Income < $10,000	70%	77%	85%	81%	0.017
Ever incarcerated since 1977	65%	51%	52%	54%	0.111
Not a high school graduate	30%	34%	37%	38%	0.158
Currently married	10%	20%	24%	17%	0.246
Never attend religious services	61%	54%	54%	47%	0.064
Roles in drug scene					
Sell syringes	28%	14%	14%	15%	0.005
Sell drugs	17%	20%	14%	23%	0.255
Commerical sex work	20%	21%	10%	13%	0.013

[a]For some cells, the denominators vary from these due to missing data or, as for race–ethnicity, the exclusion of "other" groupings from the table.
[b]Probabilities by Mantel–Haenzel test for trend.
[c]In addition, there was one Asian/Pacific Islander (in the periphery), three Native Americans (all in the two-core), and three "others" (one each in the periphery, small component, and unlinked categories).

process are of interest, since they are tied to larger social pressures. By 1990, street-level drug markets in Bushwick had gained a reputation throughout the New York City metropolitan area as a place where outsiders could easily purchase drugs. But, as the notoriety of the markets grew, so too did the attention given to these markets by the police. Intensified police pressure decreased the blatancy of street-level drug distributors, but it simultaneously increased the already lucrative business of acting as a market intermediary—a task dominated by members of the core network—who served as go-betweens (and hence, often as drug-using partners) for those drug users who were relatively "unconnected" to the market. By late 1992, as special police initiatives focused their energies on dismantling the large drug distribution organizations that dominated the neighborhood, many core network members who had formerly earned money via a wide range of "hustles" (selling syringes, sex work, selling scrap metal, shoplifting, etc.) found that it was much easier to sustain their habits by purchasing drugs for outsiders. For example, Patricia, a 34-year-old African-American IDU and member of the core network, once earned money through sex work and as a crack/heroin seller in the neighborhood, but when the market became less hospitable to outsiders, she found it much easier and less dangerous to make money by negotiating the market for them:

> The main way I make money is takin' people to go cop drugs. I got maybe eight or nine different customers. They are mostly white people from Long Island who can't afford to get busted, or they're too clean-cut to go on the block, or they're scared to death to go on the block. Usually, I would cop a bundle* or better. Dope, coke, both. When they come from Long Island, they don't come down here to buy less than a bundle. A bundle of each. That's $150. Usually, I'll get a bag of dope, a bag of coke, and $20.
>
> Most of them are older than me [34]. Most of them are 40, 38, somewhere around there. They mostly have good jobs. They all got their own houses. All of them have nice cars. There's two of them who take the train, but they do have a house out on Long Island.
>
> I have one female customer from Long Island used to be a top, top supervisor with Sony's, you know, top name TV brand. I mean, I'm talkin about top dollars. Sometimes she comes twice a week. Sometimes she comes once a week. She buys two bundles of dope and two bundles of coke. She gets off up here. Sometimes she buys syringes from me, but if I don't have any I'll go to M——— and I get it from him. She'll buy four or five at a time. She hooks it up in the gallery. She gives me a shot from it. She gives me my own one and one. But she needs me to hit her though. I'll hit her in her arm. She can't hit herself at all. I'll hit her before I do any drugs.
>
> Nobody brings syringes with them. They said that they can't find them out there. They would buy them from M——— if I don't have any. They know that I sell them, and they're coming to me to cop, so, its only right that they ask me first. But since I've been home [from the hospital; 3 weeks] I haven't had any. Sometimes I have them all the time, sometimes I don't.

While Patricia's comments suggest that risk is affected by location in network structures, they also indicate that a host of external factors can influence the risk that members of these networks experience.

Although sociometric risk location is not related to age, members of the large component (both the periphery and the two-core) are somewhat less likely to be new injectors than are unlinked drug injectors. This may imply that as people enter the drug injection scene, most of them take some time to enter fully into its social and risk relationships. This may also provide a window of time in which they can receive social and medical services that can help them either to reduce or end their

---

*A bundle of heroin was ten ten-dollar bags. A bundle of cocaine was ten five-dollar bags. A bundle of crack was 24 five-dollar vials.

involvement with the drug scene or to at least learn how to protect themselves from engaging in high-risk behaviors.

For example, Jeannie, a 25-year-old Latina who took several years to become a member of the core network, lived with her husband in the neighborhood and began sniffing heroin in 1991. Alarmed by her attraction to heroin, she came to our storefront in 1992 to get tested for HIV and confided that she had "skin popped" a couple of times. After fights with her abstinent husband who threatened to put her out of the house over her heroin use, she began spending more time at the storefront, sometimes asking for referrals to treatment, but rarely acting on any of them. Faced with steadily deteriorating kinship and friendship ties, her access to cash began to dry up and she reluctantly and unhappily began to spend more time with members of the core network from who she could sometimes "get straight." But, unable to rely on the largesse of core network members without reciprocating, Jeannie started working the sex "stroll" in late 1992 to earn money while trying her best to conceal it from her friends, including staff members at the storefront. She knew that word of her activities would travel through the neighborhood and eventually reach her husband, and in early 1994, after unsuccessful attempts at "detoxing," Jeannie found herself on the streets, a full-fledged member of the core network injecting upward of a bundle a day.

Drug injectors in the two-core of the large component are somewhat more likely to be homeless, to have spent time in jail or prison, not to attend religious services, and, particularly, to lack legal income. Almost two fifths of the two-core members had not had even a part-time or casual job or received any form of welfare benefits during the 6 months before their interview. They were also more likely to sell syringes and (along with peripheral members of the large component) to engage in commercial sex work. Perhaps as a result, they were less likely to be earning less than $10,000 per year, although it should be noted that 70% or more of all categories of drug injectors had earnings below $10,000.

HIV RISK AND SOCIOMETRIC RISK NETWORK LOCATION

Table 3 presents data on risk behaviors during the prior 30 days by drug injectors in different risk network locations. As can be seen, the general pattern is that the two-core is characterized by much high-risk drug injection behavior. Thus, several high-risk injecting practices that have been associated with a higher probability of HIV infection, including injecting drugs frequently (Marmor et al., 1987), injecting with syringes others have used (Des Jarlais et al., 1994; Metzger et al., 1993; Nicolosi et al., 1992), backloading (Jose et al., 1993), injecting in shooting galleries (Marmor et al., 1987) or in outdoor sites (Neaigus et al., 1993), and injecting cocaine or speedball (Chaisson et al., 1989a; Dasgupta et al., 1995; Novick et al., 1989), are more likely to have been engaged in by drug injectors in

Table 3. Relationships between Sociometric Risk Network Location
and High-Risk Behaviors ($N = 767$)[a]

Behaviors in last 30 days	Large connected component		Small components ($n = 210$)	Unlinked ($n = 299$)	p[b]
	Two-core ($n = 125$)	Periphery ($n = 133$)			
Injected more than once a day	77%	57%	50%	46%	0.001
Injected with a needle or syringe after someone else injected with it or that someone else may have used	47%	41%	43%	28%	0.001
"Got a taste" from someone else's syringe	40%	24%	14%	15%	0.001
Backloaded (syringe-mediated drug sharing)	38%	22%	16%	12%	0.001
Shared cooker	74%	61%	66%	43%	0.001
Shared rinse water	60%	42%	50%	29%	0.001
Injected in shooting galleries	28%	24%	11%	19%	0.013
Injected in outside places	53%	48%	29%	33%	0.001
Injected cocaine or speedball	90%	79%	66%	55%	0.001
Crack use	58%	54%	43%	37%	0.001
Had a sex partner who is an IDU	28%	45%	48%	21%	0.008
Any unprotected vaginal or anal sex	31%	52%	55%	40%	0.001[c]

[a]For some cells, the denominators vary from these due to missing data or, as for condom use, the exclusion of those who had no sex during the period from the table.
[b]Probabilities by Mantel–Haenszel test for trend.
[c]By χ^2. The probability by Mantel–Haenszel test for trend is 0.49.

the two-core (and, for some variables, in the periphery) of the large component. Crack use is also more common among subjects with a greater degree of linkage to other injectors. Data on risk behaviors during the prior 2 years, although not presented here, show a similar pattern.

Sexual risk behaviors during the prior 30 days display a more complicated pattern, with both members of the two-core and the unlinked *less* likely than peripheral members of the large component or members of small components to engage in unprotected vaginal or anal sex (or to report having a sex partner who is a drug injector). This reflects a complicated pattern. Only 55% of members of the two-core and 61% of the unlinked drug injectors reported having had sex in the prior 30 days, as compared to 76% of members of the periphery of the large component or 72% of members of the small components [p (χ^2) = 0.001].

In ethnographic interviews, a recurrent theme mentioned by many men (as well as by female sex workers) was their lack of sex drive while using heroin and feelings of hypersexuality while trying to kick the habit. But while heroin is notorious for curbing sexual appetite, another reason cited by many core network members for not having sex very often was that they were simply too busy hustling money, buying drugs, or using them to have sex. The pursuit of drugs or money to buy them was so all-consuming that core network members had little time to do anything else. For example, Bruce, an African-American shooting gallery operator and one of the few core network members who discussed having sex with his "girlfriend," was perhaps typical of the preoccupation with drug use to the exclusion of much else that core network members exhibited. Like nearly every member of the core network, Bruce devoted most of his time to maintaining his habit, but on several occasions, he came into the research storefront asking to be interviewed. At first, the ethnographer thought that he was simply looking to earn money from being interviewed, but Bruce said that he was not looking for money; the ethnographic interview was one of the only opportunities he had to escape the 24-hour grind of chasing the next bag of heroin and have a "real" conversation. It was not simply sex that Bruce had been missing as a result of his nodal position within the core network; he also missed many other facets of everyday life that other people often take for granted.

Of those who did have sex,* the unlinked (35%) were considerably less likely to report having any drug-injecting partners than two-core members (50%), periphery members (58%), or members of small components (67%) ($p = 0.003$ by Mantel–Haenszel test for trend). Also, among those who had sex, 2-core members were less likely to report having unprotected vaginal or anal sex (57% did so) than the unlinked (67%), members of the periphery (69%), or members of small components (78%) [p (χ^2) = 0.019]. Thus, the overall pattern for subjects having unprotected sex is produced by (1) two-core members and the unlinked being less likely to have sex and also by (2) their being somewhat less likely to have sex with IDUs or to engage in unprotected sex when they do have sex.

We also compared behaviors during the recent past of the 51 HIV-seronegative drug injectors in the two-core with those of the 364 other uninfected drug injectors in the data set. As can be seen from Table 4, the seronegative two-core members were more likely to have engaged in a wide range of high-risk drug injection behaviors, as well as to have smoked crack. Members of the other categories, however, may have been more likely to have engaged in unprotected vaginal or anal sex.

One of the advantages of having sociometric risk network data is that we are able to compare the extent to which the 51 seronegative two-core members took risks with linked others whom we tested and were HIV-infected with the extent to which the 194 seronegative members of the periphery of the large component or of the smaller components engaged in high-risk behaviors with linked seropositives.

---

*The data here vary from the data in Table 3, which presents data on the drug-injecting sexual partners for *all* participants (including those who did not have sex during this period).

Table 4. Comparison among 415 HIV-Seronegative Street-Recruited Brooklyn
Drug Injectors of Members of the Two-Core in the Large Connected Component
versus Other Drug Injectors on Whether or Not They Engaged
in High-Risk Behaviors in the Last 30 Day

	Two-core members ($n = 51$)	Others ($n = 364$)	p (χ^2)
Receptive syringe sharing	49%	35%	0.044
Were "given a taste" of drugs from someone else's syringe	25%	12%	0.006
Backloading (syringe-mediated drug sharing)	35%	11%	0.001
Injected in shooting galleries	20%	16%	0.473
Injected in outdoor places	57%	29%	0.001
Injected cocaine or speedball	90%	56%	0.001
Shared cooker	69%	49%	0.007
Shared rinse water	53%	32%	0.003
Used crack	65%	45%	0.008
Vaginal or anal sex without a condom	36%	51%	0.052

Seronegative members of the two-core were significantly more likely during the
last 30 days to have injected with a seropositive drug injector (61% vs. 28%), to
have shared a cooker with a seropositive drug injector (39% vs. 18%), and to have
shared rinse water with a seropositive drug injector (27% vs. 14%). They tended to
be more likely to have injected with a syringe that a seropositive drug injector had
previously injected with (16% vs. 7%; $p = 0.051$). They were not statistically
distinguishable, however, in terms of the proportion who had had any sex with a
seropositive drug injector (6% vs. 8%) or unprotected sex with a seropositive drug
injector (4% vs. 7%) in the prior 30 days.

Table 5 presents data on the egocentric networks of drug injectors in different
risk network locations. Here, it is important to remember a methods-based distinction between the sociometric and the egocentric data: Egocentric data concern the
persons the respondent describes as being in his or her network, regardless of
whether these network members take part in the study or not. The sociometric data
concern ties with other persons in the data set; furthermore, they incorporate
nominations made by either member of the pair, so a respondent "ego" can be
linked to an "alter" because alter named ego (and a linkage was made by one of the
techniques described in Chapter 5 on methods and in Chapter 13). Thus, it is
entirely logical that some unlinked drug injectors report that they have egocentric
network members who are drug injectors (because the linkage was never made).

As can be seen, two-core members are particularly likely to have members
of their egocentric network who inject drugs more than once a day, and the
members of the large component (both two-core and periphery members) are more

Table 5.   Relationships between Sociometric Risk Network Location
and High-Risk Characteristics of Drugs Injectors' Egocentric Networks (N = 767)[a]

Reports that she or he has a drug-injection network member who	Large connected component		Small components (n = 210)	Unlinked (n = 299)	p^b
	Two-core (n = 125)	Periphery (n = 133)			
Injects > 1 time per day	77%	57%	53%	36%	0.001
Injects at shooting gallery	36%	34%	18%	22%	0.001
Is ⩾5 years older than subject	53%	42%	35%	26%	0.001

[a]For some cells, the denominators vary from these due to missing data.
[b]Probabilities by Mantel–Haenszel test for trend.

likely to have egocentric network members who inject at shooting galleries. They
are also more likely to have older injectors in their networks. All three of these
characteristics—injecting more frequently, injecting in shooting galleries, and
age—have been associated with the probability that a drug injector is infected with
HIV (Marmor et al., 1987), and they are also significantly associated with HIV
serostatus in the SFHR data set. Thus, what Tables 3 through 5 mean, taken
together, is that drug injectors in the two-core and, to a lesser degree, in the
periphery of the large component are more likely than other drug injectors to
engage in various high-risk injection behaviors; also, that when they inject, they
are more likely to do so with a high-risk drug injector who is thus more likely to be
infected with HIV.

This fact was not lost on core network members, many of whom admitted
feeling somewhat fatalistic about the way in which they were using drugs. Millie, a
35-year-old shooting gallery operator, noted that "we all figure that we've got the
virus whether we really know or not. You can't live like this for long and not get
it." Bruce admitted that members of his injection network (the people who came
into his shooting gallery) did not talk about HIV/AIDS too much because to do so
would necessarily dampen the mood in the gallery and force "customers" to think
about something that, at that precise moment when risk seemed so obvious, they
would rather not face.

As a consequence, the data in Table 6 should come as little surprise. For the
687 drug injectors for whom HIV data are available, those in the two-core are
considerably more likely than others to be infected with HIV. Similarly, among the
591 drug injectors with data on hepatitis B core antibody, two-core members tend
to be more likely to be positive, an indicator that they have at some time been
exposed to hepatitis B virus (which is transmitted through sexual and drug-
injecting behaviors in the same way as HIV is, only more easily).

One very interesting implication of the data in Table 6 may not be obvious.

Table 6.   Sociometric Risk Network Location and Infection with HIV and HBV

Infections	Large connected component		Small components	Unlinked	P^a
	Two-core	Periphery			
Percent HIV+	54%	36%	37%	37%	0.019
	$(110)^b$	(117)	(189)	(271)	
Percent hepatitis B core antibody-	83%	71%	71%	70%	0.052
positive	(82)	(97)	(164)	(248)	

^{a}Probabilities by Mantel–Haenszel test for trend.
^{b}Number in parentheses indicate the sample size for which data were available for each variable for subjects in a given sociometric network location.

The analyses of sociometric risk network location are based on risk behaviors with persons who have been network members during the 30 days prior to the interview. However, few, if any, of the infections will have occurred during this 30-day period, for two reasons: First, most HIV infections among drug injectors in New York probably occurred during or before the mid-1980s (Des Jarlais et al., 1989). Second, if any of the participants did become infected during this 30-day period, the chances are high that they would not yet have developed the antibody to HIV (or, similarly, to the core of the hepatitis B virus), and thus would not have tested positive. Thus, what the table implies is that infections that probably occurred years before can be "predicted" by more-or-less current network patterns. Since, as was discussed in Chapter 7, many of the egocentric risk network ties are relatively short-term (less than 12 months duration), this suggests one of two things is probably true: Either infected drug injectors disproportionately form the kinds of linkages that lead them to be in the core after they become infected (and we have not been able to develop any credible scenario as to why and how this would happen), or the pattern of social linkages (as opposed to each linkage considered separately) is fairly robust over time, so that (1) drug injectors tend to spend considerable proportions of time in their given sociometric risk network category and (2) drug injectors in the two-core of a large component in a high-seroprevalence city like New York are particularly likely to become infected. (The reasons why this might be true are discussed more in Chapter 11.)

SOCIOMETRIC RISK NETWORK LOCATION AND PREVENTION RESOURCES

From these data, it is clear that sociometric risk network location is related to a drug injector's degree of marginalization, roles in the drug scene, behaviors, egocentric network characteristics, and probability of infection. Let us now consider whether sociometric risk network location is related to access to medical and prevention services and to discussion with other injectors about AIDS and risk reduction. Table 7 presents data on medical and prevention services. None of the drug injectors are likely to have received medical care in the past 3 months, with the exception that about one fifth were in drug abuse treatment at the time of interview.

Members of the core network loathed going to local hospitals for a variety of reasons, including the disrespectful treatment they often received there, the lack of adequate medical care they have received, outstanding warrants against them, and insufficient methadone while hospitalized. Even IDUs with the most pressing needs often avoided medical care. For example, when an abscess burst on the back of Benny's hand, he wrapped a rag around it and treated it himself, risking serious infection. After he injected a bundle of heroin that he had been entrusted to sell, Jerry's arm was broken by his angry Dominican managers. He refused to go the hospital to set the bone, saying that he did not want to spend the entire day "dope sick" in the emergency room. When Patricia experienced a high fever, she waited so long to seek medical care that an ambulance had to be called to bring her to the hospital. The only times that Bruce and Louie had seen health care professionals in the last 10 years were when they were in Rikers Island. They both discovered their HIV statuses in this jail and generally praised the quality of care in jail as compared with care that was available in the neighborhood. Of course, they were not eager to see the "good" doctors again if this required going to jail. From the data in Table 7, noncore IDUs also rarely sought medical treatment. As Table 7 also shows, drug injectors in the two-core were considerably less likely than others to be in treatment, whereas those in the small components were most likely to be in treatment.

Table 7. Sociometric Risk Network Location and Use of Medical and Prevention Services ($N = 767$)[a]

	Large connected component		Small components ($n = 210$)	Unlinked ($n = 299$)	p[b]
	Two-core ($n = 125$)	Periphery ($n = 133$)			
In drug abuse treatment	10%	20%	32%	20%	0.029
Received in last 3 months any:					
Medical treatment	3%	3%	3%	6%	0.108
Sterile syringes	48%	35%	27%	23%	0.001
Bleach	65%	61%	50%	51%	0.003
Condoms	65%	63%	54%	52%	0.004

[a]For some cells, the denominators vary from these due to missing data.
[b]Probabilities by Mantel–Haenszel test for trend.

One reason why core network members were infrequently seen by health care professionals, including drug abuse treatment specialists, was because many lacked sufficient identification and/or were ineligible at the time they needed services the most. For example, when Patricia decided that she could not sustain a habit of more than a bundle of heroin a day, she expressed interest in enrolling in a methadone program. Unable to pay for methadone, Patricia would have had to rely on Medicaid to pay for her participation. But it had been so long since Patricia had seen a health care provider that her Medicaid eligibility had expired and her card was no longer active. To reapply for Medicaid benefits proved a daunting task that brought her to at least four different social service offices over a 2-week period, each of which required a wait of several hours to speak with social workers (a difficult task even for the unaddicted). Each of these social workers asked her to produce identification, proof of residence (a lease, gas or electric bill) and proof from the Department of Labor that she had unsuccessfully sought employment. After the first week, even though she was surely eligible, Patricia began to wonder whether she would ever regain Medicaid benefits, especially since she knew that the state was trying to cut down on their number of Medicaid dependents. Sensing that her resolve to enroll in a methadone program was waning, the ethnographer agreed to pay for her participation in a program until her Medicaid benefits became effective. But even that proved to be virtually impossible to arrange. The only methadone program in Brooklyn that had vacancies was located three neighborhoods away from where Patricia was staying and would require her to take three buses to get there. Patricia, feeling "dope sick," arrived at the methadone program at 8:30 AM, together with the ethnographer, cash in hand, only to be turned away at the door by a security guard who said that it was too late to see an intake worker. The following day, arriving at the program at 6:45 AM, Patricia and the ethnographer were told that she could not participate in the program because she did not have Medicaid (their preferred method of reimbursement) and they could not accept payment for services from anyone else but the client him- or herself. To become eligible for the program's "sliding scale" payment plan, potential clients had to show a pay stub that verified their ability to pay and established an appropriate amount to be charged. They would not accept payment from a third party. Disheartened by 2 weeks of earnestly trying to enroll in a methadone program, Patricia gave up and returned to the familiarity of the shooting gallery. Parenthetically, it is worth noting that, during much of the SFHR project, the mayor of New York opposed syringe exchange because drug injectors should enter treatment instead.

Table 7 does provide some good news, however. Syringe exchanges* and outreach programs seemed to be reaching many members of the large component

---

*Syringe exchanges in Bushwick were initiated by SFHR staff (and others) in 1991 on an "illegal" basis. They were subsequently legalized.

Table 8.   Sociometric Risk Network Location
and AIDS-Related Discussion $(N = 767)^a$

In last 30 days	Large connected component		Small components ($n = 210$)	Unlinked ($n = 299$)	P^b
	Two-core ($n = 125$)	Periphery ($n = 133$)			
Another user has told subject that she or he should use bleach	68%	55%	46%	45%	0.001
Subject has told someone else to use bleach	65%	50%	49%	46%	0.002
Subject has discussed AIDS with another IDU	59%	53%	54%	42%	0.001

^{a}For some cells, the denominators vary from these due to missing data.
^{b}Probabilities by Mantel–Haenszel test for trend.

(including its core). Since HIV is particularly prevalent in the large component, HIV prevention services can help prevent transmission from the infected person to others. Of course, almost two fifths of the unlinked and members of small components are also infected, and the other members are at potentially high risk, so prevention services are also needed by members of these network locations (Friedman et al., 1997a).

Perhaps partly as a result of their contact with these services, members of the two-core are most likely to be told by other users to use bleach to decontaminate their syringes and also to convey this same message to other users (Table 8). The unlinked are least likely to discuss AIDS with other drug injectors.

SUMMARY AND DISCUSSION

This chapter has discussed sociometric networks among drug injectors in Bushwick. What stands out in the data presented is a simple point: Sociometric network locations can be measured, and both the behaviors and the personal (egocentric) networks of drug injectors seem to vary by network location. (Although we have shown this only for the sociometric risk network, it is also true for the sociometric social network and the ethnographic social network.) When we examine data on sociometric risk networks, those in the two-core of the large component seem to be at particularly high risk. In the next chapter, we will focus our analysis of the relationship of sociometric network location on the probability of HIV infection on the dichotomy between these two-core members and the other participants in the study.

Networks and HIV and Other Infections

So far, our major focus has been on the lives, activities, social relationships, and networks of drug injectors. As we have written about these issues, the HIV/AIDS epidemic has been a constant touchstone that has guided the topics that were discussed. In this chapter, we will try to tie these threads together in terms of their impact on whether or not a given drug injector who takes part in the research is or is not infected with HIV. To a lesser extent, we will also consider what factors may be related to infection with hepatitis B.

To begin, we will examine which drug injectors are infected. We will consider this by looking at how infection rates vary for drug injectors by their socio-demographic characteristics, social marginalization, behavior, and characteristics of their egocentric networks. We will then use multiple logistic regression techniques to determine the independent and significant predictors of HIV serostatus, including both egocentric network characteristics and sociometric risk network location. We will follow this by a consideration of how sociometric risk network location is related to the behavioral and egocentric network predictors of HIV.

Next, we will consider HIV infection among new injectors (defined here as those who have been injecting for less than 10 years), with a major focus on examining data that indicate that women get infected earlier in their injection careers than do men. Consideration of network variables helps us to specify that this is occurring among women with high-risk egocentric networks.

Finally, we will discuss some of the limitations in what can be concluded from these analyses, both because of methodological issues (such as the ways in which the sample was recruited and the variables measured) and because of real limitations on what can be studied using cross-sectional data.

WHICH DRUG INJECTORS ARE INFECTED?

Table 1 provides data on which of the 687 members of the sample with determinate HIV test results were infected with HIV. We were unable to obtain blood for testing for approximately 65 subjects because there was no phlebotomist on duty at the time when the subject was there, because of difficulties in finding

Table 1.   Relationships of Selected Variables to HIV and Hepatitis B Core Antibody

	Percent HIV+ (n = 272; N 687)	p (χ²)	Percent hepatitis B cAb+ (n = 426; N = 591)	p (χ²)
Background:				
Sex		0.810		0.225
Men	40		73	
Women	39		68	
Race–ethnicity		0.008		0.259
White and other	31		70	
Black/African American	44		77	
Latino/a	43		70	
Age		0.003		0.001
< 35	34		63	
≥ 35	45		80	
New injectors (< 6 years)		0.001		0.001
New	19		40	
Long term	45		81	
Social marginalization/integration:				
Residence		0.851		0.656
Homeless	40		74	
Not homeless	39		72	
Legal income in prior 6 months		0.598		0.928
No	38		72	
Yes	40		72	
Income		0.772		0.002
< $10,000	40		74	
≥ $10,000	39		59	
Education		0.551		0.897
Not a high school graduate	41		72	
High school graduate	39		72	
Incarcerated since 1977		0.001		0.001
No	33		64	
Yes	45		79	
Incarcerated in last 2 years		0.004		0.003
No	35		68	
Yes	46		80	
Marital status		0.008		0.216
Currently married or living together	29		68	
Not	42		73	
Attend religious services?		0.872		0.113
No	40		75	
Yes	39		69	
Currently in drug treatment		0.332		0.831
No	40		72	
Yes	36		73	

Table 1. *(Continued)*

	Percent HIV+ ($n = 272$; N 687)	p (χ^2)	Percent hepatitis B cAb+ ($n = 426$; $N = 591$)	p (χ^2)
Behaviors during prior 2 years:				
Receptive syringe sharing		0.111		0.358
None	36		70	
Any	42		74	
Backloading (syringe-mediated drug sharing)		0.001		0.126
None	35		70	
Any	53		77	
Injected in shooting galleries		0.001		0.056
None	35		70	
Any	50		77	
Injected in outdoor places		0.001		0.006
None	32		67	
Any	47		77	
Injected cocaine or speedball		0.001		0.001
None	25		.56	
Any	44		.78	
Crack use		0.138		0.908
None	42		.72	
Any	37		.72	
Any unprotected sex in last 30 days		0.001		0.047
None	48		76	
Any	33		69	
Use condoms among those who had sex during prior 2 years		0.023		0.069
None or some	36		.69	
Always	48		.79	
Provided sex for money or drugs		0.144		0.273
None	38		71	
Any	46		77	
Was a man who had sex with another man		0.072[a]		1.00[a]
No	39		72	
Yes	67		75	
Was a woman who had sex with another woman		0.113		0.013[a]
No	39		71	
Yes	53		95	
Role behaviors in prior 30 days:				
Sold drugs		0.271		0.693
None	40		72	
Any	35		70	

(continued)

Table 1. (*Continued*)

	Percent HIV+ (n = 272; N 687)	p (χ²)	Percent hepatitis B cAb+ (n = 426; N = 591)	p (χ²)
Sold needles or syringes		0.038		0.263
None	38		71	
Any	48		77	
Hit doctors		0.001		0.024
No	38		71	
Yes	65		90	
Reports that she or he has a drug-injection network member who:				
Injects > 1 time per day		0.271		0.086
No	37		69	
Yes	42		75	
Is 5 years older than subject		0.181		0.255
No	38		74	
Yes	43		69	
Injects drugs in shooting galleries		0.109		0.019
No	38		70	
Yes	45		79	
Subjects has known < one year		0.329		0.738
No	38		73	
Yes	42		71	
Sociometric risk network location		0.019[b]		0.052[b]
Large connected component				
Two-core	54		83	
Periphery	36		71	
Small components	37		71	
Unlinked	37		70	

[a]Probability by 2-tail Fisher's exact test.
[b]Probability by Mantel–Haenszel test for trend.

veins that had not been too damaged by drug injection for blood to be taken, or because the subjects decided, either during the interview or during pretest counseling, that they did not want to be tested for HIV. Data on the presence of hepatitis B (HBV) core antibody (which tests for prior infection but might miss new infection) were available for 591 subjects.

Groups that are particularly likely to be infected with both HIV and HBV include longer-term injectors (since they have had more time to become infected; older injectors (who tend to be longer-term ones); those who have been incarcerated (which may reflect exposure time plus being "deep" into the street scene); those who inject in high-risk locations such as shooting galleries and outside settings; those who inject cocaine and/or speedball (who may be more likely to engage in high-risk behaviors during "binges" in which they may inject several times an hour for many hours, as has been discussed in Chaisson et al. (1989b), Friedman et al. (1989d), and Vlahov et al. (1990); hit doctors (who, as discussed in Chapter 7, often inject in shooting galleries and outdoor settings, have high-risk egocentric networks, and often "share a taste" in which they get a small share of the drugs from their customer's syringe); and those in the two-core of the large connected component of the sociometric risk network. Interestingly, those drug injectors who are infected with either HIV or HBV are more likely to report that they always used condoms when having sex in the last 2 years and less likely to report engaging in any unprotected sex in the recent past. As was discussed in Chapter 9, this may well reflect efforts not to infect others and/or efforts on the part of their partners to avoid becoming infected.

Blacks and Latinos, those who engage in backloading, and needle–syringe sellers are more likely to be infected with HIV but not significantly more likely to be infected with HBV. This may reflect both the longer time that HBV has been in the New York area (such that it has had more time to diffuse across racial–ethnic barriers) and its greater ease of transmission (so that there are enough ways that it can be transmitted to make it difficult to detect any one of them as a risk factor).

Income and education variables do not seem to be related to HIV in this sample, although those with less than $10,000 annual income were more likely to be infected with hepatitis B.

Neither receptive syringe sharing nor the characteristics of egocentric networks (with the limited exception of having a shooting gallery user in the injection network being associated with a 9% increase in the proportion infected with HBV) from these data seem to be related to infection probabilities. For receptive syringe sharing, which has been shown to be a risk factor for new HIV infection (Des Jarlais et al., 1994; Friedman et al., 1995; Metzger et al., 1993; Nicolosi et al., 1992), this probably reflects the fact that there has been a considerable decrease in this behavior as a result of the HIV epidemic, including among those who are already infected. For the egocentric network variables, it may reflect the difficulties of characterizing long-term infection probabilities over many years in the past by measuring network characteristics during the past 30 days. Nonetheless, as is shown later in this chapter, egocentric variables are related to HIV seroprevalence among newer injectors, and, in the entire sample, egocentric and sociometric network variables are significant predictors of HIV with appropriate controls.

Men who have sex with men are more likely to be infected with HIV than other drug injectors, although the small number (12) of men who report same-sex sex in the last 2 years causes this result to have a p value greater than 0.05. Women who report having had sex with women in the prior 2 years are more numerous (30 with data on HIV, 22 with data on HBV), but these numbers are still small enough for a 14% difference in HIV seroprevalence between these women and other IDUs not to be statistically significant. However, as we will see, there is considerable correlation between being a woman who has sex with women and other variables; after adjustment for these other variables, women injectors who have sex with women are more likely to be infected with HIV. Even in cross-tabular analysis, women who have sex with women are more likely than other IDUs to be positive on the test for antibodies to the core of HBV.

MULTIPLE LOGISTIC REGRESSION PREDICTORS OF HIV SEROSTATUS

The data just discussed give us a picture of which drug injectors are infected. One way to attempt to determine the causal mechanisms by which this happens is to use multiple logistic regression techniques to determine the independent and significant predictors of HIV. (Limitations in this technique are included among the limitations discussed at the end of this chapter.) In particular, we want to investigate whether the association of HIV infection with (1) sociometric risk network location and (2) egocentric network characteristics are explained by these variables. Table 2 presents the results of a logistic regression analysis in which previously determined sociodemographic and behavioral risk factors for HIV among subjects in the SFHR project (Jose et al., 1993) were entered simultaneously with sociometric risk network location (two-core vs. noncore) as predictors of

Table 2. Sociodemographic, Behavioral, and Sociometric Risk Network Characteristic Logistic Regression Predictors of HIV Serostatus among 673 Street-Recruited Brooklyn Drug Injectors

	Odds ratio	95% Confidence interval
Core (vs. all other)	1.73	1.09, 2.76
Black (vs. white)	1.46	0.94, 2.28
Latino (vs. white)	1.94	1.29, 2.92
Years since started injecting	1.06	1.04, 1.08
Behaviors in last 2 years		
Any backloading	1.59	1.07, 2.36
Speedball injection frequency (scale = 10/month)	1.005	1.002, 1.007
Any woman-to-woman sex	2.42	1.08, 5.42
Any man-to-man sex	3.60	1.03, 12.6

Equation (-2 log likelihood) = 805.555.

HIV. As can be seen, all of the variables, including sociometric risk network location (odds ratio = 1.72), remain significant predictors (except "Black," which almost retains significance.)

Of three variables that describe potentially high-risk egocentric networks (having a drug-injecting network member who (1) injects drugs daily, (2) injects in shooting galleries, or (3) is 5 or more years older than the research participant), one is a significant predictor of HIV serostatus when sociodemographics and sociometric risk network location are controlled (see Table 3). A drug injector whose egocentric social network contains any drug injector who is 5 or more years older than the subject is more likely to be infected with HIV (odds ratio = 1.51). The addition of this variable does not alter the significance of any of the variables in Table 2. Risk behaviors and sociometric risk network two-core location remain significant predictors of HIV serostatus. Comparing equation statistics for Tables 2 and 3, the difference in -2 log likelihood $= 4.772$ with 1 degree of freedom, $p (\chi^2) < 0.05$.

Additional equations were estimated that included (1) interaction terms between egocentric networks variables and risk behaviors, and (2) additional risk behavioral variables; both sociometric risk network location and having a drug injector(s) in the egocentric network who is 5 or more years older than is the subject remained significant predictors (data not shown). Finally, when the number of drug injectors in a subject's egocentric network was added to the equation in Table 3, sociometric risk network location (odds ratio = 1.68) and having an

Table 3. Sociodemographic, Behavioral, Egocentric Network Characteristic, and Sociometric Risk Network-Characteristic Logistic Regression Predictors of HIV Serostatus among 673 Street-Recruited Brooklyn Drug Injectors

	Odds ratio	95% Confidence interval
Core (vs. all other)	1.65	1.04, 2.64
Black (vs. white)	1.49	0.96, 2.32
Latino (vs. white)	2.02	1.34, 3.05
Years since started injecting	1.07	1.04, 1.09
Behaviors in last 2 years		
Any backloading	1.53	1.03, 2.28
Speedball injection frequency (scale = 10/month)	1.004	1.002, 1.007
Any woman-to-woman sex	2.41	1.07, 5.42
Any man-to-man sex	3.85	1.09, 13.6
Has drug injector egocentric network member who is 5 years older than subject	1.51	1.04, 2.20

Equation (-2 log likelihood) = 800.783.

egocentric network member who is 5 or more years older than the subject (odds ratio = 1.58) remain significant predictors of HIV, and the number of drug injectors in the egocentric network is not a significant predictor ($p > 0.80$).

MULTIPLE REGRESSION ANALYSES OF RELATIONSHIPS OF SOCIOMETRIC RISK NETWORK LOCATION

Sociometric risk network location is also a significant independent predictor of the drug-injecting behaviors and of the egocentric network characteristic, which are themselves significant multivariate predictors of HIV. Being a member of the two-core was a significant independent predictor of backloading (adjusted OR = 2.01; CI, 1.27, 3.41) and of having a drug injector in the egocentric social network who is 5 or more years older than is the subject (adjusted OR = 1.93; CI, 1.16, 3.20) with multiple logistic regression controls for race–ethnicity, gender, age, homelessness, income (less than $10,000 per year or not), employment at regular full-time or part-time work, years of injection experience, and any use in the prior 2 years of injected cocaine, injected heroin, injected speedball, or crack. Being a member of the two-core is also a significant predictor of more-than-daily speedball injection (adjusted OR = 2.63; CI, 1.56, 4.43), with these same variables other than "any speedball injection" controlled, and, in ordinary least-squares multiple regression with these same variables controlled, of speedball injection frequency, with two-core members reporting approximately 1.4 more speedball injections per day than other drug injectors ($t = 5.17$; $p < 0.0001$.)

Figure 1 presents these results schematically: two-core members are more likely, than other Bushwick drug injectors to (1) engage in high-risk behaviors and to (2) have a high-risk egocentric network even after statistically adjusting for their other characteristics. They are also more likely to be infected with HIV, even after these risk behaviors and egocentric network characteristics (among other variables) are controlled.

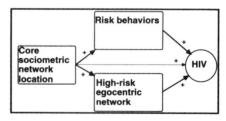

Figure 1.   Schematic diagram of relationships among key variables (control variables are omitted).

A NOTE ON THE OTHER PREDICTORS OF HIV

There were other behavioral and social predictors of HIV infection in Table 3 besides being in the two-core and having a high-risk egocentric network. Race–ethnicity, years of injection experience, frequent speedball injection, backloading, and male–male sex have all been reported as risk factors for HIV or similarly transmitted viruses in other studies (D'Aquila et al., 1989; Friedman et al., 1989a; Marmor et al., 1987; Stark et al., 1996; Vlahov et al., 1995). Woman–woman sex is interesting because it is not likely that the infections actually occurred through woman–woman sexual transmission. Even though HIV has been reported to be transmissible sexually between women (Centers for Disease Control, 1995), existing data indicate that it is a rare event (Kennedy, Scarlett, Duerr, & Chu, 1995; Schaper, Plumb, & Escoffier, 1996). Other cross-sectional studies have also found women drug injectors who have sex with women to be at enhanced risk of being infected with HIV (Cheng et al., 1997; Ross et al., 1992; but see Bevier et al., 1995; Deren et al., 1996) or of becoming infected with HIV in a cohort study (Friedman et al., 1995). Instead, what may be happening perhaps can be explained in network terms, as a possible result of engaging in high-risk injecting (or sex) in networks that contain drug-injecting men who have sex with men, or of high-risk injection practices or network dynamics among groups of women injectors who have sex with women. Thus, while there are no published studies that explain the mechanisms that explain why women injectors who have sex with women are at increased HIV risk, one hypothesis that has been advanced by us and others is that they may engage in more high-risk injecting and/or sex with gay and bisexual men than do other women drug injectors; thus, their egocentric risk networks may have higher seroprevalence than the immediate risk networks of other women injectors (Case et al., 1988; Friedman et al., 1995; Hollibaugh & Vazquez, 1994; Young 1993b). Data from the Cultural Network Study in New York (a longitudinal study of HIV risks among women in outpatient medical settings in New York) and from the AWARE project in San Francisco indicate that women who have sex with women—both drug injectors and noninjectors—do report a higher proportion of male sexual partners who have sex with other men (Mantell et al., 1995; Young et al., 1992). Furthermore, in a multicity study conducted by Battjes and his collaborators of entrants in methadone treatment programs, 20% (109/555) of the women injectors who have sex with women but only 6% (158/2762) of other women IDUs reported having shared syringes with a man whom they believed to be one who engages in male–male sex (odds ratio = 4.03; $p < 0.0001$) (R. Battjes, personal communication, July 13, 1992). In another study, in the San Francisco Bay area, 31% of 52 lesbian or bisexual women IDUs reported having shared needles with gay or bisexual men (Lemp et al., 1995). There also may be other differences between the egocentric risk networks of women drug injectors who have sex with women and other women IDUs. For example, in unpublished analyses of data from a multicity study of out-of-treatment drug injectors (the NADR study, which is described in Brown & Beschner, 1993), women IDUs who have sex with women are considerably more likely than other drug-injecting women to report having a sex partner who is an IDU (74% vs. 50%; odds ratio = 2.85; $p < 0.001$). There is as yet, however, no definitive answer to why women IDUs who have sex with women seem to be at such HIV risk. Our research team is conducting an ethnographic research project to provide the basis both for answering this question and for improving prevention efforts for these women.

DRUG-INJECTING CAREERS, NETWORKS, AND HIV

Few people who begin to inject drugs will be infected with HIV when they do so. The few exceptions to this rule will mainly be men who got infected through sex with other men or people of either sex who got infected through sex with the opposite sex. Many of these people are likely to have been crack smokers before they began to inject (Edlin et al., 1994).

Our initial analyses made it clear that women were becoming infected earlier in their injection careers than were men (see Table 4). We present these data using 10 years of drug-injecting experience as a cutoff point because this provides the clearest picture. (It is only thereafter that men's seroprevalence catches up with women's.)

In thinking about why this could be true, there were three major kinds of hypotheses that might have explained why drug-injecting women would get infected earlier in their injection careers than drug-injecting men:

1. *Biological*: Women may be more likely to become infected through sexual transmission due to asymmetrical rates of heterosexual HIV transmission by gender (Padian, Shiboski, Glass, & Vittinghoff, 1997; Padian & Shiboski, 1994).

Table 4. HIV Infection by Sex and Years of Injection

Years of injection	Percent HIV positive		p	Odds ratio (95% CI)
	Women	Men		
< 10	31	16	0.004	2.33 (1.30, 4.15)
10 or more	43	50	0.32	0.77 (.47, 1.28)

2. *Behavioral*: Drug-injecting women may engage in more high-risk behavior earlier in their injection careers. In addition, they might engage in more high-risk sex (perhaps including commercial sex work) and/or be more likely to smoke crack before beginning to inject.

3. *Risk networks*: Drug-injecting women may be more likely early in their injection careers to take risks with drug or sex partners who are themselves more likely to be infected with HIV.

Biological explanations tend to be universal, i.e., if they are true in one city, they should be true in all cities. As part of a multicity study of street-recruited and treatment-recruited drug injectors conducted under the auspices of the World Health Organization (WHO), analyses were performed to determine whether there were differences in HIV seroprevalence between men and women new injectors in these cities (Friedman et al., 1998b). (In that paper, however, the definition of new injector was persons who had been injecting 6 years or less, rather than less than 10 years as in the analyses of Bushwick data being presented in this section.) In the WHO paper, men and women seemed to have similar infection rates—about 15%—among the total sample of new injectors. Women, however, were significantly ($p < 0.05$) more likely to be infected among new injectors in Berlin (17% vs. 5%), New York (34% vs. 18%), and Athens (where 2 of 33 women and none of 147 men were infected). In the other cities—Bangkok, Glasgow, London, Madrid, Rio de Janeiro, Rome, Santos (Brazil), Sydney, and Toronto—men were not statistically distinguishable in terms of their HIV seroprevalence.

Additional data were available from the National AIDS Demonstration Research (NADR) project (which is described in Brown & Beschner, 1993). This was a multicity study of street-recruited drug injectors. In 18 of these cities, data were available on HIV serostatus for at least 40 drug injectors of each sex who had been injecting for less than 10 years. In three of these cities, women were significantly more likely to be infected, with women's and men's seroprevalence rates being 7% versus 1% in one city, 28% versus 21% in a second, and 34% versus 24% in a third. (City names are not publicly available.) In the other 15 cities, newer injectors' serostatus did not differ significantly by gender. (HIV prevalence among longer-term injectors did *not* vary significantly by gender in cities A, B, or C, but was higher among men in three of the other cities and among women in one other city.) Thus, it does not appear that the pattern of women injectors becoming infected earlier in their careers is universal, so biological explanations do not seem to be appropriate for explaining why women new injectors were at greater risk in the Bushwick sample (nor, for that matter, in the New York sample for the WHO project, which was collected in Manhattan rather than in Brooklyn).

Behavioral explanations also seem to be inadequate. We compared the risk behaviors of men new injectors with those of women new injectors. There were few behavioral differences. Men were more likely to report ever having engaged in

Table 5.   Multiple Logistic Equation to Predict HIV among 256 New Injectors[a]

Variable	Odds ratio	95% CI	p
Female vs. male	2.06	.993, 4.26	.0521
Any anal sex in lifetime	1.76	.912, 3.39	.0922
Injected with a used syringe at first injection	1.67	.781, 3.58	.1855
Behavior during prior two years			
Any same-sex sex	4.55	1.63, 12.7	.0039
Used crack more than once per day, on average	.894	.355, 2.25	.8125
Had sex to obtain money or drugs	2.05	.928, 4.51	.0758

[a]Years of injection less than 10 years. Nine of 265 observations were deleted due to missing values.

anal sex (62% vs. 40%) and tended to have been more likely to inject with a used syringe the first time they injected (23% vs. 14%). Women, on the other hand, were more likely to report that during the prior 2 years they had engaged in same-sex sex (15% vs. 3%), engaged in sex to obtain money or drugs (40% vs. 7%), and smoked crack more than once a day on the average (26% vs. 7%).

The existence of such behavioral differences, however, does not imply that these differences explain the differences in infection rate. To test this, we used multivariate techniques. First, we entered each of these variables in turn into a logistic regression equation along with sex to determine if (1) they were significant predictors of HIV with sex controlled and (2) sex lost significance when the behavior was considered. In each case, sex remained a significant predictor. We then ran a logistic regression in which all of these variables were entered, along with sex, as a predictor of HIV. The results of this equation are shown in Table 5. Women new injectors tend to be more likely to be infected even with these behaviors controlled, although the correlation between gender and commercial sex work leads to a p-value of only .0521. Finally, stepwise multiple logistic regression techniques were used to determine a "best predictor" equation for HIV (see Table 6). Here, sex is a significant predictor. Thus, these behavioral factors do not explain

Table 6.   Multiple Logistic Stepwise Equation
to Predict HIV among 261 New Injectors[a]

Variable	Odds ratio	95% CI
Women (vs. men)	2.63	1.31, 5.27
Injected in outside settings (2 years)	3.55	1.73, 7.31
Backloaded (2 years)	2.60	1.22, 5.57
Any same-sex sex (2 years)	4.28	1.42, 12.9
Injected speedball a mean of more than once per day (2 years)	2.00	0.91, 4.39

[a]Four of 265 observations were deleted due to missing values. New injectors are those with years of injection less than 10 years.

Table 7. Egocentric Risk Network Characteristics, Sex,
and HIV Infection among New Injectors

	N	Percent HIV+		$p\ (\chi^2)$
		Men	Women	
Does subject have an IDU network member who is at least 5 years older?				
No	148	17	22	0.044
Yes	117	16	42	0.002
	$p\ (\chi^2)$	0.103	0.432	
Does subject have an IDU network member whom he or she has known one year or less?				
No	157	17	21	0.55
Yes	108	16	48	0.001
	$p\ (\chi^2)$	0.697	0.479	
Does subject have an IDU network member who injects more than once a day?				
No	136	17	22	0.52
Yes	129	15	39	0.002
	$p\ (\chi^2)$	0.697	0.479	
Does subject have a high risk egocentric network?[a]				
No	82	18	7	0.195
Yes	183	15	38	0.001
	$p\ (\chi^2)$	0.664	0.002	

[a]High risk egocentric networks contain at least one IDU member who is 5 or more years older than the subject, who injects once a day or more, or whom the subject has known less than or equal to 1 year.

the differences in seroprevalence. (Our study design does not allow us to determine what impact behaviors prior to beginning to inject might have on seroprevalence, however.)

Risk network explanations were also tested. Women were more likely to report that their egocentric risk networks included someone who injects more than once a day (55% vs. 44%). First, we examined whether egocentric risk network characteristics might help us to understand which new injectors had become infected. Table 7 shows that, among new injectors, HIV infection is higher among women with high-risk drug injectors in their egocentric networks than among either men with high-risk drug injectors in their egocentric networks or among other women or men. Table 8 shows that, among long-term injectors, this pattern does not hold. Thus, for IDUs who have been injecting for less than 10 years (but not for longer-term injectors), we find that the gender-related difference in seroprevalence is specific to subjects with high-risk egocentric networks.

Each of these network variables was added to the "behavioral risk equation" in Table 6 for new injectors. None of them was significant, nor did they lead the

Table 8.   Egocentric Risk Network Characteristics, Sex,
and HIV Infection among IDUs Who Have Been Injecting at Least 10 Years

	N	Men	Women	p (χ^2)
		Percent HIV+		
Does subject have an IDU network member who is at least 5 years older?				
No	268	49	46	0.71
Yes	135	51	38	0.22
p (χ^2)		0.697	0.479	
Does subject have an IDU network member who injects more than once a day?				
No	187	51	38	0.16
Yes	216	49	49	1.00
p (χ^2)		0.621	0.370	
Does subject have a high-risk egocentric network?[a]				
No	116	50	42	0.47
Yes	294	50	44	0.47
p (χ^2)		0.972	0.834	

[a]High-risk egocentric networks contain at least one IDU member who is 5 or more years older than the subject, who injects once a day or more, or whom the subject has known less than or equal to 1 year.

relationship between gender and HIV serostatus to lose significance. This was not surprising, since the network variables by themselves do not distinguish men from women.

We thus used interaction terms that have the value 1 if the subject is a woman whose network has a given characteristic and value 0 if this is not true. These interaction terms (and the simple network variable) were entered singly into the "behavioral risk equation" in Table 6 (see Table 9). Three of the interaction terms

Table 9.   Women New Injectors with High-Risk Networks
Are More Likely to Be Infected

Variable	Adjusted odds ratio[a]	95 CI[b]
Women with an IDU network member who is at least 5 years older than she is (vs. men and vs. women without such a network member)	4.54	1.11, 18.6
Women with an IDU network member who she has known 1 year or less (vs. men and vs. women without such a network member)	5.77	1.34, 24.8
Woman with high-risk network (vs. men and other women)	13.10	1.69, 102

[a]Odds ratios are adjusted for behavioral risk variables from the prior equation: injecting in outdoor settings, backloading, same-sex sex, daily speedball injection, and gender; and for the particular network variable.
[b]Confidence intervals are wide because of the correlation between the interaction term and its component variables. Multivariate analysis including any two of these interaction terms was not feasible due to their high correlations ($r > .49$).

were statistically significant (with the other terms of the equation thus "controlled"), and subject's gender was nonsignificant ($p > 0.25$) in each of these equations.

These analyses suggest a number of conclusions. First, in some but not all cities, women new injectors have higher HIV seroprevalence than males. Second, the social and cultural variation in this relationship indicates that biologically based gender differences in rates of heterosexual transmission are not likely to explain them. If such biological differences were the cause, women injectors would be infected earlier in their careers in all of the cities in the WHO and NADR studies, not just in 3 of 15 WHO cities and 3 of 18 NADR cities. Third, women drug injector's egocentric risk networks may be particularly likely to affect their probability of becoming infected early in their injection career. This suggests the importance of the issues being discussed in this volume. It also suggests that we need to conduct research to determine why some women (and men) come to have high-risk personal networks and others do not. This research should include studies of network variation among cities and whether this is related to differences in risk behaviors and infection.

These findings also have prevention implications. In some cities—those where women get infected earlier—there is an urgent need to reach them both before they start to inject and early in their injection careers with appropriate interventions to help them protect themselves from HIV. More generally, it may be that these patterns are related to more general issues of the social status of women, whether in the relatively restricted community of drug injectors, in their wider neighborhoods and communities, and in the socioeconomic system as a whole. If so, we need to study this to determine the connections and then to consider how these elements of women's statuses and lives might be changed.

Prevention and Research

We have now seen how studying drug injectors' networks can illuminate both their behaviors and their patterns of HIV infection in ways in which studying them as isolated individuals does not. Network data allow us both to incorporate data on individuals and to go beyond it. For example, when we analyzed the predictors of receptive syringe sharing in Chapter 8, or those of consistent condom use in Chapter 9, we used data about individuals, their partners, and their relationships. In each case, we found that relationships that are very close, of long duration, or otherwise important were those in which the partners were most likely to engage in high-risk behaviors. (This can be expressed in the terms of Oscar Wilde, in "The Ballad of Reading Gaol," as "all men kill the thing they love.") Now, this was not a totally new discovery, since a number of studies both of drug injectors (Paone et al., 1995; van den Hoek et al., 1990; Watkins, et al., 1993; White et al., 1993) and others (Morris et al., 1995a) have found that condom use is less likely with primary partners than with casual partners, but it does allow us to study this phenomenon in terms of the various different aspects of closeness. For example, both the "type" of relationship (that is, whether the sex partner is spouse, ex-spouse, or lover) and the perceived degree of closeness of the relationship affect the probability that a condom will be used. Furthermore, this understanding poses an immediate set of additional questions for research and prevention: What is it about a close relationship that makes it difficult to engage in protective tactics? How can the feelings people have for their friends and lovers be mobilized as a protective resource rather than functioning as a barrier to risk reduction?

Similarly, when we studied the issue of how egocentric network characteristics affect the probability that men and women injectors who have been injecting for less than 10 years have become infected with HIV, we saw that those with high-risk members of their egocentric networks were most likely to be infected. Elsewhere, we analyzed the determinants of infection among those who had been injecting for 6 years or less and found that HIV infection is particularly likely among those who both have high-risk network members and report that they have injected with syringes that others had used (Neaigus et al., 1996). As an example, we found seroprevalence among them to be distributed as in Table 1.

Now, this pattern is relatively easy to understand from basic principles of epidemiology, even though it may be harder to understand for those who think of

Table 1. Percent HIV+ among Subjects
Who Have Injected Drugs for 6 Years

Did subject have any risk network members who are 10 or more years older than the subject?	Did subject inject with other injectors' used syringes during prior 2 years?		
	Yes	No	p
Yes	43%	10%	0.016
No	18%	16%	0.770
p	0.021	0.728	

behaviors alone are the cause of infection. Basically, infection with HIV requires two conditions to be met: (1) a risk behavior, such as injecting with someone else's syringe; and (2) this other person must be infected with HIV (and infectious), which is more likely to be true if this other person is a high-risk person such as somebody who has been injecting drugs for a longer time or who injects drugs frequently.

The research on sociometric networks had several additional implications. First, it showed that HIV is more prevalent among drug injectors in New York who are in the two-core of a large connected component. Furthermore, members of the two-core (and, to a lesser degree, other members of the large component) are more likely to engage in high-risk behaviors than are other drug injectors; and, beyond that, those two-core members who are uninfected are more likely than those outside of the two-core to engage in high-risk behaviors with infected drug injectors. Although it is somewhat difficult to generalize from this analysis since it is specific to this study, it does suggest several general hypotheses that need to be investigated:

1. Risk behaviors are shaped by the entirety of one's network environment, not just by personal characteristics, the characteristics of one's partners or relationships, or even the characteristics of one's egocentric network. Other ways of saying this are that behaviors are shaped by social structural characteristics that are not "local," or that social influence flows through network channels in ways that over time a person may be influenced by the actions or views of those she or he does not know.

2. HIV and other infectious agents also flow through network channels. This means that prevention efforts that disrupt these flows should be developed. It also means that the probability that a given instance of a high-risk behavior will turn out to be with an infected partner is shaped by where in the drug scene the virus has already penetrated and where it is rare or nonexistent.

What we have presented in this volume may seem like much information, but it is only the beginning of relevant research. An enormous amount remains unknown. Many research issues are methodological. These include determining the best ways to ask research participants about their contacts so as to minimize under-reporting and errors; how to sample index participants and how to sample from within their contacts to decide who else to interview, which measures of socio-metric network structure are most relevant for understanding what dependent variables; and what issues social networks and risk networks are most useful for. There are also some important statistical issues that need considerable study; perhaps most important is how to conduct statistical analyses when the assumption of "statistical independence of sampling" (which means that the probability that a given person will be interviewed does not depend on who else is interviewed) is violated. Sociometric network research, after all, massively violates this assump-tion by using network linkages to pick many of the people to be interviewed.

However, we want to highlight three areas as perhaps the most important for future research: (1) how networks change over time and the effects of this; (2) how sociometric network research on drug injectors and other community-based groups of people can be done quickly and cheaply; and (3) the larger-scale determinants of network structures.

HOW NETWORKS CHANGE OVER TIME AND THE EFFECTS OF THIS

In trying to apply the results of this research to prevention, we are greatly hindered by having only cross-sectional data about IDU networks in Bushwick. It would be extremely useful to know what happens as time passes. Some of this, of course, we were able to determine by asking about earlier behaviors and egocentric networks. In particular, we gathered useful information about what they did and who they did it with the first time they injected drugs. Retrospective data, however, have several problems, including the fact that we are only gathering information about a subset of those who began to inject drugs: at a minimum, those who have not died, not stopped injecting drugs, and have been engaged in enough "street" drug use to be recruited in this study. As it stands, however, we know very little about how networks change over time or about how changes in the network characteristics of individuals are related to changes in their individual behavior (or behavior within relationships), or even how and why the network locations and characteristics of drug injectors change over their careers as injectors. This can be clarified by considering Fig. 1. Figure 1 is extremely schematic. It suggests that everything at time 1 may help shape the changes in every other variable. Thus, for example, it is possible that there are patterns in how people's sociometric network location changes over time, which would imply that one's location at time 1 would

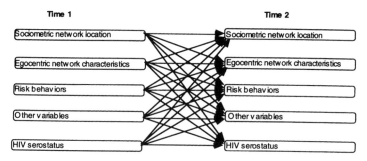

Figure 1. Schematic diagram of possible causal paths among variables.

influence one's location at time 2. Or, as we have some reason to believe, being in the two-core makes it more likely that an uninfected drug injector will become infected by time 2 and, as a consequence, engage in behavior changes by time 3 such as using condoms more consistently (at least with noninjector sex partners). The truth is, however, that we have relatively little idea about how the variables in Fig. 1 affect each other over time or how such changes are mediated by other variables. As an example of such possible mediation, the amount and kinds of changes that occur in a drug injectors' egocentric network in a year might be heavily mediated by her or his stage in an injection career: If she is a new injector, she may make many new drug injector acquaintances quite rapidly, whereas 10 years further in her career, her networks might change much more slowly. Similarly, if an injector takes on a street role as a needle seller, this might also lead to rapid changes in his or her egocentric network.

Thus, although the research presented in this volume suggests a number of possible interventions to prevent HIV spread, our ability to suggest and conduct interventions will be increased considerably when the results of longitudinal network studies become available. Such research has begun. We are aware of (and, where possible, helping with) studies of drug injectors' networks and how they change over time in Atlanta, Georgia (Richard Rothenberg, Principal Investigator); Flagstaff, Arizona (Robert Trotter, Principal Investigator); Washington, DC (Susan Su, Principal Investigator) and Houston, Texas (Isaac Montoya, Principal Investigator).

HOW SOCIOMETRIC NETWORK RESEARCH ON DRUG INJECTORS AND OTHER COMMUNITY-BASED GROUPS OF PEOPLE CAN BE DONE QUICKLY AND CHEAPLY

When we first discovered that two-cores of large components are dangerous social locations in terms of HIV, we immediately began to think about whether it would make sense to try to reduce the size of connected components and/or the size of two-cores within them. We quickly came to several realizations. First, this would be heavy-duty social engineering. Neither drug injectors nor other people form their social relationships (or their risk relationships) on the basis of sociometric understanding of their risk for HIV. Thus, it would probably be impossible to conduct such interventions without eliciting the conscious and organized support of the population at risk. [Drug injectors can organize, although the extent to which they are impoverished, stigmatized, and subjected to police repression makes this more difficult. Drug users' organizations nonetheless exist in Europe, North America, and Australia and have played important roles in forming and implementing AIDS-related policy in Australia and the Netherlands. This is discussed in Brown and Beschner (1993), Friedman (1996), and Friedman et al. (1993)]. We also realized that too little was known about why network structures are what they are in a given city or neighborhood or why and how they change over time to know how to change them.

Shortly thereafter, we realized that it is so difficult and time-consuming, using current technologies, to know where individual drug injectors fit in sociometric networks that this might make it impossible to intervene effectively. For example, Klovdahl (1985) had suggested that there might be "bottlenecks" in networks that were crucial in the potential spread of HIV from one group of high-risk persons to another group (Fig. 2).

Here, persons A and B can be viewed as a bottleneck that could prevent the spread of HIV from the drug injectors on the left side of the diagram to those on the right. Thus, it might be suggested that the prospects for HIV spread could be reduced by concentrating interventions (such as syringe exchange, drug treatment access, or outreach) on such bottlenecks.

Unfortunately, it is extremely difficult to determine the members of such bottlenecks. Consider that the project presented in this volume recruited subjects over a period of 19 months, and that it took many months thereafter to get the data into shape to analyze. In part, it took so long because we were the first project

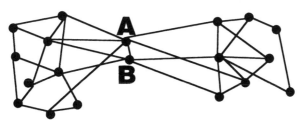

Figure 2.   Schematic diagram of a network "bottleneck." From Sklar (1995).

of this type to study drug injectors' networks and HIV risk, and in some ways we were making up methods as we went along. However, even now, it would require a year or more to recruit the subjects and conduct the interviews, and a few additional months before we would be able to ascertain and check for errors in all the linkage information and then conduct the analyses to determine the large and small components and the two-cores within any large components. This would cost hundreds of thousands of dollars. Furthermore, some of the network linkages would have changed by the time we had our results. Perhaps person A would have set up new friendship patterns altogether, for example, so that she would no longer be a potential bottleneck, and concentrating efforts on her would not yield the hoped-for benefits.

The question, then, is whether ways can be found to ascertain network structures and individual locations within these structures rapidly and inexpensively, and ideally to update our information on an ongoing basis. Several ways might help us to do this. One of these, as Trotter has discussed (Trotter, Baldwin, & Bowen, 1995), is to try to find proxy measures that are highly correlated with the relevant network measures. We found, for example, that drug injectors in the two-core are about twice as likely to be syringe sellers as are drug injectors in other network locations. However, this still meant that almost three fourths of the syringe sellers in our data were not in the two-core. Thus, although there might be great value in working with syringe sellers in prevention efforts, it would be incorrect to use this role as a proxy for sociometric network location. This does not mean that such proxies cannot be found, but it does suggest that they may be hard to locate; furthermore, they might vary between cities or even between sections of cities (which would obviate the gain in finding them, since it would have to be done through a full network study each time).

Another method to ascertain network structures and locations rapidly and at the same time to create the mechanisms for updating the information and for conducting the intervention might be to recruit well-known drug injectors as informants and collaborators. This could be done relatively quickly using ethnographic techniques, but it might best be done, where possible, by collaborating with local drug users' organizations. These collaborators would be trained in network concepts and could use their preexisting knowledge to list many people who inject drugs and trace the linkages among them. They could also fairly rapidly talk with other members of the drug scene about their behaviors and their linkages. The data they collected would undoubtedly contain many errors (although perhaps not as many as network data collected by professional research teams), but might well be more than adequate to use in interventions to prevent the spread of HIV. Furthermore, the drug injectors involved in collecting the network data could also keep track of and report changes in the networks, and perhaps work as part of the HIV intervention team using their enhanced understanding of social relationships and networks as a resource.

THE LARGER-SCALE DETERMINANTS OF NETWORK STRUCTURES

As we have discussed, it may be extremely difficult to determine the network structures that exist in a drug scene and the network locations of individual drug injectors within them in a timely and inexpensive fashion. Similarly, even if we can determine network structures and locations, it is not at all clear whether we will be able to develop ways to reshape them that can reduce HIV risk. As mentioned, people do not set up their associational patterns because of HIV, but rather because of love, convenience, or necessity. For example, some drug injectors are linked to many others in the two-core of the large component because they are shooting gallery owners or because they help others to buy drugs (in return for "sharing a taste"). Relationships with these persons are based on the necessities of the drug life and are difficult to change.

On the other hand, if we understood how the social environments of drug injectors (or other groups at risk) shape their networks, we might be able to affect network-based risk by changing these environments. A couple of examples may make this clear. First, policing patterns probably affect patterns of relationships among drug users. When policing is stringent and/or vicious, users will have stronger motivation to inject indoors. In Bushwick, this has led to increased use of shooting galleries and consequently to shooting gallery managers and habitués becoming part of more drug injectors' networks. For example, Louie boasted that once he took over the tire shop shooting gallery, he injected "like crazy man with all kinds of guys, black, white, Spanish." When the sociometric data about Louie's injection network were examined, 28 people named Louie as a partner. Several of those who named Louie belonged to the ethnographically defined core network of injectors (see Chapter 10), but significantly, 18 of the 28 were injectors who came from outside the area—from at least nine different neighborhoods—who used the tire shop because there were no other places to try their drugs before returning home.

Second, more general characteristics of cities may affect network structures. Although no data exist on it, we have been impressionistically struck by the extent to which most cities in the United States with high-seroprevalence rates among drug injectors are cities in which the major drug injection neighborhoods are pedestrian-oriented rather than automobile-oriented. Thus, in New York, Newark, San Juan, Miami, and Chicago—cities in which 30% or more of drug injectors are infected—drug scenes are places where many people walk rather than drive. Many of the drug scenes in Los Angeles and Houston (cities with seroprevalences less than 10%), on the other hand, are places people drive to when they want to buy drugs. This difference probably affects both the social networks and the risk networks of drug injectors. For example, it may mean that connected components of risk networks turn out to be larger in New York than in Los Angeles, and this in turn could mean that HIV spreads more widely in New York. Of course, this speculation could easily be completely false. If it should be true, on the other hand, this might have implications in terms of prevention (either by changing accessibility of drug scenes to automobiles or in terms of concentrating prevention resources such as syringe exchanges on pedestrian drug scenes) or in terms of forecasting which cities might be most vulnerable to future epidemics of HIV (if they are not yet so cursed) or other similar diseases.

There are many other possible relationships between larger social structures and network structures. For example, urban redevelopment programs probably affect networks (Curtis et al., 1995; Wallace, 1990, 1991a,b, 1992). This was exemplified by the way in which gentrification of the Williamsburg section of Brooklyn led to large-scale "migration" of drug injectors from there to Bushwick, with consequent reshaping of Bushwick networks (and breaking up of preexisting network ties, for example, between people who moved to Bushwick, those who remained in Williamsburg, and those who moved to other drug scenes such as those in East New York).

Understanding these relationships might help us to develop programs, or at least to forecast potential disasters based on urban redevelopment, economic downturns, or other factors. One way in which such understandings might be institutionalized would be to require police departments, developers, and others to produce "AIDS Impact Statements" prior to taking actions that might have dangerous consequences (Lurie, Hintzen, & Lowe, 1995).

Thus, one strong recommendation that we would make out of this study is that enough other network studies be funded and conducted so that it becomes possible to study the determinants of network structures across cities and/or neighborhoods.

PAST RESEARCH

Even though network-based research does not yet provide us with a full picture of what might be done to prevent the spread of HIV and other infectious agents like hepatitis B and C, network concepts have been used and evaluated to a small degree, and other projects or suggestions have been proposed. Here, we will briefly describe a few of them.

As was discussed in the first chapter, Latkin and his colleagues (Latkin, 1995; Latkin et al., 1995a,b, 1996) have experimented with egocentric network intervention techniques. They ask a drug injector to bring in members of his or her egocentric network for a series of group sessions. In these sessions, they discuss HIV and how they can work together to protect themselves from infection. Underlying this is the theory that the group has norms and bonds. Thus, they will mutually reinforce one another in their efforts to avoid risk behaviors. In their evaluation, they found that it "worked" in that participants in the network intervention changed a variety of risk behaviors (sharing syringes, injecting in shooting galleries, carrying and using bleach to clean syringes) more than did drug injectors who received an individually focused intervention. Furthermore, unlike some interventions where the stimulus to safer behaviors wears off in a few months, the continued mutual reinforcement seems to have produced long-lasting effects. In a long-term follow-up, Latkin et al. (1996) found that, even 18 months after the program, uninfected participants in the network intervention were much less likely than uninfected recipients of the individually-oriented intervention to share syringes or to share cookers (adjusted odds ratios in multiple logistic regression were 0.36 and 0.37, respectively) (pp. 341–364).

In a successor study, Latkin turned the focus of research to a more community-oriented intervention. He located and recruited peer leaders among Baltimore drug injectors and trained them (over ten 90-minute sessions) to understand social norms, social influence, and such leadership skills as goal setting, effective communication, modeling, and conflict resolution. Role-playing was used to teach how to disseminate information to others with whom they regularly interacted and thereafter to others. The project evaluation indicates that the peer leaders became active in outreach activities within their networks, and also that the peer leaders themselves became more careful to avoid HIV risk (Latkin, 1998).

In spite of the enormous amount of research that is needed and the difficulties in collecting sociometric network data quickly enough to use it to target interventions to individuals or network components, it is probably useful to provide a "shopping list" of some of the ideas for network interventions that we have considered. This appears in Table 2 [an earlier version of this table appeared in Friedman et al. (1997d)].

This shopping list should be taken as a spur to creative thought and research rather than as a serious proposal for specific programs. Nevertheless, it does suggest some of the potential power of network-based interventions.

BROADER ISSUES

To conclude this volume, however, we want to step back from considerations of social and risk networks to discuss broader issues that deal with the intersection of drug use and the HIV epidemic. On the one hand, HIV seems to serve as a mirror that shows many of the ills of society in truly graphic ways. In the United States, we have a long history of social division and stratification based on race–ethnicity, class, and sex. The entire society is divided by these differences, and the history of the country reflects conflicts over them. The HIV/AIDS epidemic in the United States particularly has shown the importance of race–ethnicity and of sex (in the form of sexual orientation). Class would also be very visible in the disease statistics except for the fact that it is almost never measured. For example, nowhere

Table 2. "Shopping List" of Types of Network Interventions[a]

Interventions can focus on

1. Helping individuals navigate within and between risk network structures so that they avoid relationships that might put them at extra risk of becoming infected.

2. Helping individuals reshape their egocentric risk networks to be less dangerous. This might present them with some very hard choices between friendship or love and health.

3. Using social network pressures to change individuals' behavior, including getting them contact with syringe exchanges or drug abuse treatment.

4. Using large-scale network pressures to change behaviors of small groups. This might best be done through working with drug users' organizations where they exist (Friedman, 1996, 1998).

5. Shaping the movement patterns within networks:
   a. Reducing turnover, so as to isolate pockets of infection.
   b. Helping new injectors (and others) to avoid two-cores of large components.

6. Changing sociometric network structures:
   a. Before HIV becomes widespread in a large component, perhaps work with its members to (1) reduce its size; (2) change the intensity of relationships among members; (3) change the culture of risk within them; and (4) become a center for outreach (and needle exchange) for others who come into contact with the core.
   b. Before HIV becomes widespread in large components, change policy (e.g., away from police repression of users) so as to reduce pressures to be members of large components or cores.
   c. Conceivably, before HIV becomes widespread in large components, use police to disrupt large components. There is, however, considerable reason to suspect that this will fail, and indeed will drive drug injectors even further into large components or cores.
   d. After HIV becomes widespread in a component, it becomes a possible source of infection for others. Possible approaches include (1) helping a component bifurcate by serostatus into infected and uninfected parts with no or little risk behavior involving members of both parts; (2) reducing interaction between component and other IDUs/network structures; and (3) helping component reduce its behavioral risk.

7. Programs aimed at risk reduction that are differentiated by network location. That is, it might be useful to use somewhat different prevention approaches for cores and peripheries of large components, for small and large components, and for unlinked drug injectors.

[a]As we come to understand the population dynamics of recruitment to components or cores, of weak ties between cliques and other subgroupings, of the role of multi–user settings and the associated changes in use of these settings, of individual leavings and group secessions from network structures, of formation of egocentric networks, and so forth, we may be able to deepen this categorization and make it more processible.

does the official AIDS surveillance data ask about the incomes, occupations, or relationships to production and distribution processes of people who are diagnosed with AIDS.

Race–Ethnicity

Consider the figures on United States AIDS diagnoses by race–ethnicity through June 1996 (see Table 3). Clearly, blacks and Hispanics are at considerably

Table 3. Adult and Adolescent AIDS Cases in the United States by Race–Ethnicity through June 1996

	Non-Hispanic white	Non-Hispanic black	Hispanic	Asian/Pacific Islander	American Indian/ Alaska Native
AIDS cases	255,147	184,803	94,910	3,786	1,417
Percent of total AIDS cases (540,806)[a]	47.2	34.2	17.5	0.700	0.262
Percent of total US population[b]	73.7	12.0	10.3	3.32	0.735
Relative risk	0.64	2.85	1.70	0.21	0.356
(second row divided by third row)					

[a]Centers for Disease Control and Prevention(1996).
[b]Bureau of the Census (1996–1997, p. 22).

higher risk than are whites, Asian/Pacific Islanders, or American Indian/Alaskan Natives.

Among drug injectors, there are similar variations in the AIDS data. Furthermore, similar patterns are true for HIV infection. This was clearly shown in the previous chapter. For the drug injectors in this study, infection rates were 31% for whites, 44% for blacks, and 43% for Latinos. When we controlled for other variables such as years of injection, specific risk behaviors, and sociometric network location, both blacks and Latinos were more likely to be infected (with adjusted odds ratios of 1.46 for blacks and 1.94 for Latinos, as compared with whites). As we have elsewhere discussed (Friedman et al., 1998b), drug injectors who report that they are both black and Latino can be conceived of as doubly subordinated (as both blacks and Latinos); they are also particularly likely to be infected with HIV (56% HIV+), to be homeless (30%), to be in the two-core of the large connected component (33%), and less likely to be in drug abuse treatment (only 8%, as opposed to 21% of other blacks and Latinos).

Class

The relationship of social class and AIDS has been much harder to study since no data are collected on it. To get around this problem, people have studied small geographic areas (zip codes or census tracts) and compared data on median income in the area with the proportion of the local population who have been diagnosed with AIDS (Fife & Mode, 1992; Hu et al., 1994; Simon, Hu, Diaz, & Kerndt, 1995). For example, in a study of zip code areas in the Newark, NJ metropolitan area, Hu et al. (1994) found that areas with a low median income had a cumulative AIDS incidence almost five times higher than that of higher income zip codes (controlling for family structure and race–ethnicity). Simon et al. (1995) used zip code data for Los Angeles County, CA, and found similar results, with AIDS rates highest in low income areas, intermediate in intermediate income areas, and lowest in high income areas. They also found this inverse relationship to hold separately for blacks, whites, and Latinos. Furthermore, AIDS rates were highest in low-income areas, intermediate in intermediate-income areas, and lowest in high-income areas when looking only at specific exposure categories for male/male sex cases, for drug injector cases, for cases who reported both drug injection and male/male sex, and for persons with other exposure categories.

Sex

The relationship of sex and HIV/AIDS is greatly complicated by the fact that in the United States (unlike in much of Africa) male–male sex has been a major transmission behavior for the disease. Thus, 51% (274,192) of the 540,806 AIDS cases diagnosed in the United States through June 1996, were among men who reported having had sex with men (and there were another 35,218, or 7%, who reported both male–male sex and drug injection). (The rates of male–male sex and male–male sex and drug injection cases have been declining over time, as is shown by the fact that the proportions of AIDS cases in these categories for the year July 1995 through June 1996 were only 41% and 4%, respectively.) In our study, however, the complexities of sex–gender issues are illustrated by the fact that women drug injectors seem to be getting infected earlier in their injection careers than men who inject drugs and also by the finding that women injectors who have sex with women were more likely to be infected than other drug injectors (see Chapter 8). For both of these findings, we have some reason to believe that the higher infection rates may be due to network phenomena in terms of the high-risk women being more likely to have other high-risk people in their egocentric networks.

Drug Policy

The United States has long had a policy of criminalizing drug use. During the AIDS era, this has reached extremes, with "Drug War" rhetoric being a major staple of political campaigns, prime-time TV shows, and public policies. Yet this drug war policy has not succeeded in solving the drug problems of the participants in this research. Drug treatment has not significantly expanded during the AIDS era. In New York City, the number of treatment slots has increased little; as Medicaid programs are under attack and medical services in general go to managed care cost saving approaches, current budget issues may reduce the number of treatment slots available and/or lead to their being available only to those with private resources or insurance to pay for them; that is, to those who both have social class background that provides them with such resources and also are sufficiently in control of their drug use to be able to retain jobs. Furthermore, the drug war has disrupted the lives of drug injectors through making them subject to frequent arrest and to police harassment. In this study, 37% of the participants reported having been in jail or prison during the previous 2 years and 55% since 1977. Nor does such imprisonment save these drug injectors from HIV infection or HIV risk behaviors: Those who have been incarcerated during the 2 years prior to their interview were more likely than those who had not to be infected with HIV (46% vs. 35%), to have been exposed to hepatitis B (80% vs. 68%), and to have engaged (during this 2-year period) in receptive syringe sharing (58% vs. 42%), backloading (35% vs. 20%), and injecting in shooting galleries (41% vs. 22%) and outdoor settings (62% vs. 40%). Furthermore, their current risk networks are more likely to include high-risk injectors (shooting gallery users, those older by 5 or more years, those who inject more than once a day on average, and those whom they have known for less than a year).

During the course of our fieldwork, the project ethnographic staff frequently saw police harassment of drug users and other local residents. Below, Jerry talks about the increased policing in the area:

> The policing of the area has gotten a lot more thorough. It's like they're using this area as some kind of testing ground, I don't know; but they're determined to clean it up; and they're not leaving one stone unturned—if you're white especially. If you're white, you're automatically a candidate to be pulled over and shook down because you're from—in their view you have no business being in the area; and, if you can't show any address of any place here, they make you clean out your pockets and everything.

While it is hardly surprising that police officers would harass drug users in the area, they often had difficulty distinguishing the "bad guy" from people who were not involved with drugs. For example, during the summer of 1991, Maria's 18-year-old daughter was married. A large wedding reception was held in the front-yard of her house on crack row. The front yard was festooned with streamers and balloons, while a patched-together sound system blared golden oldies and Salsa. As the guests arrived, food was generously dished out. The commotion from the party drew the attention both of several drug users, who sat politely on the sidewalk across the street enjoying the music so as not to be disrespectful of the occasion, and of the police, who had difficulty believing that anyone would hold a party in such a place. Once the guests were fed, Maria asked one of her sons to offer plates of food to the small but conspicuous crowd of drug users across the street. When the police saw food being given to the growing crowd of drug users, it was apparently too much for them to tolerate. Approaching the front gate in anger, one officer demanded, "What's going on here?" When one of the guests (dressed in a tuxedo) replied that it was "obviously a wedding reception," the officer threatened the drug users with arrest if they did not move off the street. The officer then returned to the front gate and told Maria's son that "I don't live here. I live in Long Island and I could care less what happens to this neighborhood. As far as I'm concerned, they should drop an atomic bomb on this place." With that, he got back in his car and sped away; but throughout the evening, patrol cars regularly passed in front of the house to make sure that the festivities did not get out of hand and that no one made the drug users feel too welcome.

When the police could not find drug distributors to arrest, they often went to well-known shooting galleries in search of "numbers." After Maria's house burned, it became one of the primary shooting galleries in the neighborhood. The police loathed going inside because there were too many dark hiding places; and they believed that to get to the gallery on the second floor, they would have to negotiate an obstacle course of discarded HIV-infected syringes. To flush drug users out, some officers used to throw large rocks through the windows. Indeed, they were caught in the act by a prize-winning reporter for the Los Angeles Times, who had been interviewing heroin injectors when the projectiles whizzed by his head (Bearak, 1992). While some injectors had been struck by rocks, others showed the research team large welts across their torsos that officers had inflicted with whips of thick television cable as they fled the galleries.

In the summer, some local police officers often mercilessly and systematically harassed drug users who loitered near the major drug selling locales. Early in the morning, foot patrol officers would routinely rouse with kicks users who had fallen asleep on the sidewalk. Sometimes the kick simply nudged them awake; at other times it was meant to cause pain. So habituated were they to the pastime that police officers continued to do it even when the ethnographic team used video cameras to photograph them.

One of the authors of this volume captured the atmosphere in Bushwick, as observed by the ethnographic team, as part of a poem, "Snapshots of the Drug War" (Friedman, 1997):

> Brooklyn, 1992.
> Troutman and Jefferson Streets.
> Touts hawk their wares:
>> "No Exit"
>> "Dead Presidents"
>> "Cutthroat" "Royalty"
>> "Body Bag"
>> and
>> "American Airlines."
>
> Cars
> from New Jersey, Connecticut and Manhattan
> fill nearby curbs.
> Their drivers buy a bag
> of No Exit or Body Bag,
> hustle a needle
> and walk to a dumpster
> by a decaying loading dock
> for their shot.
> A post-modern Portobello Market,
> bustling;
> taking care of business.
>
> Screams at both ends of the street.
> Wall to wall cops screech
> "Eat the cement!"
> "Down on your bellies!"
> and everyone lies in the street
> for hours,
> 6-year-olds,
> junkies,
> dealers,
> hit doctors.
> A pregnant neighborhood mom
> coming home from the grocery
> lies next to her sister
> who hustles blow jobs down the block
> to buy her smack.

Furthermore, the drug wars have not succeeded in making drugs more expensive or less available. The price of a bag of heroin or cocaine has remained more or less constant for the last 15 years. Purity of drugs available in the streets has gone up, not down. Heroin purity in New York City and surrounding areas in 1992 was described by Frank, Galea, and Simeone (1992) as being "exceptionally high" (25 to 30%). Purity increased by 1994 to 72% (Frank & Galea, 1996). Current reports from the police laboratories continue to show purities in the range of 60 to 70% (Neaigus et al., 1997). Similarly, in Chicago, Ouellet et al. (1993, 1995) report that the purity of street heroin rose from about 2% in the early 1980s to 10% in 1990 and about 30% by the beginning of 1993. Cocaine purity is also high. Indeed, the 1980s and 1990s have seen widespread smoking of crack cocaine, which is a very high-purity product.

The drug wars have greatly hindered risk reduction. As has been discussed, police practices disrupt networks in ways that may reduce the (limited) reduction in HIV spread between networks whose members do not interact with each other. Furthermore, the fear of arrest can lead to increased shooting gallery use (which means that one's potential partners are likely to be infected, since 50% of those who have used shooting galleries are HIV-positive as compared to 35% of those who have not used them in the prior 2 years. See Chapter 8, and also Marmor et al. (1987).) On other occasions during the 1990s, police activity has succeeded in temporarily closing most of the shooting galleries in Bushwick. During these periods, many of the usual patrons of shooting galleries inject in outdoor settings. As we have seen in Chapter 8, injecting in outdoor locations is a predictor of HIV infection among participants in this study who have been injecting for less than 10 years. (It is also a predictor of HIV seroconversion among street recruited drug injectors in ten low-seroprevalence cities. See Friedman et al., 1995.)

Furthermore, the policy atmosphere of a drug war has greatly hindered the adoption of harm reduction and other strategies to reduce the spread of HIV among drug injectors in the United States. This is most clearly indicated by syringe exchange policy. [Syringe exchanges have been shown to reduce new HIV infections among New York City drug injectors (Des Jarlais et al., 1996); to be associated with fewer acute hepatitis B and hepatitis C infections in Tacoma, Washington (Hagan, Des Jarlais, Friedman, Purchase, & Alter, 1995); and to be part of the policies that prevented HIV epidemics among drug injectors in six cities around the world after some drug injectors in these cities became infected (Des Jarlais et al., 1995b). They have also been endorsed by national reviews of their effects (Lurie et al., 1993; Normand et al., 1995).] In many industrialized nations, such as Great Britain, the Netherlands, Switzerland, and Australia, syringe exchanges were implemented as part of national public health policy once it became clear that HIV among drug injectors was a major threat. In the United States, however, there has been a ban on the use of any federal funds for syringe exchange services. Federal officials have publicly opposed syringe exchanges and have urged states not to set them up. Some states, such as Hawaii, Washington, Connecticut, and New York, have nonetheless set up syringe exchange networks. In New York, however, syringe exchange was not legalized until 1992, although underground syringe exchanges were established in several boroughs in 1991. (One of the consequences of the SFHR project of which its staff members, as individuals, have been most proud is that some of the field staff decided to spend nonworking hours establishing and volunteer staffing an underground—and illegal—syringe exchange in Bushwick starting in 1991). Lurie and Drucker (1997) have estimated that this opposition to syringe exchanges by the United States government resulted, between 1987 and 1995, in 4000 to 10,000 unnecessary HIV infections and consequent sickness and death among drug injectors, and additional avoidable infections among the sex partners and newborn children of these drug injectors.

CAUGHT IN THE GRIPS OF A DECAYING SOCIETY

Drug injectors live in communities within nations. National and local drug policies are expressions, in part, of the societies in which governments function. Thus, it is important to realize that Bushwick is somewhat of an economic backwater, and that American drug policy is not unrelated to broader changes in the national and world economy and politics.

As was discussed in Chapter 2, Bushwick has undergone a decades-long process of capital flight that included both the closing of factories and massive amounts of arson in which housing burned down without the insurance proceeds being reinvested in new housing or in local business. Bushwick has not been isolated in this, of course. It has undergone this as part of the changes that have wracked New York City, which has experienced considerable transformation as manufacturing has left the city [due to a mixture of economic forces and to questionable economic planning decisions by the city and by corporate decision-makers (Fitch, 1993)]. In mid-century, the working class in the city, including blacks and Latinos, were able to get jobs in industries including the garment and printing–publishing. Now, such youths look forward to part-time jobs in service and retail industries with low pay and benefits. Many are currently unemployed. The market in illegal drugs is one of the few places where youths in Bushwick and other impoverished, minority areas of the city can earn money. This situation is reflected in the fact that, in a small pilot survey of household youths (aged 18 to 21) that we conducted in Bushwick after the SFHR project ended, we found that 31% had received government benefits and 62% were in households that had received such benefits in the last year. Almost half (46%) neither were employed nor attended school. Drug-related income was one source of money: 18% (20/109) reported that they had engaged in selling cocaine or heroin at some time in their lives.

Nor is New York unique. Similar economic changes have been occurring nationally. Data show that income inequality has been increasing, and both union membership and the proportion of employees engaged in manufacturing have been

Table 4.   United States Economy: Inequality Increases[a]

Ratio of pay of chief executive officers pay to pay of factory workers
    1980:   41
    1992: 157
Percent change in average after-tax family real income, 1977–1989

Bottom fifth	−10.4%
Lower middle fifth	−10%
Middle fifth	−5.2%
Upper middle fifth	+2.2%
Top fifth	+28.1%
Top 5%	+52.6%
Top 1%	+102.2%

From: Sklar (1995).

decreasing (see Table 4 and Fig. 3). Manufacturing employment as a percent of total employment has fallen from 26% in 1970 to 16% in 1994 (Bureau of the Census, 1996–1997, p. 640).

In a society that has been divided by racial–ethnic inequalities and subordinations since its birth, and where blacks and Latinos continue to be at the bottom of the economy and disproportionately harassed, arrested, and imprisoned by police and the rest of the legal system (Friedman et al., 1998b; Steinberg, 1995), time periods in which the rich get richer and the great majority have a hard time making ends meet face a high probability of social conflict. This can take the form of class against class, which reflects the overall economic reality. Alternatively, it can take the form of racial–ethnic conflict. Political hay can be made from claims that "the other race–ethnicity" is doing well and that this is why "you" are not. This was, for example, an important part of what happened in Germany in the 1920s and 1930s that brought the Nazis to power on a program of hatred toward Jews; racial

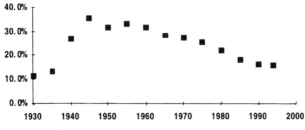

Figure 3.   Union members as percent of labor.

hatred politics toward blacks was also a powerful current in the United States during this time until it was greatly weakened by the labor-based social movements of 1932–1946. And there has been no shortage of racial hate politics in the 1980s and 1990s.

Drug injectors, in Bushwick and elsewhere, are caught up in these much larger issues. Media and political depictions of drug injectors as black or Latino serve, whether deliberately or not, to fuel stigmatization of blacks and Latinos. These depictions also serve to increase divisions among blacks and Latinos, in which drug injectors and other drug users are seen as legitimate targets of hatred by other members of these groups. In New York, this response has been most visible perhaps among political elites and part of the middle class within African American communities, who have responded with a mixture of status-based, shame-aversive distancing, as well as with what they see as the good of their community at heart (Quimby & Friedman, 1989). The direct neighbors of the drug users, particularly those who live in the immediate vicinity of drug supermarkets like that in Bushwick, sometimes join in this distancing due to the crime and unsightliness that accompany street drug addiction in a drug war society and due to fear that their own children or other relatives will be drawn into drug use.

Thus, the participants in this study are enmeshed, like it or not, in large-scale "social issue politics" of the kind that Phillips (1969) has written about. This meant that syringe exchange got short shrift when it was first proposed. Indeed, in New York, leaders of the African-American community were very visible opponents of syringe exchange for several years (Anderson, 1991; Lurie et al., 1993).

These racial–ethnic divisions also made it easier to pass welfare reform and changes in Medicaid, both of which are likely to affect drug injectors in important ways. One important set of research issues for the future is how these changes in health and welfare will shape drug users' access to drug abuse treatment and to medical care for HIV and other injection-related infections. More germane to the topic of this volume is research on how changes in welfare policy will affect income availability for drug injectors. One strong possibility is that the evictions of drug users from public (and other) housing and the reduction in the availability of welfare money will lead to:

1. More high-risk injecting behavior (due to lack of homes to inject in with some privacy, and due to more difficulty getting money to buy drugs, and thus to being more likely to be in a state of withdrawal when drugs are purchased).

2. More trading of sex for money and drugs, perhaps with less ability to negotiate for condoms to be used, and as a consequence more STDs (which may be less likely to be treated due to changes in the medical system), which will increase the probability of HIV transmission per sexual act and more HIV being transmitted.

3. More income-producing crime of other kinds, including robbery and shoplifting.

4. Changes in the egocentric and sociometric networks of drug injectors. These could include more injecting in shooting galleries and outdoor settings and more pressure to band together in denser networks for mutual aid.

Thus, times are bad for drug injectors, and may well get worse. Research is clearly needed to understand these impending changes and their consequences and to figure out ways to prevent negative consequences.

It would be a mistake to underestimate the problems. Although as discussed in Chapter 1, we have succeeded in bringing down the rate of new HIV infection and indeed even levels of prevalent infection among drug injectors in New York (Des Jarlais et al., in press), this has not been easy. Major economic, policy, and political changes could yet disable or destroy the syringe exchanges and other prevention programs; make drug injectors less able to protect themselves; and change their networks in ways that could lead to considerable additional spread of HIV. These social changes might also lead to a large influx of discouraged and alienated youths into the habit of drug injection, with a high risk of their subsequently becoming HIV infected. Furthermore, the economic and political forces that have fed drug war policies, cuts in welfare, and racial hate politics are deeply entrenched and difficult to reverse or transform. Indeed, to transform these larger forces would probably take social movements of the size, perspicacity, and determination of the black civil rights movement of the United States in the 1960s, the labor movement of the 1930s, and the Solidarnosc movement of Poland in 1980–1981 rolled into one.

FINAL THOUGHTS

This volume has focused on social networks, risk behaviors, and HIV by a group of drug injectors recruited in Bushwick. Their pasts have been difficult, their lives at the moments when we were interviewing them were difficult, and their futures, as just discussed, will be difficult. Forty percent of them are infected with HIV, and most of those men and women will die from AIDS—in many cases, with much less access than is true for wealthier and less stigmatized patients to the expensive treatments that are being researched and developed for this disease and its associated opportunistic infections. For example, in addition to lack of money to pay for care and stigmatizing treatment that drives many away from care even for acute tuberculosis (Curtis et al., 1994), many of these treatments require the storage of medications in refrigerators and the careful timing of taking pills in complicated regimens; but many of these men and women are homeless and/or lack wrist-watches.

Indeed, it is sobering and horrifying to think about what has happened to the six people who were highlighted at the end of Chapter 2. When we began writing, five of the six were alive and we had little reason to believe that they would succumb so quickly, since they appeared to be fairly robust despite their lifestyles and, in four of the five, their HIV statuses. As of February 1998, however, four of the six are dead—and each of them died in a way that punctuates the problems in current drug control strategies and disease prevention efforts. Celia's body was grotesquely swollen from sepsis that she developed in Bushwick shooting gallery. Pat died of heart failure, but her condition was aggravated by a host of other health problems and a very low T-cell and CD4 count. Honey has cervical cancer, but it was detected late; and Honey's failure to follow up on treatment means that she probably would not live long. She was determined to spend her last days on the street, desperately fighting off the growing pain. Jerry died of renal failure barely 2 months after heart surgery at a major New York City hospital. As only one who did not have HIV (and he was proud of it), Jerry nevertheless punished his body (and let others abuse it too) until he went comatose in a local shooting gallery and was taken to the hospital. Louie was in some ways more fortunate than the rest. After getting arrested and doing several jail terms at Rikers Island, he was treated for various illnesses (particularly TB) and was eventually accepted as a client by the Division of AIDS Services. They found him an apartment in the Bronx where he continues to live, only visiting Bushwick when he wants to binge for a few days. Bruce is the only one of the six who remains in Bushwick. With the street-level drug scene dramatically reduced, he runs the only shooting gallery in the neighborhood and complains that he has become so well-known by the police that he has become the "celebrity criminal of the 83rd Precinct." Recently, he has begun to show symptoms of deteriorating health—pneumonia, skin lesions, wasting—and he grows increasingly pessimistic about his future.

Nonetheless, as has been discussed, the drug injectors of Bushwick helped us greatly. They answered intimate questions about their sex lives and friendship patterns; questions about drug behaviors that are reviled by society; and provided daily assistance to the ethnographic staff of the project. In many cases, they did this in between bouts of disease or even while feeling extremely sick.

As discussed throughout this volume, they and other drug injectors have changed their behaviors to protect themselves against HIV. They also seem to have changed their behaviors to protect others against HIV, so that those who are infected are more likely to use condoms and less likely to let others inject with their used syringes than are drug injectors who are not yet infected.

Drug injectors in many countries have formed organizations that work to reduce the spread of HIV and other infections among drug injectors as well as from drug injectors to sexual partners or unborn children. Increasingly, and even in the face of the stigmatization and police repression of drug war America, this is occurring in New York and other cities in the United States.

Thus, our final words are a note of appreciation for the thousands of drug-injecting men and women who have helped us in our research, and who have trusted us to keep their secrets and to use the knowledge we obtained to help them protect their own and others' health; and to the hundreds of thousands of drug injectors in Bushwick and around the world who have worked to protect themselves and others against this horrible plague.

Appendix
Methods for Assigning Linkages in Studies of Drug Injector Networks

with *GILBERT ILDEFONSO*

INTRODUCTION

Many network studies have examined "bounded" universes such as prisons or schools. The social factors and HIV risk (SFHR) project, in contrast, studied drug injectors' unbounded social and risk networks in community settings. Data were collected in Bushwick, Brooklyn, from July 1991 through January 1993.

The basic building blocks that are used to study social networks are respondents' reports about their social relationships and behaviors with other people. In unbounded networks in communities, the lack of any preexisting list of members with whom subjects can have such links presents many problems in ascertaining whether the "Mary Smith" named by one respondent is the same as the "Mary Smith" named by another, and whether either is the same "Mary Smith" who the study interviewed six months before. The difficulties in making such links are compounded in social groupings such as drug injectors or commercial sex workers in which secrecy is an important norm, in which members who engage in high-risk behavior together may know each other only by street names, and in which many members are homeless.

This chapter will map out and discuss the methodological procedures the SFHR project used in determining which subjects who were interviewed were actually linked with each other. Here, then, we discuss the "nuts and bolts" of a process that is an essential component of network studies of IDUs. Although these procedures are a crucial part of such network studies, they are complex. Developing more effective, more accurate, and more efficient ways to ascertain such links is an important part of developing methodologies, which can be used in future network studies. We present our procedures here for two reasons: First, because they may help others who are planning network studies to avoid many hours of reinventing the wheel; and second, in order to spark debate and further methodological research into an important but undeveloped aspect of network research.

OVERVIEW OF THE METHODOLOGY

A purposive sampling technique, which was ethnographically directed, was used primarily during the first 5 months of the project. The sample was street-recruited drug injectors (in and out of treatment), 18 years of age or older, injecting in the year before the interview, who gave informed consent for a structured interview. Consent was also obtained from most subjects (after pretest counseling) for blood tests for HIV, hepatitis B, and syphilis. Subjects were interviewed about their sociodemographics, biography, drug and sex risk behaviors (current and historical), medical history, health beliefs, and peer culture. Information on up to 10 network members was gathered, which included how long they had known them, the nature of their relationship, their risk behaviors with the network members, and other risk behaviors by the network members.

Given the observed transience of IDUs in Bushwick and the fact that IDUs are often reluctant to name other IDUs as such, it was imperative that we obtain the best possible identifying information to ensure that the linkage process was as accurate as possible. In order to facilitate cooperation by respondents, the ethnographic team and interviewers were trained to emphasize to the respondent our commitment to and successful record in keeping confidentiality, the implications of our federal certificate of confidentiality, the nature of our work, how and by whom the information was to be handled, where and how the information was stored, and what their participation in the project meant.

In systematically recruiting IDUs for a study of their social networks, the ethnographic staff had to grapple with practical, methodological, and theoretical issues that only could have been appreciated fully while actually conducting the exercise. The problem of the representativeness of our respondents was at the root of many of our concerns. Because of the hidden nature of the population, true random probability sampling was not possible. However, it was still possible to use ethnographically directed, purposive sampling, which is similar to the targeted sampling technique described by Watters & Biernacki (1989).

The ethnographic team spent the first 5 months in the field, identifying different varieties of IDUs and in some cases their respective networks as they naturally occur in real life. We began by identifying networks of IDUs through ethnographic field observations and qualitative interviews and selecting a network member to be interviewed first. This person became an "index case." Initially we selected index cases on the basis that (1) they had several members in their social network with whom they injected and (2) they were clearly willing to cooperate in identifying network members. At this time, some IDUs were not considered good candidates for being index cases because they were too private about their affairs; others were avoided because they would see that role—being an index case—as an opportunity to scam the staff or other respondents in their network; and still others were not considered because the ethnographic team had found them too difficult to locate to be sure that they would be available to assist in recruiting the other members of their network. Later, however, IDUs were recruited who were less cooperative or who were "loners."

Specifically, the criteria for the selection of index cases changed over the duration of the SFHR Project in response to various needs and issues identified by project staff. In the first several months of operation, the ethnographers–recruiters, who were still relatively unknown to many IDUs in the neighborhood, recruited heavily among IDUs who were later identified as belonging to the "core network" of neighborhood injectors. There were several reasons why these injectors were targeted first. Since these IDUs had such large injection networks, their recruitment immediately built a large pool of potential interviewees. By tapping into large networks early in the project, the staff was able to develop a highly visible routine of daily interviewing at the project's storefront and generate a flow and schedule of IDUs to be interviewed. The ethnographers felt that it was important in the early stages of the project to establish a sense within the IDU community that interviews in the storefront were "routine" so that they did not generate a sense of concern or resistance among potential interviewees. By interviewing those IDUs with the most contacts with other injectors, word of the project spread much more rapidly and eased our eventual entry into the more discreet networks that were targeted later. The ethnographers also found that IDUs who had more connections to other IDUs (for example, shooting gallery operators) were better able and more willing to help the ethnographers locate IDUs who were harder to reach. Thus, their recruitment earlier rather than later was important to the success of the project.

By the midpoint of the project, once the ethnographers were well known among IDUs in the neighborhood, the project became less dependent on core network members to serve as index cases. Those types of IDUs were always available to be interviewed if "business" became slow, but staff members began to realize that there were many smaller networks of IDUs whose members were far more discreet in their behavior than the injectors who were encountered in local shooting galleries. Bolstered by the reputation that the SFHR project had earned among core network members, the ethnographers also began to target white injectors and working people.

Senior staff members on the SFHR project were particularly interested in examining the differences between "new" and "old" injectors with respect to HIV risk behaviors. However, with the project nearing completion, very few new injectors had been recruited. In a very real sense, the lack of new injectors among interviewees did not reflect a recruitment bias on the part of the ethnographers: There were simply very few new injectors to be found in the neighborhood.

Nevertheless, special efforts were made in the last few months of the project to recruit new injectors and youthful injectors (who might be old injectors themselves, but might have friends who were relatively new injectors) so that comparisons could be made with old injectors. As such, this segment of the IDU population was perhaps oversampled.

NETWORK MEMBERSHIP

Network membership was defined through a list of contacts provided by index subjects during structured interviews in which they listed up to 10 people. The network was generated during the "30-day" network section of the questionnaire, in which we obtained names by using a sequence of prompts to obtain the first name or street name and the last initial of people with whom the index case had more than casual contact. The prompts stressed relationships with nominees with whom HIV risk behaviors might have occurred: In sequence, the subject was asked to nominate (1) people he or she used drugs with, (2) had sex with, (3) other persons whom the subject was "closest" to, (4) whom the subject lived with, (5) who were relatives of the subject, (6) whom the subject met socially or hung out with, (7) whom the subject knew at work or hustled with, and (8) any other people the subject had close contact with during the last 30 days.

At the conclusion of the interview, these data were used to create a 30-day check-off form (as shown in Fig. 1), which included identifiers for the respondent and for the respondent's nominated subjects. The respondent's identifiers included respondent's identification number, first name, last initial, street name, interview date, date of birth, gender, and race–ethnicity. The nominee's identifiers included first or street name, last initial, age, race–ethnicity, gender, height, skin color, the date when the nominee was brought to the storefront by the index subject (as described below in the discussion of validating linkages), and whether the nominee was eligible to enter the study, i.e., whether the nominee had injected drugs in the last year. The information on the 30-day check-off form was then entered by a member of the ethnographic team into recruiting databases using the Foxbase database program (described below). The forms were also stored alphabetically by respondent's first name and last initial in a locked file cabinet that was kept separate from the questionnaire and consent forms to ensure confidentiality.

MULTIPLE EGOCENTRIC NETWORK MEMBERSHIP

Many IDUs, especially those who are on the street all day ("24/7") are members of the networks of many other IDUs. Since each IDU was eligible to be interviewed only once, the staff needed to find a way to quickly determine if a

Respondent

First or	Last	ID #		Sex	Race/Ethnicity
street name	Initial	Date of Birth	1=M,	1=Bl,2=Lat,3=Wh
		Mo./Day/Year	2=F	4=Asn, 5=Oth

Contacts:

Line #	First or	Last	Age	Race/Ethnicity	Sex	Height	Skin Color	Date	Eligible?
	street	Initial		1=Bl,2=Lat,	1=M,	(ft' in')	1=Wh, 2=Bl.	Brought In	0=no; 1=yes
	name			3=White	2=F		3=Brn, 4= Olive	Mo./Day/Yr	
				4=Asn, 5=Oth			5=Other		

1 _____

2 _____

3 _____

4 _____

5 _____

6 _____

7 _____

8 _____

9 _____

10 _____

It is essential that the names on this list be in the same order, and on the same lines, as on the 30-day lists in the questionnaire.

Figure 1.   30-Day check-off form.

person named on one index subject's 30-day network members' list had already been interviewed.

The problem with respect to multiple egocentric network membership centered around the problem of linking each individual subject to the respective egocentric networks in which he or she had been nominated. For example, A, an index subject, mentions B on his or her 30-day network members' list, and B is subsequently interviewed. One year later, C also mentions B on his or her 30-day network members' list. Once the ethnographic staff is able to ascertain that these two people are the same B, B's interview from a year earlier must be retrieved (since subjects can only be interviewed once) and an entry made that records the connection to C.*

In order to facilitate the search for subjects' membership in multiple egocentric networks, a "respondent" database of interviewed subjects was set up using the Foxbase database program. Subject information was retrieved from the database by using a series of identifiers: first name or street name, last initial, age, race–ethnicity, gender, height, skin color, and number of months injecting.

FOXBASE DATABASES

Foxbase is a relational database program (which we used on a Macintosh desktop computer). The relational aspects of Foxbase allow for opening and managing up to 10 databases at any one time, which can be merged with one another through the use of key index variables, for example, a respondent's identification number. The program has multiple data management functions, which include entry, storage, retrieval, import and export, and database query. It also contains some analysis features, for example, frequencies. Export data sets can be created in different formats, for example, ASCII, which can then be used in other computer systems.

Three recruiting data sets were developed in Foxbase:

1. The *network list* data set, which contained entries for all the members (up to 10) listed by index subjects in their 30-day check-off form (see Fig. 1). A network member was identified by the index subject's identification number ("RESID") and the line number (from 1 to 10) on the index subject's network members list on which his or her name was listed.

2. The *respondent* data set contained entries for interviewed subjects. Entries in this data set can be related to the network list data set through the index subject's identification number on the 30-day check-off form and the line number of the subject on the index subject's network members list. For example, assume subject B, whose identification number is 54, was named by subject A, whose identification number is 49. Subject B was the fourth person nominated by B and so is listed on line number 4 on subject A's network member list. Thus, subject B on the respondent database can be related to subject A's network member list in the network list database through the index key, which combines A's identification number, 0049, with B's line number on A's network member list, 04, which is coded as an index key value of "004904."

3. The *network referral* database allowed a person to be linked to many networks. For example, at the time she or he is interviewed, a respondent

---

*Throughout this appendix, the names of respondents have been changed to alphabetic letters to preserve confidentiality.

may be linked to one network, or if he or she is an index subject to no networks. However, subjects who are interviewed later may nominate the previously interviewed subject as a member of their networks. In order to keep track of subsequent nominations and of multiple network contacts, a data set was developed that contained an entry for each link to an index subject's network. Thus, this data set recorded every dyadic link among interviewed subjects.

The network referral data set lay the basis for a subsequent data set, the *dyadic* data set, which was used to link the structured interview data of index subjects and of their nominated network members (this was done using SAS statistical analysis software on an IBM mainframe computer). In the dyadic data set, linked dyads were identified by their interview identification number and by their line number on each other's network list, as well as by demographic identifiers for each subject. For example, subject 49 became A's "RESID" and subject 54 became B's "RESID." In order to link B to A's network member list, a data field entry would contain B's line number on A's list. Similarly if B had nominated A (in other words, there was a bidirectional link), then another data field would contain A's line number on B's network member's list. (If B did not nominate A, i.e., there was only a unidirectional link from A to B, then A's line number on B's list would be assigned the value of 99). This data set was the mechanism by which we linked (by using the SAS *sort* procedure and *merge* function) interviewed subjects' reports about their own characteristics and behaviors and their reports about each other (identified by the network member's line number).

An essential first step in setting up these databases, however, was to validate the links between network members. The details of this process are described next.

VALIDATING NETWORK MEMBER LINKS

Four methods for validating network links were utilized. These were: (1) the *storefront link* (the respondent brings in his or her 30-day network member); (2) the *field link* (different from the storefront link, in that the respondent physically identified a member on his or her 30-day network list to the ethnographic team in the field); (3) the *ethnographic link* (linking respondents through ethnographic field observations); and (4) the *data set link* (links made through the use of data set identifiers).

We believe that the validity of the links proceeds in descending order of strength, with the storefront link being the strongest and the data set link the weakest. The four types of links were not mutually exclusive, i.e., a respondent could be linked in any or up to all four links. A detailed description of the four types of linkages follows below.

Storefront Network Linkages

We engaged respondents who had already been interviewed to act as auxiliary recruiters. This was done at the end of the interview by asking respondents to ask their nominees to be interviewed and to physically accompany them to the storefront. The interviewed respondent already would have provided us with some identifiers for the drug-injecting members during the interview. These, plus the additional identifiers of height and skin color, were entered on the 30-day check-off form (Fig. 1), which was administered at the end of the interview. (These forms were kept at the storefront, in a locked file cabinet, to ensure confidentiality.) Then, the respondent was paid a fee for his or her time and effort during the interview and referred to the ethnographic team. The team then encouraged the respondent to bring in their drug-injecting network members, and told her or him that he or she would be paid an additional $3 for each eligible network member he or she brought to the storefront. (We also inquired about any additional new injectors—defined as someone 18 years or older who had been injecting drugs for less than 5 years and had injected drugs within the last year—whom the respondent might know.)

Once a respondent came to the storefront with a network member, the field data manager would first pull out the respondent's 30-day check-off form to determine if the network member was on the 30-day list and then search the respondent data base to determine if the nominated person already had been interviewed. If there was doubt about the identity of the nominee, project staff used identifiers (first name or street name, last initial, age, race–ethnicity, gender, height, skin color, and number of months injecting) from the respondent database to make a determination of eligibility. If the nominee had not been interviewed, an interview was scheduled and identifying information was entered on the potential subject form (see Fig. 2). This form contained information about the nominee, scheduled interview dates, and the numeric identifier of the auxiliary recruiter(s) and the network line number of the nominee. The nominee was then given an appointment card with date, time, recruiter's first name, and the storefront telephone number, which could be used toll free to reschedule or cancel an interview appointment or for general information. The appointment card did not include the potential subject's name to preserve the potential subject's anonymity and confidentiality, since he or she might not want others to know of his or her involvement with our project. The appointment card was to be brought in on the date of the scheduled interview, at which time it was destroyed.

Field Network Linkages

This method of establishing network linkages relied on our ethnographic team who worked in the field plus respondents who already had been interviewed. These respondents assisted our ethnographic team in locating people whom they

First Name   Initial

Date of birth   Race/Ethnicity

Sex   Number of years injecting

Is the potential subject eligible?   No   Yes

    If **NO**:   Age:

        Has she/he ever injected drugs? No   Yes

        How many months since last injection? __ __ __

RESID (when assigned):   __ __ __ __

Date of scheduled interview, if any: __ __/__ __/__ __

                                                              Month Day Year

Re-scheduled interview dates: __ __/__ __/__ __

                                                              Month Day Year

                                                              __ __/__ __/__ __

                                                              Month Day Year

People who have recruited this subject:

A.   RESID __ __ __ __   First Name   _____

Their Line # for Potential Subject: __ __   Date   __ __/__ __/__ __

                                                          Month Day Year

B.   RESID __ __ __ __   First Name   _____

Their Line # for Potential Subject: __ __   Date   __ __/__ __/__ __

                                                            Month Day Year

C.   RESID __ __ __ __   First Name   _____

Their Line # for Potential Subject: __ __   Date   __ __/__ __/__ __

                                                           Month Day Year

Figure 2. Potential subject form.

had nominated as members of their injecting network. In return for helping our team, respondents were paid a small stipend ($3) for each person from the 30-day check-off form whom the respondent was able to locate. (The ethnographic team carried no money into the field. Payment was done through a chit system that worked as follows: once a linkage was established, the respondent was given a

National Development and Research Institutes (NDRI) business card signed by a member of the ethnographic team. Each signed business card was worth $3 and could be redeemed only at the storefront. When a respondent presented a signed business card(s) at the storefront, he or she was asked to sign a receipt for the payment of linkage fees. The signed business card(s) were then destroyed.

We began by locating respondents in the field and verifying their identity. Verification was done by asking the respondent to provide us with identifying information, including first name or street name, last initial, birthdate, approximate date of interview, and the name of at least one person they nominated as a member of their injecting network. Once this identifying information had been obtained from the respondent, the ethnographic team telephoned the storefront and spoke to the field data manager, who would then retrieve that respondent's list of network members on the 30-day check-off form. The field data manager read off all of the names (and their identifying information, e.g., sex, age, ethnicity, height, and skin color) of the network members the respondent had nominated. After verifying the identity of the respondent from the information the respondent had provided to the ethnographic team in the field, the field data manager would provide the names of only those nominees who were eligible to be interviewed (i.e., IDUs) and for whom linkages to the respondent had *not* already been made. These names were relayed to the respondent by the ethnographic team in the field in order to refresh the respondent's memory of whom he or she had named during the interview. All of the identifying information was read over the telephone from a closed office where no one could hear the conversation to preserve confidentiality.

The ethnographic team then asked the respondent to assist us in locating as many of these people as possible within a reasonable period of time. Given the transience of much of the drug-injecting the population in this area, we often had to work with the same respondent on several occasions—especially those who nominated many IDUs or whose lists included people who might not be immediately available (e.g., white working men from Queens who bought or used drugs in this predominantly Latino/a neighborhood).

Once a respondent introduced us to someone who was listed on his or her 30-day check-off form, the ethnographic team first verified the identity of that person. This was done by asking the person his or her first name and last initial and by using the other identifying information which was listed on the 30-day check-off form, including age (plus or minus 5 years), ethnicity, height, skin color and drug injection behavior ("eligibility").

When the identity of the network member had been verified, the ethnographic team then asked if she or he had already been interviewed. If she or he claimed to have been interviewed, the ethnographic team asked for further identifying information (birthdate, approximate date of interview, and the name of at least one person she or he named on her or his 30-day check-off form) so that we could make a positive link with our dyadic data set by telephoning the storefront for verifica-

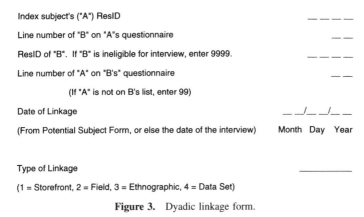

Index subject's ("A") ResID   _ _ _ _

Line number of "B" on "A"s questionnaire   _ _

ResID of "B". If "B" is ineligible for interview, enter 9999. _ _ _ _

Line number of "A" on "B's" questionnaire   _ _

　　　　　(If "A" is not on B's list, enter 99)

Date of Linkage   _ _/_ _/_ _

(From Potential Subject Form, or else the date of the interview)　Month Day Year

Type of Linkage   _____

(1 = Storefront, 2 = Field, 3 = Ethnographic, 4 = Data Set)

Figure 3. Dyadic linkage form.

tion. The field data manager then filled out a dyadic linkage form (see Fig. 3) linking the two respondents. Once a positive linkage had been made between the two network members, the ethnographic team in the field gave the network member a signed business card which he or she redeemed ($3 linkage fee) at the storefront via the same procedures described above.

If the respondent introduced the ethnographic team to a person who was a network member listed on their 30-day check-off form who had not been interviewed, we tried to recruit this person for an interview. If this person agreed to be interviewed, the ethnographic team telephoned the storefront and an appointment was scheduled for him or her.

Ethnographic Network Linkages

This linkage method was developed by our staff and used by our ethnographic field team. After a respondent was interviewed, the ethnographic team would ask about their hangout spots, where they "do their thing" (e.g., setting(s) where an injection event(s) might take place).

Ethnographic observations alone might confirm that respondent A (who had already been interviewed) was connected to respondent B, on his or her 30-day network list. The following techniques were used as a basis for assigning such a link: (1) the ethnographic team observing them hanging out together or participating in an injection event (whether sharing injection equipment or not); and (2) triangulation, i.e., through independent confirmation from several sources that potential respondent B had close contact with, injected with, or had a sexual relationship with respondent A. Ethnographic links could be made retroactively, on the basis of interactions between A and B that occurred no sooner than 30 days prior to A's interview, or prospectively, if the interactions occurred reasonably soon after B's interview. Clearly, research would be helpful on the temporal criteria to be used for ethnographic validation of time-defined relationships.

Data Set Network Linkages

The data set link established links among interviewed subjects by using the respondent database. An interviewed respondent was linked with another interviewed respondent by comparing his or her identifiers in the respondent database with the network member identifiers provided by another respondent that were recorded on that respondent's 30-day check-off form. For example, A's identifiers in the respondent database were matched against A's identifiers as provided by B on B's 30-day check-off form. Similarly, B's identifiers in the respondent database are matched against B's identifiers on A's 30-day check-off form. This type of validation of links was retrospective. It could be used when, although both respondents nominated each other, their link had not been validated by any of the three other methods (they had not brought each other to the storefront, they did not identify each other in the field, and they were not observed in the field by the ethnographic team). It was particularly useful in unidirectional links where the network list of A (interviewed prior to B) may not have contained B's name (and therefore there was no reason to actively recruit B and validate a storefront, field, or ethnographic link). Subsequently, when B (who may have been either an index subject or alternatively may have been nominated by another index subject, e.g., C) was interviewed, B listed A's name. One way to validate B's link to A was through a database link (although the other types of validation could also occur).

Using a respondent's 30-day check-off form, a determination was made of whether or not a nominee on the form had been interviewed. To answer this question, the respondent database was searched by using a subset of the identifiers of the nominees on the 30-day check-off form. The identifiers that were used for the search were first name and/or street name, age within 5 years, race–ethnicity, gender, and number of months since started injecting. In addition, the identifiers on the 30-day check-off form also included the nominee's last initial, height within 3 inches, and skin color. An identifier linkage priority criterion was set up to try and make as accurate a link as possible. In order for a data set link to be assigned, the following identifiers on the respondent database and 30-day check-off form had to match: first name and/or street name, age within 5 years, race–ethnicity, and gender. The field data manager searched the respondent database regularly, at least once a week, in order to ensure that the recruiters were not seeking someone who had already been interviewed and in order to maintain a current list of dyadic links.

Within this minimal set of identifiers, there were occasions when the identifiers provided a close but not an exact match. For example, the first name given by the respondent may have been somewhat different from that on the network list given by another respondent (although the other identifiers matched), such as when the respondent refers to himself as "John" and another respondent lists this person as "Johnny." Overall, we found that subjects were able to accurately describe each other (Goldstein et al., 1995). In those situations when there was a close but not an exact match or when there was a tie (which affected only a few respondents), we utilized ethnographic information to confirm the database link.

EGOCENTRIC NETWORK LINKAGE CASE STUDY

The following case study of an egocentric drug injector network and the linkage process, from start (subject recruitment and interview) to finish (network nomination and the types of links assigned or not within the network structure), may help clarify what was done.

Ethnographic field observations defined the respondent's parameters, that is, hangout spots (copping and injecting), drug (s) of choice, and running partners. Consider a respondent I, who was a 33-year-old Puerto Rican male and was recruited as an index subject by the ethnographic team. This individual was well known in the neighborhood, ran a shooting gallery, and had been injecting speedball (cocaine and heroin) for 14 years. I was interviewed in September 1991, and originally named 14 contacts as part of his social network. However, because we limited the number of contacts to 10, information was obtained only about the first 10 nominees.

We were able to interview eight network members, with the first one taking place in August 1991 and the last in June 1992. Of these eight network members, two also named I. Thus, there were two bidirectional links and six unidirectional links (from I). The linkage validation process for this particular egocentric network used all four types of linkage processes (see Table 1). Members C, E, and F were linked to I by all four types of links (storefront, field, ethnographic, and data set links); members B, D, G, and H were linked via ethnographic and data set links; and member A was linked only via a data set link. Members J and K were never interviewed (insofar as we could determine), and thus never linked. In addition to the two members of his IDU egocentric network who named him, I was also named by 25 other different subjects as a member of their IDU egocentric networks. It thus appears that I is a central person among the IDU networks in Bushwick.

To some extent our ability to recruit IDUs' network members was limited by contingent factors. For example, I was interviewed early in the project, and thus our knowledge of IDU networks in the community was still developing. Again, there was a seasonal effect as winter set in: IDUs were not as easily contacted on the street since they were on the move, seeking warmth and shelter. Police sweeps were also a factor to deal with, which may have slowed down our recruiting efforts. In fact, we found out that in April 1992 five of I's network members (A, E, F, G, and H) were incarcerated due to an increase in the level of police sweeps in

Table 1. Linkages of an Egocentric Network
of a 33-Year-Old, Male Drug Injector

Network member[a]	Storefront link[b]	Field link	Ethnographic link	Data set link
A	0	0	0	1
B	0	0	1	1
C	1	1	1	1
D	0	0	1	1
E	1	1	1	1
F	1	1	1	1
G	0	0	1	1
H	0	0	1	1
J	0	0	0	0
K	0	0	0	0

[a]The names of respondents have been changed to alphabetic letters to preserve confidentiality.
[b]Coding: 0, no link; 1, yes, there is a link.

Bushwick. Fortunately, however, we had already interviewed and linked all five of these members.

LINKAGE STATISTICS

The study identified 515 unique dyads through 662 linkages; 368 (71%) of these dyads were linked one-way and the remaining 147 (29%) were linked both ways (two-way linkages). Since considerable time sometimes elapsed between the interviews of two dyad members and the naming stimuli asked about interactions over the previous 30 days, some of the one-way links may reflect changes in the existence or strength of social ties between the interviews.

Every linkage was established through one more of the four methods mentioned earlier. Thus, of the 662 total linkages, 444 (67%) were identified through only one method, 172 (26%) through two methods, 29 (4%) through three methods, and 17 (3%) through all four methods.

CONCLUSIONS

Doing network research among IDUs requires specialized methodologies, not only in conception and analysis, but also in the implementation of research protocols. We have discussed the methods we used to locate IDU networks in a street setting and to recruit members of their drug injecting network. These methods require a combination of techniques, including ethnography, structured interviews, and interviewing techniques that gain the confidence of subjects so that they will reveal the names of the people they inject drugs with; the careful recording of network recruiting data; and computer-assisted techniques for database management and retrieval that can be used for recruiting in the field. Of particular importance are the methods for validating network linkages. When dealing with hidden populations, such as drug injectors, establishing the validity of links may not be possible using identifiers such as full name, street address, telephone number, place of employment, and so on. The validation of links requires methods that are appropriate for the population. We have outlined four methods we used: the store-front link, field link, ethnographic link, and database link. In the case of the first two links, the method of validating links required the physical identification of the index subject and the nominee at the same time. Of particular importance was the assistance of index subjects as auxiliary recruiters in locating and identifying members of their injecting networks. To obtain such assistance, it may be necessary to provide a nominal payment for the index subject's time. The second two links were more indirect, relying on ethnographic observation and on the creation and utilization of relational databases.

Since the conditions under which drug injectors and members of their injecting networks operate may vary from neighborhood to neighborhood and from city to city, it may be necessary to develop other methods, appropriate for the particular location, for recruiting drug injector networks and for validating links. The accumulation of knowledge about these methods also may assist in the further development of the conceptualization and analysis of drug injector networks.

References

Abdul-Quader, A. S., Tross, S., Friedman, S. R., Kouzi, A. C., & Des Jarlais, D. C. (1990). Street-recruited intravenous drug users and sexual risk reduction in New York City. *AIDS, 4,* 1075–1079.

Abdul-Quader, A., Des Jarlais, C., Tross, S., McCoy, E., Morales, G., & Velez, I. (1992). Outreach to injecting drug users and female sexual partners of drug users on the Lower East Side of New York City. *British Journal of Addiction, 87,* 681–688.

Agar, M. H. (1973). *Ripping and running: A formal ethnography of urban heroin addicts.* New York: Seminar Press.

Agresti, A. (1990). *Categorical data analysis.* New York: John Wiley & Sons.

Ajzen, I., & Fishbein, M. (1980). *Understanding attitudes and predicting social behavior.* Englewood Cliffs, NJ: Prentice-Hall.

Ajzen, I., & Timko, C. (1986). Correspondence between health attitudes and behavior. *Basic and Applied Social Psychology, 7*(4), 259–276.

Amaro, H. (1995). Love, sex, and power. Considering women's realities in HIV prevention. *American Psychologist, 50*(6), 437–447.

Anderson, W. (1991). The New York Needle Trial: The politics of public health in the age of AIDS. *American Journal of Public Health, 81,* 1506–1517.

Anthony, J., Vlahov, D., Nelson, K., Cohn, S., Astemborski, J., & Solomon, L. (1991). New evidence on intravenous cocaine use and the risk of infection with human immunodeficiency virus type 1. *American Journal of Epidemiology, 134,* 1175–1189.

Ashley, R. L., Militoni, J., Lee, F., Nahmias, A., Corey, L. (1988). Comparison of Western blot and glycoprotein G-specific immunodot enzyme assay for detecting HSV-1 and HSV-2 antibodies in human sera. *Journal of Clinical Microbiology, 26,* 662–667.

Atwood, K. (1998). *The social, behavioral and structural features of first injection.* Unpublished dissertation, Harvard School of Public Health.

Auerbach, D. M., Darrow, W. W., Jaffe, H. W., & Curran, J. W. (1984). Cluster of cases of the acquired immune deficiency syndrome: patients linked by sexual contact. *American Journal of Medicine, 76,* 487–492.

Auerbach, J. D., Wypijewska, C., & Brodie, H. K. H. (Eds.). (1994). *AIDS and behavior: An integrated approach.* Washington, DC: Institute of Medicine/National Academy Press.

Ball, A. L., Rana, S., & Dehne, K. (1998). HIV prevention among injecting drug users: A global perspective. *Public Health Reports, 113*(supplement 1), 170–181.

Bandura, A. (1977). *Social learning theory.* Englewood, NJ: Prentice-Hall.

Bandura, A. (1993). Social cognitive theory and exercise of control over HIV infection. In J. Peterson & R. DiClemente (Eds.), *Preventing AIDS: Theory and practice of behavioral interventions* (pp. 25–59). New York: Plenum Press.

Barnard, M. (1993). Needle sharing in context: Patterns of sharing among men and women injectors and HIV risks. *Addiction, 88,* 805–812.

Bassiri, M., Hu, H., Domeika, M., Burczak, J., Svensson, L. O., Lee, H. H., & Mardh, P. A. (1995). Detection of *Chlamydia trachomatis* in urine specimens from women by ligase chain reaction. *Journal of Clinical Microbiology, 33,* 898–900.

Bastos, F. I., & Barcellos, C. (1995). A geografia social da AIDS no Brasil (The social geography of AIDS in Brazil). *Revista de Saude Publica, 29*(1), 52–62.

Bearak, B. (1992, September, 27). A room for heroin and HIV. *Los Angeles Times*, p. A1.

Becker, M. H., & Joseph, J. G. (1974). *The health belief model and personal health behavior*. Thorofare, NJ: Slack.

Becker, M. H., & Joseph, J. G. (1988). AIDS and behavioral change to reduce risk: A review. *American Journal of Public Health, 78*(4), 394–410.

Bevier, P., Chiasson, M. A., Heffernan, R. T., & Castro, K. G. (1995). Women at a sexually transmitted disease clinic who reported same-sex contact. *American Journal of Public Health, 85*, 1366–1371.

Binion, V. (1982). Sex differences in socialization and family dynamics of female and male heroin users. *Journal of Social Issues, 38*(2), 43–57.

Blower, S. (1991). Behaviour change and stabilization of seroprevalence levels in communities of injecting drug users: Correlation or causation? *Journal of Acquired Immune Deficiency Syndrome, 4*(9), 920–923.

Brown, B. S., & Beschner, G. M. (Eds.). (1993). *Handbook on risk of AIDS: Injection drug users and sexual partners*. Westport, CT: Greenwood Press.

Brunswick, A., Messeri, P., Dobkin, J., Flood, M., & Yang, A. (1995). Sibling homophily in HIV infection: Biopsychosocial linkages in an urban African-American sample. In R. H. Needle, S. L. Coyle, S. G. Genser, & R. T. Trotter (Eds.), *Social networks, drug abuse, and HIV transmission* (pp. 20–37). Rockville, MD: National Institute on Drug Abuse.

Casadonte, P., Des Jarlais, D. C., Friedman, S. R., & Rotrosen, J. P. (1990). Psychological and behavioral impact among intravenous drug users of learning HIV test results. *The International Journal of the Addictions, 25*(4), 409–426.

Casriel, C., Des Jarlais, D. C., Rodriguez, R., Friedman, S. R., Stepherson, B., & Khuri, E. (1990). Working with heroin sniffers: Clinical issues in preventing drug injection. *Journal of Substance Abuse Treatment, 7*, 1–10.

Catania, J., Coates, T., Stall, R., Bye, L., Capell, F. et al. (1989, June). *Changes in condom use among gay men: predictors and methodological issues*. Paper presented at the Vth International Conference on AIDS, Montreal, Canada.

Catania, J. A., Kegeles, S. M., & Coates, T. J. (1990). Towards an understanding of risk behavior: An AIDS risk reduction model (AARM). *Health Education Quarterly, 17*, 53–72.

Caussy, D., Weiss, S., Blattner, W., French, J., Cantor, J., Ginzburg, H., Altman, R., & Goedert, J. (1990). Exposure factors for HIV-1 infection among heterosexual drug abusers in New Jersey treatment programs. *AIDS Research and Human Retroviruses, 6*, 1459–1467.

Centers for Disease Control and Prevention. (1993). Update: Barrier protection against HIV infection and other sexually transmitted diseases. *Morbidity and Mortality Weekly Report, 42*, 589–591, 597.

Centers for Disease Control and Prevention, Health Resources and Services Administration, National Institute on Drug Abuse, and Administration, Substance Abuse and Mental Health Services Administration. (1997). *HIV prevention bulletin: Medical advice for persons who inject illicit drugs*. U.S. Department of Health and Human Services.

Centers for Disease Control. (1995). *Report on lesbian HIV issues meeting*. CDC National Center for HIV, STD and TB Prevention, Division of HIV/AIDS Prevention. Atlanta, GA.

Chaisson, M. A., Stoneburner, R. L., Telzak, E., Hildebrandt, D., Schultz, S., & Jaffe, H. (1989a). Risk factors for HIV-1 infection in STD clinic patients: Evidence for crack-related heterosexual transmission. Presented at *5th International Conference on AIDS*, Montreal, Canada. June.

Chaisson, R., Baccheti, P., Osmond, D., Brodie, B., Sande, M., & Moss, A. (1989b). Cocaine use and HIV infection in intravenous drug users in San Francisco. *Journal of American Medical Association, 261*, 561–565.

Cheng, F., Ford, W. L., Weber, M. D., Cheng, S.-Y., & Kerndt, P. R. (1997). A probability-based approach for predicting HIV infection in a low prevalent population of injection drug users. *Annals of Epidemiology, 7,* 28–34.

Chernesky, M. A., Lee, H. H., Schachter, J., Burczak, J. D., Stamm, W. E., McCormack, W. M., & Quinn, T. C. (1994). Diagnosis of *Chlamydia trachomatis* urethral infection in symptomatic and asymptomatic men by testing first-void urine in a ligase chain reaction assay. *Journal of Infectious Diseases, 170,* 1308–1311.

Cherubin, C. (1967). The medical sequelae of narcotic addiction. *Annals of Internal Medicine, 67,* 23–33.

Cherubin, C., & Sapira, J. (1993). The medical complications of drug addiction and the medical assessment of the intravenous drug user: 25 years later. *Annals of Internal Medicine, 119,* 1017–1028.

Clayton, R., & Voss, H. (1981). *Young men and drugs in Manhattan: a causal analysis.* National Institute on Drug Abuse Research Monograph 39. Rockville, MD: US Department of Health and Human Services.

Colón, H., Robles, R., Marrero, C., Reyes, J., & Sahai, H. (1996). Behavioral effects of receiving HIV test results among injecting drug users in Puerto Rico. *AIDS, 10*(10), 1163–1168.

Corby, N., & Wolitski, R. (1996). Condom use with main and other sex partners. *Drugs and Society, 9*(1/2), 75–96.

Crofts, N., Louie, R., Rosenthal, D., & Jolley, D. (1996). The first hit: Circumstances surrounding initiation into injecting. *Addiction, 91*(8), 1187–1196.

Curtis, R., Friedman, S. R., Neaigus, A., Jose, B., Goldstein, M., & Des Jarlais, D. C. (1994). Implications of directly observed therapy in tuberculosis control measures among IDUs. *Public Health Reports, 109,* 319–327.

Curtis, R., Friedman, S., Neaigus, A., Jose, B., Goldstein, M., & Ildefonso, G. (1995). Street level drug market structure and HIV risk. *Social Networks, 17,* 219–228.

D'Aquila, R., Peterson, L., Williams, A., & Williams, A. (1989). Race/ethnicity as a risk factor for HIV-1 infection among Connecticut intravenous drug users. *Journal of Acquired Immune Deficiency Syndrome, 2,* 503–513.

Dasgupta, S., Friedman, S. R., Jose, B., Neaigus, A., Rosenblum, A., Goldsmith, D. S., Kleinman, P. H., & Des Jarlais, D. C. (1995). Using retrospective behavioral data to determine HIV risk factors among street-recruited drug injectors. *Journal of Drug Issues, 25*(1), 161–171.

De la Fuente, L., Saavedra, P., Barrio, G., Royuela, L., Vicente, J., & Spanish Group for the Study of the Purity of Seized Drugs. (1996). Temporal and geographic variation in the characteristics of heroin seized in Spain and their relation with the route of administration. *Drug and Alcohol Dependence, 40*(3), 185–194.

Deren, S., Goldstein, M., Williams, M., Stark, M., Estrada, A., Friedman, S., Young, R., Needle, R., Tortu, S., & Saunders, L. (1996). Sexual orientation, HIV risk behavior and serostatus in a multi-site sample of drug injecting and crack using women. *Women's Health: Research, Behavior, and Policy, 2,* 35–48.

Des Jarlais, D. C., & Friedman, S. R. (1989). Ethnic differences in HIV seroprevalence rates among intravenous drug users. In R. W. Pickens (Ed.), *AIDS and intravenous drug abuse among minorities* (pp. 24–33). Rockville, MD: National Institute on Drug Abuse.

Des Jarlais, D. C., & Friedman, S. R. (1992). AIDS and legal access to sterile drug injection equipment. *The Annals of the American Academy of Political and Social Science, 521,* 42–65.

Des Jarlais, D. C., Friedman, S. R., & Hopkins, W. (1985). Risk reduction for the acquired immunodeficiency syndrome among intravenous drug users. *Annals of Internal Medicine, 103,* 755–759.

Des Jarlais, D. C., Friedman, S. R., Novick, D., Sotheran, J. L., Thomas, P., Yancovitz, S., Mildvan, D., Weber, J., Kreek, M. J., Maslansky, R., Bartelme, S., Spira, T., & M., M. (1989). HIV-1 infection among intravenous drug users in Manhattan, New York City, from 1977 through 1987. *Journal of the American Medical Association, 261,* 1008–1012.

Des Jarlais, D. C., Casriel, C., Friedman, S. R., & Rosenblum, A. (1992). AIDS and the transition to illicit drug injection: Results of a randomized trial prevention program. *British Journal of the Addictions*, *87*, 493–498.

Des Jarlais, D. C., Choopanya, K., Vanichseni, S., Plangsringarm, K., Sonchai, W., Carballo, M., Friedmann, P., & Friedman, S. R. (1994). AIDS risk reduction and reduced HIV seroconversion among injection drug users in Bangkok. *American Journal of Public Health*, *84*(3), 452–455.

Des Jarlais, D. C., Friedman, S. R., Friedmann, P., Wenston, J., Sotheran, J. L., Choopanya, K., Vanichseni, S., Raktham, S., Goldberg, D., Frischer, M., Green, S., Lima, E. S., Bastos, F. I., & Telles, P. R. (1995a). HIV/AIDS-related behavior change among injecting drug users in different national settings. *AIDS*, *6*, 611–617.

Des Jarlais, D. C., Hagan, H. H., Friedman, S. R., Friedman, P., Goldberg, D., Frischer, M., Green, S., Tunving, K., Ljungberg, B., Wodak, A., Ross, M., Purchase, D., Millson, M. E., & Myers, T. (1995b). Maintaining low HIV seroprevalence in populations of injecting drug users. *Journal of the American Medical Association*, *274*(15), 1226–1231.

Des Jarlais, D., Marmor, M., Paone, D., Titus, S., Shi, Q., Perlis, T., & Friedman, S. (1996). HIV incidence among syringe exchange participants in New York City. *Lancet*, *348*, 987–991.

Des Jarlais, D. C., Perlis, T., Friedman, S., Deren, S., Sotheran, J., Tortu, S., Beardsley, M., Paone, D., Torian, L., Beatrice, S., DeBernardo, E., Monterroso, E., & Marmor, M. (in press). Declining seroprevalence in a very large HIV epidemic: Injecting drug users in New York City, 1991–1996. *American Journal of Public Health*.

Edlin, B. R., Irwin, K. L., & Faruque, S. (1994). Intersecting epidemics: Crack cocaine use and HIV infection among inner-city young adults. *New England Journal of Medicine*, *331*, 1422–1427.

El-Bassel, N., Gilbert, L., & Schilling, R. (1991, June). *Social support and sexual risk taking among female recovering IV drug users*. Paper presented at the VIIth International Conference on AIDS, Florence, Italy.

Eldred, C., & Washington, M. (1976). Interpersonal relationships in heroin use by men and women and their role in treatment outcome. *International Journal of the Addictions*, *11*(1), 117–130.

Ellinwood, E., Smith, W., & Vaillant, G. (1966). Narcotic addiction in males and females: A comparison. *International Journal of the Addictions*, *1*, 33–45.

Farmer, P. (1992). *AIDS and accusation. Haiti and the geography of blame*. Berkeley: University of California Press.

Farmer, P., Connors, M., & Simmins, J. (1996). *Women, poverty, and AIDS*. Monroe, Maine: Common Courage Press.

Fife, D., & Mode, C. (1992). AIDS incidence and income. *Journal of Acquired Immune Deficiency Syndrome*, *5*, 1105–1110.

Fishbein, M., & Ajzen, I. (1975). *Belief, attitude, intention and behavior: An introduction to theory and research*. Boston: Addison-Wesley.

Fishbein, M., & Middlestadt, S. E. (1987). Using the theory of reasoned action to develop educational interventions: Applications to illicit drug use. *Health Education Research*, *2*(4), 361–371.

Fitch, R. (1993). *The assassination of New York*. New York: Verso.

Frank, B., & Galea, J. (1996). Cocaine trends and other drug trends in New York City, 1986–1994. *Journal of Addictive Diseases*, *15*, 1–12.

Frank, B., Galea, J., & Simeone, R. S. (Eds.). (1992). *Current drug use trends in New York City*. Rockville, MD: National Institute on Drug Abuse.

Freeland, J., & Campbell, R. (1973). The social context of first marijuana use. *International Journal of the Addictions*, *8*(2), 317–324.

Freeman, R., Rodriguez, G., & French, J. (1994). A comparison of male and female intravenous drug users' risk behaviors for HIV infection. *American Journal of Drug and Alcohol Abuse*, *20*(2), 129–157.

Frey, F. W., Abrutyn, E., Metzger, D. S., Woody, G. E., O'Brien, C. P., & Trusiani, P. (Eds.). (1995).

Focal networks and HIV risk among African-American male intravenous drug users (IDUs). Rockville, MD: National Institute on Drug Abuse.

Friedman, S. R. (1991). Supportive environments for risk reduction by drug injectors: A call for innovation [editorial]. *AIDS Health Promotion Exchange, 2*, 1–3.

Friedman, S. R. (1992). AIDS as a sociohistorical phenomenon. In G.L. Albrecht & R. Zimmerman (Eds.), *Advances in medical sociology, vol. III: The social and behavioral aspects of AIDS* (pp. 1–35). Greenwich, CT: JAI Press.

Friedman, S. (1995). Promising social network research results and suggestions for a research agenda. In R. H. Needle, S. L. Coyle, S. G. Genser, & R. T. Trotter (Eds.), *Social networks, drug abuse and HIV transmission* (pp. 144–180). NIDA Research Monograph 151. Rockville, MD: National Institute on Drug Abuse.

Friedman, S. R. (1996). Theoretical bases for understanding drug users' organizations. *The International Journal of Drug Policy, 7*(4), 212–219.

Friedman, S. (1997, Winter). Snapshots of the drug war. *Dionysos, 7*, 18–22.

Friedman, S. R. (1998). The political economy of drug-user scapegoating and the philosophy and politics of resistance. *Drugs: Education, Prevention, and Policy, 5*(1), 15–32.

Friedman, S. R. (1998). HIV-related politics in long-term perspective. *AIDS Care, 10*(supplement 2), S93–S103.

Friedman, S., & Wypijewska, C. (1995). Social science intervention models for reducing HIV transmission. In *Assessing the social and behavioral science base for HIV/AIDS prevention and intervention: Workshop summary—Background papers* (pp. 53–74). Washington, DC: National Academy Press.

Friedman, S. R., de Jong, W. M., Des Jarlais, D. C., Kaplan, C. D., & Goldsmith, D. S. (1987a). Drug users' organizations and AIDS prevention: Differences in structure and strategy. Presented at Third International AIDS Conference. Washington, D.C. June.

Friedman, S. R., Des Jarlais, D. C., Sotheran, J. L., Garber, J., Cohen, H., & Smith, D. (1987b). AIDS and self-organization among intravenous drug users. *International Journal of the Addictions, 22*, 201–219.

Friedman, S. R., Sotheran, J. L., Abdul-Quader, A., Primm, B. J., Des Jarlais, D. C., Kleinman, P., Mauge, C., Goldsmith, D. S., El-Sadr, W., & Maslansky, R. (1987c). The AIDS epidemic among blacks and Hispanics. *Milbank Quarterly, 65*, 455–499.

Friedman, S. R., de Jong, W. M., & Des Jarlais, D. C. (1988). Problems and dynamics of organizing intravenous drug users for AIDS prevention. *Health Education Research, 3*, 49–57.

Friedman, S., Des Jarlais, D., Neaigus, A., Abdul-Quader, A., Sotheran, J., Sufian, M., Tross, S., & Goldsmith, D. (1989a). AIDS and the new drug injector. *Nature, 339*, 333–334.

Friedman, S. R., Des Jarlais, D. C., & Goldsmith, D. S. (1989b). An overview of AIDS prevention efforts aimed at intravenous drug users circa 1987. *Journal of Drug Issues, 19*(1), 93–112.

Friedman, S. R., Rosenblum, A., Goldsmith, D. S., Des Jarlais, D. C., Neaigus, A., & Sufian, M. (1989c). Risk factors for HIV-1 infection among street-recruited intravenous drug users in New York City. Presented at 5th International Conference on AIDS. Montreal, Canada. June.

Friedman, S. R., Sterk, C., Sufian, M., & Des Jarlais, D. C. (1989d). Will bleach decontaminate needles during cocaine binges in shooting galleries? *Journal of the American Medical Association, 262* (11), 1467.

Friedman, S. R., Des Jarlais, D. C., Sterk, C. E., Sotheran, J. L., Tross, S., Woods, J., Sufian, M., & Abdul-Quader, A. (1990). AIDS and the social relations of intravenous drug users. *Millbank Quarterly, 68*(Suppl. 1), 85–110.

Friedman, S. R., Sufian, M., Curtis, R., Neaigus, A., & Des Jarlais, D. C. (1991). AIDS-related organizing of intravenous drug users from the outside. In E. Schneider & J. Huber (Eds.), *Culture and social relations in the AIDS crisis* (pp. 115–130). Newbury Park, CA: Sage.

Friedman, S. R., Des Jarlais, D. C., Neaigus, A., Jose, B., Sufian, M., Stepherson, B., Mota, P. M., &

Manthei, D. (1992). Organizing drug injectors against AIDS: Preliminary data on behavioral outcomes. *Psychology of Addictive Behaviors, 6*(2), 100–106.

Friedman, S. R., de Jong, W., & Wodak, A. (1993a). Community development as a response to HIV among drug injectors. *AIDS, 7,* S263–S269.

Friedman, S. R., Wiebel, W., Jose, B., & Levin, L. (1993b). Changing the culture of risk. In B. S. Brown, G. M. Beschner, & National AIDS Demonstration Research Consortium (Ed.), *Handbook on risk of AIDS: Injection drug users and sexual partners* (pp. 499–516). Westport, CT: Greenwood Press.

Friedman, S. R., Des Jarlais, D. C., & Ward, T. P. (1994a). Social models for changing health-relevant behavior. In R. DiClemente & J. Peterson (Eds.), *Preventing AIDS: Theories and methods of behavioral interventions* (pp. 95–116). New York: Plenum Press.

Friedman, S. R., Doherty, M. C., Paone, D., & Jose, B. (1994b). *Notes on research on the etiology of drug injection.* Washington, DC: National Academy of Science.

Friedman, S. R., Jose B, Neaigus A, Goldstein M, Curtis R, Ildefonso G, Mota P, & Des Jarlais., D. C. (1994c). Consistent condom use in relationships between seropositive injecting drug users and sex partners who do not inject drugs. *AIDS, 8,* 357–361.

Friedman, S. R., Des Jarlais, D.C., Ward, T.P., Jose, B., Neaigus, A., & Goldstein, M.F. (1994d). Drug injectors and heterosexual AIDS. In L. Sherr (Ed.), *AIDS and the heterosexual population* (pp. 41–65). Chur, Switzerland: Harwood Academic Publishers.

Friedman, S., Jose, B., Deren, S., Des Jarlais, D., Neaigus, A., & National AIDS Demonstration Research Consortium. (1995). Risk factors for HIV seroconversion among out-of-treatment drug injectors in high and low-seroprevalence cities. *American Journal of Epidemiology, 142*(8), 864–874.

Friedman, S., Perlis, T., Atillasoy, A., Goldsmith, D., Neaigus, A., Gu, X. C., Sotheran, J. L., Curtis R., Jose, B., Telles, P., Des Jarlais, D. C. (1996a). Changes in modes of drug administration and in the drugs that are administered: Implications for retrovirus transmission. *Publicacion Oficial de la Sociedad Espanola Interdisciplinaria de S.I.D.A., 7*(4), 167–169.

Friedman, S., Neaigus, A., Perlis, T., Jose, B., Sotheran, J., Curtis, R., Goldstein, M., Ildefonso, G., Rockwell, R., & DC., D. J. (1996b). Personal, relation-specific, and event-specific influences on risk behaviors by drug injectors. *Publicacion Oficial de la Sociedad Espanola Interdisciplinaria de S.I.D.A., 7*(4), 184–186.

Friedman, S. R., Curtis, R., Jose, B., Neaigus, A., Zenilman, J., Culpepper-Morgan, J., Borg, L., Kreek, M. J., Paone, D., & Des Jarlais, D. C. (1997a). Sex, drugs, and infections among youth: Parenterally- and sexually-transmitted diseases in a high-risk neighborhood. *Sexually Transmitted Diseases, 24*(7), 322–326.

Friedman, S. R., Des Jarlais, D. C., Neaigus, A., Perlis, T., Jose, B., & Paone, D. (1997b). Epidemics of HIV among drug injectors can be "reversed." *Publicacion Oficial de la Sociedad Espanola Interdisciplinaria del S.I.D.A., 8*(4), 183–184.

Friedman, S. R., Neaigus, A., Jose, B., Curtis, R., Goldstein, M., Ildefonso, G., Rothenberg, R. B., & Des Jarlais, D. C. (1997c). Sociometric risk networks and HIV risk. *American Journal of Public Health, 87*(8), 1289–1296.

Friedman, S. R., Neaigus, A., Jose, B., Curtis, R., Goldstein, M., Sotheran, J. L., Wenston, J., Latkin, C. A., & Des Jarlais, D. C. (1997d). Network and sociohistorical approaches to the HIV epidemic among drug injectors. In J. Catalán, L. Sherr, & B. Hedge (Eds.), *The impact of AIDS. Psychological and social aspects of HIV infection* (pp. 89–113). Amsterdam: Harwood Academic Publishers.

Friedman, S., Furst, R., Jose, B., Curtis, R., Neaigus, A., Jarlais, D. D., Goldstein, M., & Ildefonso, G. (1998a). Drug Scene Roles and HIV Risk. *Addiction, 93,* 1403–1416.

Friedman, S., Neaigus, A., & Jose, B. (1998b). AIDS research and social theory: selected enigmas and contributions from a long-duration program of applied research. *Research in Social Policy, 6,* 137–157.

Friedman, S. R., Friedmann, P., Telles, P., Bastos, F., Bueno, R., Mesquita, F., & Des Jarlais, D. C. (1998c). New injectors and HIV risk. In G. V. Stimson, D. C. Des Jarlais, & A. Ball (Eds.), *Drug injecting and HIV infection: Global dimensions and local responses* (pp. 76–90). London: Taylor and Francis.

Friedman, S. R., Jose, B., Neaigus, A., Goldstein, M., Mota, P., Curtis, R., Ildefonso, G., & Des Jarlais, D. C. (1998d). Multiple racial/ethnic subordination and HIV among drug injectors. In M. Singer (Ed.), *The political economy of AIDS* (pp. 105–127). Amityville, NY: Baywood Press.

Garfein, R. S., Vlahov, D., Galai, N., Doherty, M., & Nelson, K. E. (1996). Viral infections in short-term drug users: The prevalence of the hepatitis C, hepatitis C, human immunodeficiency, and human T-lymphtropic viruses. *American Journal of Public Health, 86*(5), 655–661.

Goldstein, M. F., Friedman, S. R., Neaigus, A., Jose, B., Ildefonso, G., & Curtis, R. (1995). Self-reports of HIV risk behavior by injecting drug users: Are they reliable? *Addiction, 90*(8), 1097–1104.

Gossop, M., Griffiths, P., Powis, B., & Strang, J. (1993). Severity of heroin dependence and HIV risk. I. Sexual behavior. *AIDS Care, 5*(2), 149–157.

Griffiths, P., Gossop, M., Powis, B., & Strang, J. (1992). Extent and nature of transitions of route among heroin addicts in treatment. *British Journal of Addiction, 87*, 485–491.

Griffiths, P., Gossop, M., Powis, B., & Strang, J. (1994). Transitions in patterns of heroin administration: A study of heroin chasers and heroin injectors. *Addiction, 89*, 301–309.

Grund, J.-P. C., Friedman, S. R., Stern, L. S., Jose, B., Neaigus, A., Curtis, R., & Des Jarlais, D. C. (1996). Syringe-mediated drug sharing among injecting drug users: Patterns, social context and implications for transmission of blood-borne pathogens. *Social Science and Medicine, 45*(5), 691–703.

Hagan, H., Des Jarlais, D. C., Friedman, S. R., Purchase, D., & Alter, M. J. (1995). Reduced risk of hepatitis B and hepatitis C among injecting drug users participating in the Tacoma Syringe exchange program. *American Journal of Public Health, 85*(11), 1531–1537.

Hartgers, C., van den Hoek, A., Krijnen, P., van Brussel, G. H. A., & Coutinho, R. A. (1991). Changes over time in heroin and cocaine use among injecting drug users in Amsterdam, the Netherlands, 1985–1989. *British Journal of Addiction, 86*, 1091–1098.

Heimer, R., Khoshnood, K., Stephens, P., Jariwala Freeman, B., & Kaplan, E. (1996). Evaluating a needle exchange program in a small city: Models for testing HIV-1 risk reduction. *International Journal of Drug Policy, 7*, 123–129.

Helpern, M., & Rho, Y.-M. (1966). Deaths from narcotism in New York City. *New York State Journal of Medicine, 66*(18), 2391–2408.

Hser, Y.-I., Anglin, M., & McGlothlin, W. (1987). Sex differences in addict careers. 1. Initiation of use. *American Journal of Drug and Alcohol Abuse, 13*(1&2), 33–57.

Hu, D. J., Frey, R., Costa, S. J., Massey, J., Ryan, J., Fleming, P. L., D'Errico, S., Ward, J. W., & Buehler, J. (1994). Geographical AIDS rates and sociodemographic variables in the Newark, New Jersey, metropolitan area. *AIDS and Public Policy, 9*, 20–25.

Huang, K. H. C., Watters, J., & Case, P. (1989a). Compliance with AIDS prevention measures among intravenous drug users: Health beliefs or social/environmental factors? Presented at *Vth International Conference on AIDS*. Montréal. June.

Huang, K. H. C., Watters, J. K., & Lorvick, J. (1989b). Relationship characteristics of heterosexual IV drug users. Presented at *117th Annual Meeting of the American Public Health Association*. Chicago, Illinois. October.

Jose, B. (1996). *Racial/ethnic differences in the prevalence of HIV-1 infection among injecting drug users: Social and behavioral risk factors*. Doctoral dissertation, Fordham University.

Jose, B., Friedman, S. R., Neaigus, A., Curtis, R., & Des Jarlais, D. C. (1992). "Frontloading" is associated with HIV infection among drug injectors in New York City. Presented at *8th International Conference on AIDS*. Amsterdam. July.

Jose, B., Friedman, S. R., Curtis, R., Grund, J.-P. C., Goldstein, M. F., Ward, T. P., & Des Jarlais, D. C. (1993). Syringe-mediated drug-sharing (backloading): A new risk factor for HIV among injecting drug users. *AIDS, 7*, 1653–1660.

Jose, B., Friedman, S. R., Neaigus, A., Curtis, R., Sufian, M., Stepherson, B., & Des Jarlais, D. C. (1996). Collective organization of injecting drug users and the struggle against AIDS. In T. Rhodes & R. Hartnoll (Eds.), *AIDS, drugs and prevention* (pp. 216–233). London: Routledge.

Kandel, D. (1973). Adolescent marijuana use: Role of parents and peers. *Science, 181*(104), 1067–1070.

Kandel, D. B. (1985). On the process of peer influences in adolescent drug use. *Advances in Alcohol and Substance Abuse, 4*, 139–163.

Kelly, J. A., St. Lawrence, J. S., Diaz, Y. E., Stevenson, L. Y., Hauth, A. C., Brasfield, T. L., Kalichman, S. C., Smith, J. E., & Andrew, M. E. (1991). HIV risk behavior reduction following intervention with key opinion leaders of population: An experimental analysis. *American Journal of Public Health, 81*(2), 168–171.

Kelly, J., St. Lawrence, J. S., Stevenson, L. Y., Hauth, A. C., Kalichman, S. C., Diaz, Y. E., Brasfeld, T. L., Koob, J. J., & Morgan, M. G. (1992). Community AIDS/HIV risk reduction. *American Journal of Public Health, 82*, 1483–1489.

Kennedy, M., Scarlett, M., Duerr, A., & Chu, S. (1995). Assessing HIV risk among women who have sex with women: Scientific and communication issues. *Journal of the American Medical Women's Association, 50*(3&4), 103–107.

Kleinman, P. H., Goldsmith, D. S., Friedman, S. R., Maugé, C. E., Hopkins, W., & Des Jarlais, D. C. (1990). Knowledge about and behaviors affecting the spread of AIDS: A street survey of IDUs and their associates in New York City. *International Journal of the Addictions, 25*(4), 345–361.

Klovdahl, A. (1985). Social networks and the spread of infectious diseases: The AIDS example. *Social Science and Medicine, 21*, 1203–1216.

Klovdahl, A. S., Potterat, J. J., Woodhouse, D. E., Muth, J. B., Muth, S. Q., & Darrow, W. W. (1994). Social networks and infectious disease: The Colorado Springs study. *Social Science and Medicine, 38*(1), 79–88.

Koester, S. (1989). Water, cookers, and cottons: Additional risks for intravenous drug abusers. In Community Epidemiology Work Group, *Epidemiologic trends in drug abuse*. Rockville, MD: National Institute on Drug Abuse.

Koester, S., & Hoffer, L. (1994). "Indirect sharing": Additional HIV risks associated with drug injection. *AIDS and Public Policy, 9*(2), 100–105.

Koester, S., Booth, R. E., & Zhang, Y. (1996). The prevalence of additional injection-related HIV risk behaviors among injection drug users. *Journal of Acquired Immune Deficiency Syndromes and Human Retrovirology, 12*, 202–207.

Lart, R., & Stimson, G. V. (1990). National survey of syringe exchange schemes in England. *British Journal of Addiction, 85*, 1433–1443.

Latkin, C. (1995). A personal network approach to AIDS prevention: An experimental peer group intervention for street-injecting drug users: The SAFE study. In R. H. Needle, S. L. Coyle, S. G. Genser, & R. T. Trotter, (Eds.), *Social networks, drug abuse and HIV transmission* (pp. 181–195). Rockville, MD: National Institute on Drug Abuse.

Latkin, C. A. (1998). Outreach in natural settings: The use of peer leaders for HIV prevention among injection drug users' networks. *Public Health Reports, 113*(supplement 1), 151–159.

Latkin, C., Mandell, W., Oziemkowska, M., Celentano, D., Vlahov, D., & Ensminger, M. (1995a). Using social network analysis to study patterns of drug use among urban drug users at high risk for HIV/AIDS. *Drug and Alcohol Dependence, 38*(1), 1–9.

Latkin, C., Mandell, W., Vlahov, D., Knowlton, A., Oziemkowska, M., & Celentano, D. (1995b). Personal network characteristics as antecedents to needle-sharing and shooting gallery attendance. *Social Networks, 17*(3–4), 219–228.

Latkin, C. A., Mandell, W., Vlahov, D., Oziemkowska, M., & Celentano, D. D. (1996). The long-term outcome of a personal network-oriented HIV prevention intervention for injection drug users: The SAFE study. *American Journal of Community Psychology, 24*, 341–364.

Lewis, D. K., & Watters, J. K. (1991). Sexual risk behavior among heterosexual intravenous drug users: Ethnic and gender variations. *AIDS*, 5(1), 77–83.

Lima, E. S., Friedman, S. R., Bastos, F. I., Telles, P. R., Friedmann, P., Ward, T. P., & Des Jarlais, D. C. (1994). Risk factors for HIV-1 seroprevalence among drug injectors in the cocaine-using environment of Rio de Janeiro. *Addiction*, 89, 689–698.

Lorvick, J., Estilo, M., & Watters, J. (1993). Risk behavior among heterosexual injection drug users. Presented at Ninth International Conference on AIDS. Berlin. June.

Louria, D., Hensle, T., & Rose, J. (1967). The major medical complications of heroin addiction. *Annals of Internal Medicine*, 67(1), 1–22.

Lurie, P., & Drucker, E. (1997). An opportunity lost: HIV infections associated with lack of a national needle-exchange programme in the USA. *Lancet*, 349, 604–608.

Lurie, P., Reingold, A. L., & Bowser, B. (Eds.). (1993). *The public health impact of needle-exchange programs in the United States and abroad, vol. 1*. Atlanta, GA: Centers for Disease Control and Prevention.

Lurie, P., Hintzen, P., & Lowe, R. A. (1995). Socioeconomic obstacles to HIV prevention and treatment in developing countries: The roles of the International Monetary Fund and the World Bank. *AIDS*, 9(6), 539–546.

Magura, S., Grossman, J. I., Lipton, D. S., Siddiqi, Q., Shapiro, J., Marion, I., & Amann, K. R. (1989). Determinants of needle sharing among intravenous drug users. *American Journal of Public Health*, 79(4), 459–460.

Magura, S., Shapiro, J., Siddiqi, Q., & Lipton, D. S. (1990). Variables influencing condom use among IV drug users. *American Journal of Public Health*, 80, 82–84.

Malow, R., Corrigan, S., Cunningham, S., West, J. A., & Pena, J. M. (1993). Psychosocial factors associated with condom use among African-American drug abusers in treatment. *AIDS Education and Prevention*, 5, 244–254.

Mandell, W., Vlahov, D., Latkin, C., Oziemkowska, M., & Cohn, S. (1994). Correlates of needle sharing among injection drug users. *American Journal of Public Health*, 84(6), 920–923.

Marmor, M., Des Jarlais, D. C., Cohen, H., Friedman, S. R., Beatrice, S. T., Dubin, N., El-Sadr, W., Mildvan, D., Yancovitz, S., Mathur, U., & Holzman, R. (1987). Risk factors for infection with human immunodeficiency virus among intravenous drug abusers in New York City. *AIDS*, 1, 39–44.

Metzger, D., Woody, G., McLellan, A., O'Brien, C., Druley, P., Navaline, H., DePhilippis, D., Stolley, P., & Abrutyn, E. (1993). Human immunodeficiency virus seroconversion among in- and out-of-treatment drug users: An 18 month prospective follow-up. *Journal of the Acquired Immune Deficiency Syndromes*, 6, 1049–1056.

Miller, M., Paone, D., & Friedmann, P. (1998). Social network characteristics as mediators in the relationship between sexual abuse and HIV risk. *Social Science and Medicine*, 47, 765–777.

Minkin, W., & Cohen, H. (1967). Dermatologic complications of heroin addiction. *New England Journal of Medicine*, 277(9), 473–475.

Morris, M. (1991). A log-linear modeling framework for selective mixing. *Mathematical Biosciences*, 107(2), 349–377.

Morris, M. (1993). Epidemiology and social networks. *Sociological Methods and Research*, 22, 99–126.

Morris, M., Pramualratana, A., Podhisita, C., & Wawer, M. (1995a). The relational determinants of condom use with commercial sex partners in Thailand. *AIDS*, 9, 507–515.

Morris, M., Zavisca, J., & Dean, L. (1995b). Social and sexual networks: Their role in the spread of HIV/AIDS among young gay men. *AIDS Education and Prevention*, 7(Suppl.), 24–35.

Musto, D. (1991). Opium, cocaine, and marijuana in American history. *Scientific American*, 265, 40–47.

Neaigus, A., Sufian, M., Friedman, S. R., Goldsmith, D. S., Stepherson, B., Mota, P., Pascal, J., & Des Jarlais, D. C. (1990). Effects of outreach intervention on risk reduction among intravenous drug users. *AIDS Education and Prevention, 2*(4), 253–271.

Neaigus, A., Friedman, S. R., Stepherson, B., Jose, B., & Sufian, M. (1991). Declines in syringe sharing during the first drug injection. Presented at *7th International Conference on AIDS.* Florence, Italy. June.

Neaigus, A., Friedman, S., Jose, B., Goldstein, M., Curtis, R., & Des Jarlais, D. C. (1993). Risk factors for HIV infection among new drug injectors. Presented at *IXth International Conference on AIDS.* Berlin. June.

Neaigus, A., Friedman, S. R., Curtis, R., Des Jarlais, D. C., Furst, R. T., Jose, B., Mota, P., Stepherson, B., Sufian, M., Ward, T., & Wright, J. W. (1994). The relevance of drug injectors' social and risk networks for understanding and preventing HIV infection. *Social Science and Medicine, 38*(1), 67–78.

Neaigus, A., Friedman, S. R., Jose, B., Goldstein, M. F., Curtis, R., Ildefonso, G., & Des Jarlais, D. C. (1996). High-risk personal networks and syringe sharing as risk factors for HIV infection among new drug injectors. *Journal of Acquired Immune Deficiency Syndromes and Human Retrovirology, 11,* 499–509.

Neaigus, A., Atillasoy, A., Friedman, S. R., Andrade, X., Miller, M., Ildefonso, G., & Des Jarlais, D. C. (1997). Trends in the non-injected use of heroin and factors associated with the transition to injecting. In J. Inciardi & L. D. Harrison (Eds.), *Heroin in the age of crack cocaine* (pp. 131–159). Thousand Oaks, CA: Sage.

Needle, R. H., Coyle, S. L., Genser, S. G., & Trotter, R. T. (Eds.). (1995). *Social networks, drug abuse and HIV transmission.* Rockville, MD: National Institute on Drug Abuse.

New York City Division of Planning. (1993). *Community district needs, Fiscal year 1993.* New York: New York City Department of City Planning.

Nicolosi, A., Leite, M. L. C., Musicco, M., Molinari, S., & Lazzarin, A. (1992). Parenteral and sexual transmission of human immunodeficiency virus in intravenous drug users: A study of seroconversion. *American Journal of Epidemiology, 135*(3), 225–233.

Normand, J., Vlahov, D., & Moses, L. E. (Eds.). (1995). *Preventing HIV transmission: The role of sterile needles and bleach.* Washington, DC: National Academy Press/National Research Council/ Institute of Medicine.

Novick, D. M., Trigg, H. L., Des Jarlais, D. C., Friedman, S. R., Vlahov, D., & Kreek, M. J. (1989). Cocaine injection and ethnicity in parenteral drug users during the early years of the human immunodeficiency virus (HIV) epidemic in New York City. *Journal of Medical Virology, 29,* 181–185.

Novick, D., Joseph, H., Croxson, S., Salsitz, E., Wang, G., Richman, B., Poretsky, L., Keefe, J., & Whimbey, E. (1990). Absence of antibody to human immunodeficiency virus in long-term, socially rehabilitated methadone maintenance patients. *Archives of Internal Medicine, 150*(1), 97–99.

Nyamathi, A., Lewis, C., Leake, B., Flaskerud, J., & Bennett, C. (1995). Barriers to condom use and needle cleaning among impoverished minority injection drug users and partners of injection drug users. *Public Health Reports, 110,* 166–172.

O'Donnell, J. (1965). The relapse rate in narcotic addiction: A critique of follow-up studies,. In D. Wilner & G. Kassenbaum (Eds.), *Narcotics* (pp. 226–246). New York: McGraw-Hill.

Ouellet, L., Jimenez, A. D., & Wiebel, W. (1993). *Heroin again: New users of heroin in Chicago.* Miami, FL: Society for the Study of Social Problems.

Ouellet, L. J., Wiebel, W. W., & Jimenez, A. D. (1995). Team research methods for studying intranasal heroin use and its HIV risks. In R. Needle & E. Lambert (Eds.), *Qualitative methods and drug abuse and HIV* (pp. 182–211). Rockville, MD: National Institute on Drug Abuse.

Ouellet, L. J., Rahimian, A., & Wiebel, W. W. (1998). The onset of drug injection among sex partners of injecting drug users. *AIDS Education and Prevention, 10,* 341–350.

Padian, N. S., & Shiboski, S. C. (1994). Partner studies in the heterosexual transmission of HIV. In A. Nicolosi (Ed.), *HIV epidemiology: Models and methods* (pp. 87–98). New York: Raven Press.

Padian, N., Shiboski, S., Glass, S., & Vittinghoff, E. (1997). Heterosexual transmission of human immunodeficiency virus (HIV) in Northern California: Results from a ten-year study. *American Journal of Epidemiology, 146,* 350–357.

Paone, D., Caloir, S., Shi, Q., & Des Jarlais, D. C. (1995a). Sex, drugs, and syringe exchange in New York City: Women's experiences. *Journal of the American Medical Women's Association, 50* (3&4), 109–114.

Paone, D., Des Jarlais, D. C., Gangloff, R., Milliken, J., & Friedman, S. R. (1995b). Syringe exchange: HIV prevention, key findings, and the future directions. *International Journal of Addictions, 30*(12), 1647–1683.

Parker, R. G. (1991). *Bodies, pleasures, and passions: Sexual culture in contemporary Brazil.* Boston: Beacon.

Patrick, D., Strathdee, S., Archibald, V., Ofner, M., Craib, K., Cornelisse, P., Schecter, M., Reckart, M., & O'Shaughnessy, M. (1997). Determinants of HIV seroconversion in injection drug users during a period of rising prevalence in Vancouver. *International Journal of STD and AIDS, 8,* 437–445.

Phillips, K. (1969). *The emerging republican majority.* New Rochelle, NY: Arlington House.

Potterat, J. J., Woodhouse, D. E., Rothenberg, R. B., Muth, S. Q., Darrow, W. W., Muth, J. B., & Reynolds, M. U. (1993). AIDS in Colorado Springs: Is there an epidemic? *AIDS, 7,* 1517–1521.

Prather, J., & Fidell, L. (1978). Drug use and abuse among women. An overview. *International Journal of the Addictions, 13*(6), 863–885.

Preble, E., & Casey, J. (1969). Taking care of business: The heroin user's life on the street. *International Journal of the Addictions, 4,* 1–4.

Price, C. (1992). AIDS, Organization of drug users, and public policy. *AIDS and Public Policy Journal, 7*(3), 141–144.

Price, R. K., Cottler, L. B., Mager, D., & Murray, K. S. (1995). Injecting drug use, characteristics of significant others, and HIV risk behaviors. In R. H. Needle, S. L. Coyle, S. G. Genser, & R. T. Trotter, (Eds.), *Social networks, drug abuse and HIV transmission* (pp. 38–59). Rockville, MD: National Institute on Drug Abuse.

Quimby, E., & Friedman, S. R. (1989). Dynamics of black mobilization against AIDS in New York City. *Social Problems, 36*(4), 403–415.

Ramsey, R., Gunnar, R., & Tobin, J. (1970). Endocarditis in the drug addict. *American Journal of Cardiology, 25,* 608–618.

Rhodes, T. (1996). Culture, drugs and unsafe sex: Confusion about causation. *Addiction, 91*(6), 753–758.

Rietmeijer, C., Kane, M., Simons, P., Corby, N., Wolitski, R., Higgins, D., Judson, F., & Cohn, D. (1996). Increasing the use of bleach and condoms among injecting drug users in Denver. *AIDS, 10*(3), 291–298.

Rittenhouse, J. (1977). Selected themes of the discussion. In J. Rittenhouse (Ed.), *The epidemiology of heroin and other narcotics* (pp. 16–20). Rockville, MD: National Institute on Drug Abuse.

Rockwell, R., Des Jarlais, D., Friedman, S., Perlis, T., & Paone, D. (submitted). Residential proximity and use of syringe exchanges.

Rodríguez Arenas, M. A., Zunzunegui, M. V., Friedman, S. R., Romero Bellido, J. C., & Ward, T. P. (1996). Sharing syringes in Madrid: A social phenomenon. *European Journal of Public Health, 6*(1), 11–14.

Rosenbaum, M. (1979). Becoming addicted: The woman addict. *Contemporary Drug Problems, 8,* 141–167.

Rosenbaum, M. (1981). *Women on heroin.* New Brunswick, NJ: Rutgers University Press.

Ross, M., Wodak, A., Gold, J., & Miller, M. E. (1992). Differences across sexual orientation on HIV risk behaviours in injecting drug users. *AIDS Care, 4,* 139–148.

Rothenberg, R., Woodhouse, D., Potterat, J., Muth, S., Darrow, W., & Klovdahl, A. (1995). Social networks in disease transmission: The Colorado Springs study. In: R. H. Needle, S. L. Coyle, S. G. Genser, & R. T. Trotter (Eds.), *Social networks, drug abuse and HIV transmission* (pp. 3–19). Rockville, MD: National Institute on Drug Abuse.

Samuels, J., Vlahov, D., Anthony, J., & Chaisson, R. E. (1992). Measurement of HIV risk behaviors among intravenous drug users. *British Journal of Addiction, 87*(3), 417–428.

Schaper, P., Plumb, M., & Escoffier, J. (1996). *HIV transmission risk of cunnilingus: A review.* New York: New York City Office of Gay and Lesbian Health.

Schilling, R., El-Bassel, N., Schinke, S., Nichols, S., Botvin, G., & Orlandi, M. (1991). Sexual behavior, attitudes toward safer sex, and gender among a cohort of 244 recovering IV drug users. *International Journal of the Addictions, 26*(8), 859–877.

Schoenbaum, E. E., Hartel, D., Selwyn, P. A., Klein, R. S., Davenny, K., Rogers, M., Feiner, C., & Friedland, G. (1989). Risk factors for human immunodeficiency virus infection in intravenous drug users. *New England Journal of Medicine, 321*(13), 874–879.

Scott, J. (1991). *Social network analysis.* Newbury Park, CA: Sage.

Seeff, L., Zimmerman, H., Wright, E., Schiff, E., Kiernan, T., Leevy, C., Tamburro, C., & Ishak, K. (1975). Hepatic disease in asymptomatic parenteral narcotic drug abusers: A Veterans Administration collaborative study. *American Journal of the Medical Sciences, 270*(1), 41–47.

Selwyn, P., Feiner, C., Cox, C., Lipshutz, C., & Cohen, R. (1987). Knowledge about AIDS and high-risk behavior among intravenous drug abusers in New York City. *AIDS, 1*, 247–254.

Sherr, L. (Ed.). (1997). *AIDS among adolescents.* Chur, Switzerland: Harwood Academic Press.

Sibthorpe, B. (1992). The social construction of sexual relationships as a determinant of HIV risk perception and condom use among injection drug users. *Medical Anthropology Quarterly, 6*(3), 255–270.

Siegel, D., Golden, E., Eugene Washington, A., Morse, S. A., Fullilove, M. T., Catania, J. A., Marin, B., & Hulley, S. B. (1992). Prevalence and correlates of herpes simplex infections: The population-based AIDS in multiethnic neighborhoods study. *Journal of the American Medical Association, 268*, 1702–1708.

Simon, P. A., Hu, D. J., Diaz, T., & Kerndt, P. R. (1995). Income and AIDS rates in Los Angeles County. *AIDS, 9*(3), 281–284.

Sklar, H. (1995). *Jobs, income, and work.* Philadelphia: American Friends Service Committee.

Snyder, F. R., & Myers, M. H. (1989). *Risk behaviors of IV cocaine users vs. IV heroin users.* Chicago: American Public Health Association.

Solomon, L., Astemborski, J., Warren, D., Muñoz, A., Cohn, S., Vlahov, D., & Nelson, K. E. (1993). Differences in risk factors for human immunodeficiency virus type 1 seroconversion among male and female intravenous drug users. *American Journal of Epidemiology, 137*, 892–898.

Stark, K., Müller, R., Bienzle, U., & Guggenmoos-Holzmann, I. (1996). Frontloading: A risk factor for HIV and hepatitis C virus infection among injecting drug users in Berlin. *AIDS, 10*, 311–317.

Steinberg, S. (1995). *Turning back.* Boston: Beacon.

Stimmel, B., Vernace, S., & Heller, E. (1973). Hepatitis B antigen and antibody in former heroin addicts on methadone maintenance: Correlation with clinical and histological findings. In *Fifth National Conference on Methadone Treatment* (pp. 501–506). Washington DC: NAPAN.

Stimson, G. (1994). Reconstruction of sub-regional diffusion of HIV infection among injecting drug users in South-East Asia: Implications for prevention. *AIDS, 8*, 1630–1632.

Stimson, G. V., Adelekan, M. L., & Rhodes, T. (1996). The diffusion of drug injection in developing countries. *International Journal of Drug Policy, 7*(4), 245–255.

Stimson, G. V., Des Jarlais, D. C., & Ball, A. (Eds.). (1998). *HIV and injecting drug use: Global perspectives.* London: Taylor and Francis.

Strang, J., Des Jarlais, D. C., Griffiths, P., & Gossop, M. (1992a). The study of transitions in the route of drug use: The route from one route to another. *British Journal of Addiction, 87*, 473–483.

Strang, J., Griffiths, B., Powis, B., & Gossop, M. (1992b). First use of heroin: Changes in the route of administration over time. *British Medical Journal, 304,* 1222–1223.

Strathdee, S., Patrick, D., Archibald, C., Ofner, M., Cornelisse, P., Rekart, M., Schechter, M., & O'Shaughnessy, M. (1997). Social determinants predict needle-sharing behavior among injection drug users in Vancouver, Canada. *Addiction, 92*(10), 1339–1347.

Sudman, S. (1976). *Applied sampling.* New York: Academic Press.

Sviridoff, M., Sadd, S., Curtis, R., & Grinc, R. (1992). *The neighborhood effects of street-level drug enforcement: Tactical narcotics teams in New York.* New York: Vera Institute of Justice.

Thorton, W., & Thorton, B. (1974). Narcotic poisoning: A review of the literature. *American Journal of Psychiatry, 131*(8), 867–869.

Tross, S., Abdul-Quader, A., Silvert, H., Rapkin, B., Des Jarlais, D. C., & Friedman, S. R. (1991). Determinants of needle sharing change in street-recruited New York City IV drug users. Presented at *VIIth International Conference on AIDS.* Florence, Italy. June.

Tross, S., Abdul-Quader, A., Silvert, H., & Des Jarlais, D.C. (1992). Condom use among male injecting-drug users—New York City, 1987–1990. *Morbidity and Mortality Weekly Report, 41*(34), 617–620.

Trotter, R., Baldwin, J., & Bowen, A. (1995a). Network structure and proxy network measures of HIV, drug and incarceration risks for active drug users. *Connections, 18,* 89–104.

Trotter, R., Bowen, A., & Potter, J. (1995b). Network models for HIV outreach and prevention programs for drug users. In R. Needle, S. Coyle, S. Genser, & R. Trotter (Eds.), *Social networks, drug abuse and HIV transmission* (pp. 144–180). Rockville, MD: National Institute on Drug Abuse.

UNAIDS/WHO (1997). *Report on the global HIV/AIDS epidemic.* Geneva: UNAIDS/WHO.

U.S. Bureau of the Census. (1996–1997). Statistical abstract of the United States. Washington: Government Printing Office.

van Ameijden, E. J. C., van den Hoek, J. A. R., van Haastrecht, H. J. A., & Coutinho, R. A. (1992). The harm reduction approach and risk factors for human immunodeficiency virus (HIV) seroconversion in injecting drug users, Amsterdam. *American Journal of Epidemiology, 136,* 236–243.

van Ameijden, E. J. C., van den Hoek, J. A. R., & Coutinho, R. A. (1996). Large declines in sexual risk behavior with noncommercial partners among heterosexual injection drug users in Amsterdam, 1989–1995. *American Journal of Epidemiology, 144,* 772–781.

van den Hoek, J., van Haastrecht, H., & Coutinho, R. (1990). Heterosexual behavior of intravenous drug users in Amsterdam: implications for the AIDS epidemic. *AIDS, 4,* 449–453.

Vanichseni, S., Des Jarlais, D. C., Choopanya, K., Friedmann, P., Wenston, J., Sonchai, W., Sotheran, J. L., Raktham, S., Carballo, M., & Friedman, S. R. (1993). Condom use with primary partners among injecting drug users in Bangkok, Thailand and New York City, United States. *AIDS, 7,* 887–891.

Vlahov, D., Munoz, A., Anthony, J. C., Cohn, S., Celentano, D. C., & Nelson, K. E. (1990). Associations of drug injection patterns with antibody to HIV type 1 among intravenous drug users in Baltimore, Maryland. *American Journal of Epidemiology, 132,* 847–856.

Vlahov, D., Anthony, J., Celentano, D., Solomon, L., & Chowdhury, N. (1991a). Trends of HIV-1 risk reduction among initiates into intravenous drug use 1982–1987. *American Journal of Drug and Alcohol Abuse, 17,* 39–48.

Vlahov, D., Celentano, D. D., Muñoz, A., Cohn, S., Anthony, J. C., & Nelson, K. E. (1991b). Bleach disinfection of needles by intravenous drug users: Association with HIV seroconversion. Presented at *Seventh International Conference on AIDS.* Florence, Italy. June.

Vlahov, D., Khabbaz, R., Cohn, S., Galai, N., Taylor, E., & Kaplan, J. (1995). Incidence and risk factors for human T-lymphotropic virus type II seroconversion among injecting drug users in Baltimore, Maryland. *Journal of Acquired Immune Deficiency Syndrome, 9,* 89–96.

Wallace, R. (1990). Urban decertification, public health and public order: "Planned shrinkage," violent death, substance abuse and AIDS in the Bronx. *Social Science and Medicine, 31*(7), 801–813.

Wallace, R. (1991a). Social disintegration and the spread of AIDS, part II: Meltdown of sociogeographic structure in urban minority neighborhoods. *Social Science and Medicine, 37,* 887–896.

Wallace, R. (1991b). Social disintegration and the spread of AIDS: Thresholds for propagation along "sociographic" networks. *Social Science and Medicine, 33*(10), 1155–1162.

Wallace, R. (1992). The geography of AIDS and sociogeographic networks. *C/CRWG Newsletter, 3,* 1–32.

Wasserman, S., & Faust, K. (1994). *Social network analysis: Methods and applications.* Cambridge, UK: Cambridge University Press.

Watkins, K., Metzger, D., Woody, G., & McLellan, A. (1993). Determinants of condom use among intravenous drug users. *AIDS, 7,* 719–723.

Watters, J. K., & Biernacki, P. (1989). Targeted sampling: Options for the study of hidden populations. *Social Problems, 36*(4), 416–430.

White, A. (1973). Medical disorders in drug addicts. *Journal of the American Medical Association, 223,* 1469–1471.

White, D., Phillips, K., Mulleady, G., & Cupitt, C. (1993). Sexual issues and condom use among injecting drug users. *AIDS Care, 5*(4), 427–437.

Woodhouse, D. E., Rothenberg, R. B., & Potterat, J. J., (1994). Mapping a social network of heterosexuals at high risk for human immunodeficiency virus infection. *AIDS, 8,* 1331–1336.

Zapka, J. G., Stoddard, A., & McCusker, J. (1993). Social network, support and influence: Relationships with drug use and protective AIDS behavior. *AIDS Education and Prevention, 5*(4), 352–366.

Zierler, S., & Krieger, N. (1997). Reframing women's risk: Social inequalities and HIV infection. *Annual Review of Public Health, 18,* 401–436.

Index

An "*f*" or "*t*" after a page number indicates that the term can be found in a figure or table.

Africa, 177
African Americans: *see* Blacks
Age
  condom use and, 165, 168
  in drug injecting dyads, 145, 150
  at first injection, 92, 96, 151, 154, 155, 176–177
  for first vaginal sex, 158
  likelihood of infection and, 204, 208
  serostatus and, 207
  in sociometric risk network location, 196
  of study participants, 120–121
AIDS: *see* HIV entries
AIDS Impact Statements, 224
AIDS outreach workers, 45–46, 48, 50
AIDS risk reduction model, 9, 173
AIDS talk, 84–86
Alaskan Natives, 228
Alter, 164, 195
Altruism-solidarity, 165, 175
American Foundation for AIDS Research, 6
American Indians, 228
Anonymous works, 126, 127*f*, 133
Argentina, 2
Arson-related fires, 53–54, 64
Asians, 228
Athens, 211
Atlanta, 220
Australia, 232
Automobile-oriented neighborhoods, 223–224
AWARE, 209

Backloading, 6, 8, 122, 192
  descripion of, 78–80
  likelihood of infection and, 205, 208, 209
  in shooting galleries, 45
"Ballad of Reading Gaol, The" (Wilde), 217
Baltimore, 104, 141, 225
Bangkok, 5, 11, 211

Barney, 77–79, 109
Beat bags, 72
Bedford Stuyvesant, 55, 57
Benny, 198
Berlin, 211
Biological factors in infection, 210, 211, 215
Bisexuals, 2
Blackout, 54, 55
Blacks, vi, 4, 10, 119, 226–228
  condom use by, 165, 168
  in drug injecting dyads, 150, 151, 154, 155–156
  in drug trafficking, 55
  first injection by, 92
  inequality and, 233, 234–235
  likelihood of infection in, 205
  as percentage of Bushwick population, 54
  in risk networks and high-risk settings, 138–139*t*
  serostatus predictors in, 207
  in sexual networks, 177, 178
Bleach kits, 11, 46, 48, 50, 70
Blockbusting, 53
Blood banks, 108–109
Blue-tip syringes, 70
Blunts, 179
Booker, 71
Booting, 73
Bottlenecks, 221
Brazil, 2
Broadway, 55
Bruce, 36, 61, 83–84, 111, 155, 194, 196
  current status of, 237
  on drug trafficking, 57
  imprisonment of, 36, 37, 198
  medical care received by, 198
  story of, 33–38
Burned house shooting gallery, 31, 48–49, 65–80, 230
  description of drug practices in, 72–75